Updates in HIV and AIDS: Part I

Editors

MICHAEL S. SAAG
HENRY MASUR

INFECTIOUS DISEASE CLINICS OF NORTH AMERICA

www.id.theclinics.com

Consulting Editor
HELEN W. BOUCHER

September 2014 • Volume 28 • Number 3

ELSEVIER

1600 John F. Kennedy Boulevard • Suite 1800 • Philadelphia, Pennsylvania, 19103-2899.

http://www.theclinics.com

INFECTIOUS DISEASE CLINICS OF NORTH AMERICA Volume 28, Number 3
September 2014 ISSN 0891-5520, ISBN-13: 978-0-323-32327-7

Editor: Jessica McCool
Developmental Editor: Donald Mumford

Infectious Disease Clinics of North America (ISSN 0891-5520) is published in March, June, September, and December by Elsevier Inc., 360 Park Avenue South, New York, NY 10010-1710. Periodicals postage paid at New York, NY and additional mailing offices. Subscription prices are $295.00 per year for US individuals, $510.00 per year for US institutions, $145.00 per year for US students, $350.00 per year for Canadian individuals, $638.00 per year for Canadian institutions, $420.00 per year for international individuals, $638.00 per year for international institutions, and $200.00 per year for Canadian and international students. To receive student rate, orders must be accompanied by name of affiliated institution, date of term, and the *signature* of program/residency coordinator on institution letterhead. Orders will be billed at individual rate until proof of status is received. Foreign air speed delivery is included in all *Clinics* subscription prices. All prices are subject to change without notice. **POSTMASTER**: Send address changes to *Infectious Disease Clinics of North America*, Elsevier Health Sciences Division, Subcription Customer Service, 3251 Riverport Lane, Maryland Heights, MO 63043. **Customer Service: 1-800-654-2452 (US). From outside of the US and Canada, call 1-314-447-8871. Fax: 1-314-447-8029. E-mail: JournalsCustomerService-usa@elsevier.com (print support) or JournalsOnlineSupport-usa@elsevier.com (online support).**

Infectious Disease Clinics of North America is also published in Spanish by Editorial Inter-Médica, Junin 917, 1er A 1113, Buenos Aires, Argentina.

Reprints. For copies of 100 or more, of articles in this publication, please contact the Commercial Reprints Department, Elsevier Inc., 360 Park Avenue South, New York, New York 10010-1710. Tel. 212-633-3874, Fax: 212-633-3820, E-mail: reprints@elsevier.com.

Infectious Disease Clinics of North America is covered in MEDLINE/PubMed (Index Medicus), Current Contents/Clinical Medicine, Science Citation Alert, SCISEARCH, and Research Alert.

Contributors

CONSULTING EDITOR

HELEN W. BOUCHER, MD, FACP, FIDSA
Director, Infectious Diseases Fellowship Program, Associate Professor of Medicine, Division of Geographic Medicine and Infectious Diseases, Tufts Medical Center, Boston, Massachusetts

EDITORS

MICHAEL S. SAAG, MD
Jim Straley Chair in AIDS Research, Professor, Division of Infectious Disease; Director, Center for AIDS Research, University of Alabama at Birmingham, Birmingham, Alabama

HENRY MASUR, MD
Chief, Critical Care Medicine Department, NIH, Bethesda, Maryland

AUTHORS

HELEN W. BOUCHER, MD, FACP, FIDSA
Director, Infectious Diseases Fellowship Program, Associate Professor of Medicine, Division of Geographic Medicine and Infectious Diseases, Tufts Medical Center, Boston, Massachusetts

GREER A. BURKHOLDER, MD
Assistant Professor, Department of Medicine, University of Alabama at Birmingham School of Medicine, Birmingham, Alabama

KATYA R. CALVO, MD
Assistant Professor of Medicine, Division of HIV Medicine, Department of Internal Medicine, Harbor-UCLA Medical Center, David Geffen School of Medicine at UCLA, Torrance, California

ERIC S. DAAR, MD
Professor of Medicine, Chief, Division of HIV Medicine, Department of Internal Medicine, Harbor-UCLA Medical Center, David Geffen School of Medicine at UCLA, Torrance, California

ELLEN F. EATON, MD
Fellow, Division of Infectious Disease, University of Alabama, Birmingham, Birmingham, Alabama

JADE FETTIG, MS
Epidemiology and Strategic Information Branch, Division of Global HIV/AIDS, Center for Global Health, Centers for Disease Control and Prevention (CDC), Atlanta, Georgia

RAJESH T. GANDHI, MD
Infectious Diseases Division and Ragon Institute, Massachusetts General Hospital; Associate Professor, Harvard Medical School, Boston, Massachusetts

JOMY M. GEORGE, PharmD
Associate Professor, Department of Pharmacy Practice and Administration, Philadelphia College of Pharmacy, University of the Sciences in Philadelphia, Philadelphia, Pennsylvania; Manager, Virology US Medical Strategy, US Pharmaceuticals Medical Affairs, Bristol-Myers Squibb, Plainsboro Township, New Jersey

MICHAEL A. HORBERG, MD, MAS, FACP, FIDSA
National Director, HIV/AIDS; Executive Director, Mid-Atlantic Permanente Research Institute, Kaiser Permanente, Rockville, Maryland

DONALD M. JENSEN, MD
Professor, Department of Medicine, Center for Liver Disease, University of Chicago Medical Center, Chicago, Illinois

JENNIFER A. JOHNSON, MD
Division of Infectious Diseases, Brigham and Women's Hospital, Instructor in Medicine, Harvard Medical School, Boston, Massachusetts

JONATHAN E. KAPLAN, MD
HIV Care and Treatment Branch, Division of Global HIV/AIDS, Center for Global Health, Centers for Disease Control and Prevention (CDC), Atlanta, Georgia

MICHAEL MUGAVERO, MD
Associate Professor, Division of Infectious Disease, University of Alabama, Birmingham, Birmingham, Alabama

CHRISTOPHER S. MURRILL, PhD, MPH
Epidemiology and Strategic Information Branch, Division of Global HIV/AIDS, Center for Global Health, Centers for Disease Control and Prevention (CDC), Atlanta, Georgia

EDGAR TURNER OVERTON, MD
Associate Professor, Department of Medicine, University of Alabama at Birmingham School of Medicine, Birmingham, Alabama

ALICE K. PAU, PharmD
Staff Scientist (Clinical), Division of Clinical Research, National Institute of Allergy and Infectious Diseases, National Institutes of Health, Bethesda, Maryland

LINDSAY A. PETTY, MD
Fellow, Department of Infectious Diseases and Global Health, University of Chicago Medical Center, Chicago, Illinois

KENNETH PURSELL, MD
Professor, Department of Infectious Diseases and Global Health, University of Chicago Medical Center, Chicago, Illinois

CARLA V. RODRIGUEZ, PhD, MPH
Research Scientist, Mid-Atlantic Permanente Research Institute, Kaiser Permanente, Rockville, Maryland

MICHAEL S. SAAG, MD
Jim Straley Chair in AIDS Research, Professor, Division of Infectious Disease; Director, Center for AIDS Research, University of Alabama at Birmingham, Birmingham, Alabama

PAUL E. SAX, MD
Clinical Director, Division of Infectious Diseases, Brigham and Women's Hospital, Professor of Medicine, Harvard Medical School, Boston, Massachusetts

CHRISTOPHER J. SELLERS, MD
Division of Infectious Diseases, School of Medicine, University of North Carolina, Chapel Hill, North Carolina

JENNIFER L. STEINBECK, MD
Fellow, Department of Infectious Diseases and Global Health, University of Chicago Medical Center, Chicago, Illinois

MAHESH SWAMINATHAN, MD
Epidemiology and Strategic Information Branch, Division of Global HIV/AIDS, Center for Global Health, Centers for Disease Control and Prevention (CDC), Atlanta, Georgia

AMY H. WARRINER, MD
Assistant Professor, Department of Medicine, University of Alabama at Birmingham School of Medicine, Birmingham, Alabama

DAVID A. WOHL, MD
Division of Infectious Diseases, School of Medicine, University of North Carolina, Chapel Hill, North Carolina

BRIAN C. ZANONI, MD, MPH
Clinical and Research Fellow, Infectious Diseases Division, Massachusetts General Hospital; Harvard Medical School, Boston, Massachusetts

Contents

The number of persons living with HIV worldwide reached approximately
35.3 million in 2012. Meanwhile, AIDS-related deaths and new HIV infections have declined. Much of the increase in HIV prevalence is from rapidly
increasing numbers of people on antiretroviral treatment who are now
living longer. There is regional variation in epidemiologic patterns, major
modes of HIV transmission, and HIV program response. It is important
to focus on HIV incidence, rather than prevalence, to provide information
about HIV transmission patterns and populations at risk. Expanding HIV
treatment will function as a preventive measure through decreasing horizontal and vertical transmission of HIV.

HIV testing and incidence are stable, but trends for certain populations are
concerning. Primary prevention must be reinvigorated and target vulnerable populations. Science and policy have progressed to improve the
accuracy, speed, privacy, and affordability of HIV testing. More potent
and much better tolerated HIV treatments and a multidisciplinary approach
to care have increased adherence and viral suppression. Changes to
health care law in the United States seek to expand the affordability and
access of improved HIV diagnostics and treatment. Continued challenges
include improving long-term outcomes in people on lifetime regimens,
reducing comorbidities associated with those regimens, and preventing
further transmission.

Effective human immunodeficiency virus (HIV) care in the modern antiretroviral therapy (ART) era requires early entry into and retention in care.
Early initiation and adherence to ART therapy improves outcomes. Many
evidence-based tools and behavioral interventions are available to

optimize adherence to care and ART and can be implemented in clinical settings. Monitoring care engagement and ART adherence creates the opportunity to intervene and prevent virologic failure or loss to follow up. Special HIV-infected populations, such as pregnant and mentally ill patients, require enhanced surveillance and care.

The rapid advances in drug discovery and the development of antiretroviral therapy is unprecedented in the history of modern medicine. The administration of chronic combination antiretroviral therapy targeting different stages of the human immunodeficiency virus' replicative life cycle allows for durable and maximal suppression of plasma viremia. This suppression has resulted in dramatic improvement of patient survival. This article reviews the history of antiretroviral drug development and discusses the clinical pharmacology, efficacy, and toxicities of the antiretroviral agents most commonly used in clinical practice to date.

In this article, the scientific evidence and professional guidelines regarding the timing of antiretroviral therapy initiation are reviewed, with discussion of the increasingly persuasive evidence in favor of starting treatment early in the course of human immunodeficiency virus disease.

In this article, we review the options for initial antiretroviral therapy, including the data from clinical trials to support these choices and the factors to consider in selection of a regimen to best fit each patient.

Antiretroviral therapy (ART)–experienced individuals may choose to modify their regimens because of suboptimal virologic response, poor tolerability, convenience, or to minimize interactions with other medications or food. Constructing a new regimen for any of these reasons requires a thorough review of prior antiretroviral drug use and available drug resistance results. This article summarizes the strategies used in managing the ART-experienced individual who is considering a modification in therapy at the time of suboptimal virologic response or while virologically suppressed on a stable regimen.

Despite effective antiretroviral therapy (ART), HIV-infected individuals have residual chronic immune activation that contributes to the pathogenesis of HIV infection. This immune system dysregulation is a pathogenic state manifested by very low naïve T-cell numbers and increased terminally differentiated effector cells that generate excessive proinflammatory cytokines with limited functionality. Immune exhaustion leaves an individual at risk for accelerated aging-related diseases, including renal dysfunction, atherosclerosis, diabetes mellitus, and osteoporosis. We highlight research that clarifies the role of HIV, ART, and other factors that contribute to the development of these diseases among HIV-infected persons.

In HIV-infected individuals, coinfection with HBV and/or HCV is common because of shared modes of transmission. It is known that HIV accelerates progression of liver disease and results in increased morbidity and mortality associated with viral hepatitis, but it is less clear if viral hepatitis has a direct effect on HIV. Treatment of viral hepatitis improves outcomes and should be considered in all HIV-infected patients. Treatment of HBV without concurrent treatment of HIV is risky because resistance can occur in both viruses if regimens are not carefully chosen.

Despite enormous improvements in effectiveness of treatment for HIV infection, opportunistic infections continue to occur in those who have not yet been diagnosed with HIV and in those who are not receiving antiretroviral therapy. This review focuses on tuberculosis and cryptococcal infections, the most common opportunistic infections (OIs) in patients living with human immunodeficiency virus infection around the world, as well as on new developments in progressive multifocal leukoencephalopathy and pneumocystis pneumonia. In the sections on these conditions, updates on diagnosis, treatment, and complications, as well as information on when to start antiretroviral therapy is provided. The article concludes with a discussion of new data on 2 vaccine-preventable OIs, human papillomavirus and varicella-zoster virus.

INFECTIOUS DISEASE CLINICS OF NORTH AMERICA

Erratum

The title of the preface for volume 28, number 2 (June 2014) of *Infectious Disease Clinics of North America* should be "The Need for Antimicrobial Stewardship Programs".

Infect Dis Clin N Am 28 (2014) xi
http://dx.doi.org/10.1016/j.idc.2014.06.006
0891-5520/14/$ – see front matter © 2014 Published by Elsevier Inc.

id.theclinics.com

Dedication

A Tribute to Dr Robert C. Moellering Jr (1937–2014)

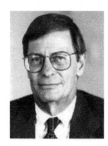

Robert C. Moellering Jr, MD

This issue of *Infectious Disease Clinics of North America* is dedicated to the memory of Dr Robert C. Moellering Jr, an outstanding teacher, clinician, researcher, mentor, friend, and colleague, who served as the first Consulting Editor of this series from 1986 to 2012. He died on February 24, 2014, after a long illness. Under Dr Moellering's leadership, *Infectious Disease Clinics of North America* became the "go-to" source for reviews and updates on the newest advances in clinical infectious diseases and therapies. A renowned clinician and researcher, he attracted world leaders in infectious diseases as authors and ensured that the most relevant issues of the time were presented. Dr Moellering was given numerous prestigious opportunities, yet retained the role of Consulting Editor for 26 years. This fact speaks volumes about who he was and what he valued.

Born in Lafayette, Indiana, Dr Moellering attended Valparaiso University before moving to Boston to attend Harvard Medical School, where he earned his MD degree *cum laude* in 1962. He continued training in Boston as a medical intern, resident, and fellow in infectious diseases at Massachusetts General Hospital where he joined the staff and Harvard Medical School faculty in 1970. He served as chairman of the Department of Medicine at the New England Deaconess Hospital from 1981 until its merger with Beth Israel Hospital in 1996. In 1998, he was named Physician-in-Chief and Chairman of the Department of Medicine at Beth Israel Deaconess Medical Center. He also served as President and CEO of Harvard Medical Faculty Physicians at Beth Israel Deaconess Medical Center. Dr Moellering was Shields Warren-Mallinckrodt Professor of Medical Research at Harvard Medical School from 1981 to 1998 and from 2005 onward; from 1999 to 2005, he assumed the Herrman Blumgart Professorship of Medicine at Harvard Medical School.

Dr Moellering's research focused on mechanisms of antibiotic action and bacterial resistance to antimicrobial agents; he and his colleagues made major advances in the investigation, treatment, and prevention of infectious diseases, including bacterial endocarditis and other serious infections. His work resulted in over 400 publications in

Infect Dis Clin N Am 28 (2014) xiii–xiv
http://dx.doi.org/10.1016/j.idc.2014.07.002
0891-5520/14/$ – see front matter © 2014 Published by Elsevier Inc.

id.theclinics.com

journals, including the *New England Journal of Medicine, Antimicrobial Agents and Chemotherapy*, and *Clinical Infectious Diseases*, and led to the development of therapies and laboratory tests that are now used worldwide. His work on the pharmacokinetics of vancomycin, including development of a dosing nomogram, immediately preceded the wide use of this agent with the rapid emergence of methicillin-resistant *Staphylococcus aureus* as a major nosocomial pathogen. He was also the first to show the clinical effectiveness of penicillin-gentamicin combination therapy for enterococcal endocarditis, which became the standard of care for this infection. "He was an internationally recognized authority on antibiotics, including how they work, how resistance to them develops, and how to use them wisely in treating patients," said George Eliopoulos, MD, who worked alongside Dr Moellering for many years.

He held numerous leadership positions in the fields of infectious diseases and microbiology and was the recipient of numerous awards. Dr. Moellering was a Fellow of the Infectious Diseases Society of America, Master of the American College of Physicians, an Honorary Fellow of the Royal College of Physicians, and was elected to membership in the American Society for Clinical Investigation and the Association of American Physicians. In addition to his role as Consulting Editor of *Infectious Disease Clinics of North America*, he served as Editor-in-Chief of *Antimicrobial Agents and Chemotherapy* and on the editorial boards of several important journals in the field. Awards included an honorary Doctor of Science degree from Valparaiso University, the Garrod Medal from the British Society for Antimicrobial Chemotherapy, the Feldman Award and the Maxwell Finland Award from the Infectious Diseases Society of America, the Hoechst-Roussel Award from the American Academy for Microbiology, and in 2006, the Maxwell Finland Award for Scientific Achievement from the National Foundation for Infectious Diseases. In 2008, he was the recipient of the Alexander Fleming Award for Lifetime Achievement from the Infectious Diseases Society of America, and in 2009, he received the Yen Memorial Award from the International Society for Chemotherapy.

While internationally recognized for his ground-breaking and prolific research, Dr Moellering valued and cherished his role as teacher and mentor to hundreds of medical residents and fellows over the past four decades. He spent many hours every week attending resident morning report and professor rounds and was intimately involved with student teaching. Despite many demands on his time, Dr Moellering took time to get to know each person and to make him or her feel important in their role as a physician. At the celebration of his retirement as Chairman of the Department of Medicine, Dr Moellering offered that "Teaching…is the most important thing we do. Imparting knowledge to the next generation of physicians is incredibly important. It's a privilege we are given in the academic setting. Not only does it give you a tremendous sense of satisfaction in that you've done something worthwhile, but it gives you some immediate gratification because you can watch students who go on to successful careers." We are most grateful for his mentorship and are inspired to try to contribute to the next generation of infectious disease physicians even a fraction of what he did for the current one.

Helen W. Boucher, MD, FACP, FIDSA
Division of Geographic Medicine and Infectious Diseases
Tufts Medical Center
800 Washington Street, Box 238
Boston, MA 02111, USA

E-mail address:
hboucher@tuftsmedicalcenter.org

Preface

HIV/AIDS

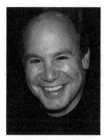 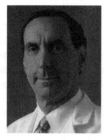

Michael S. Saag, MD   Henry Masur, MD
Editors

The last issue of the *Infectious Disease Clinics of North America* devoted specifically to HIV/AIDS was published in 1988. Edited by Merle Sande and Paul Volberding, that landmark issue provided a state-of the-art snapshot of the newly defined epidemic, its epidemiology, and the basic principles of treatment and care. Much has happened since then. In 2012, the number of persons living with HIV infection worldwide reached an all-time high of 35.3 million. The medical, social, and economic consequences of this global disaster have reached all continents, presenting society with a health-related challenge unlike any other.

Remarkably, the scientific community has investigated this epidemic and made dramatic discoveries with impressive speed. Considering that the first cases of the acquired immunodeficiency syndrome were reported in 1981, the ability of investigators to identify the causative agent in 1983, to develop a blood test in 1985, license the first active antiviral agent in 1987, and have durably lifesaving therapy a decade later is stunning. The partnership between clinicians, investigators, academic centers, government agencies, and the pharmaceutical industry has resulted in a life expectancy for HIV-infected patients with access to care that rivals that of their HIV-uninfected counterparts. In the 25 years since the publication of the last issue of *Infectious Disease Clinics of North America* on this topic, HIV has been transformed from a near-certain death sentence to a chronic, manageable condition.

Despite the remarkable scientific discoveries, the global community has not learned how to deliver effective therapy to the majority of infected patients in either the developing world or developed countries, such as the United States. Too many patients on all continents are not successfully engaged in care or provided treatment due to complex social, economic, and educational reasons. Thus, clinicians continue to be faced with patients presenting for care late in the course of infection, much as they did when HIV was first recognized in the 1980s, with a discrete constellation of opportunistic infections and neoplasms originally defined as "AIDS." Yet, modern clinicians also face a newer set of challenges by patients who are virologically well controlled on

Infect Dis Clin N Am 28 (2014) xv–xvi
http://dx.doi.org/10.1016/j.idc.2014.07.001
0891-5520/14/$ – see front matter © 2014 Elsevier Inc. All rights reserved.

id.theclinics.com

antiretroviral therapy, but who suffer long-term metabolic, neoplastic, and infectious pathologies that limit the quality and duration of their survival.

These two issues of *Infectious Disease Clinics of North America* provide a comprehensive snapshot of the HIV/AIDS clinical field as it exists today. Like the last issue in 1988, these volumes focus on epidemiology, testing, and linkage to care, as well as antiretroviral therapy and therapy for the opportunistic processes. Some of these fields, such as the management of AIDS-related opportunistic infections, have changed a bit. However, other fields have changed much more dramatically, including what antiretroviral agents to start and when to start, metabolic and chronic viral co-morbidities, and strategies for the prevention of HIV infection, including pre-exposure and postexposure HIV prophylaxis, microbicides, and the concept of "treatment as prevention."

The authors of these articles are internationally recognized experts who summarize information that clinicians who care for HIV-infected persons should know in 2014 and beyond. Much has changed in the past 25 years in terms of manifestations, diagnosis, and therapy, but much more needs to change so that the number of infected persons globally shrinks, and so that long-term morbidity and mortality are reduced and ultimately eliminated.

Michael S. Saag, MD
Center for AIDS Research
University of Alabama at Birmingham
845 19th Street South/BBRB 256
Birmingham, AL 35294-2170, USA

Henry Masur, MD
Critical Care Medicine Department
NIH–Clinical Center 2C145
Bethesda, MD 20892, USA

E-mail addresses:
msaag@uab.edu (M.S. Saag)
hmasur@cc.nih.gov (H. Masur)

Global Epidemiology of HIV

Jade Fettig, MS[a], Mahesh Swaminathan, MD[a], Christopher S. Murrill, PhD, MPH[a], Jonathan E. Kaplan, MD[b],*

KEYWORDS

• HIV • Global health • Epidemiology • Antiretroviral therapy • Risk behavior

KEY POINTS

• HIV prevalence is increasing in nearly every geographic region in the world, mostly because of deaths averted from antiretroviral treatment.
• The main mode of HIV transmission in sub-Saharan Africa is heterosexual contact; mother-to-child transmission rates are decreasing.
• Injection drug use is a major risk factor for HIV acquisition in Eastern Europe, Central Asia, North Africa, and the Middle East.
• Men who have sex with men remain at highest risk for infection in many countries of North America, Western Europe, and Oceania.
• Expanding access to HIV treatment will reduce vertical and horizontal transmission of HIV and decrease HIV morbidity and mortality globally.

INTRODUCTION

The HIV epidemic has shifted over the past 30 years, from the first reported cases in the early 1980s, to an estimated high of 3.7 million new infections in 1997, to declining new infections and AIDS-related mortality throughout the 2000s.[1] In 2012, approximately 9.7 million people in low- and middle-income countries were on antiretroviral drugs (ART).[2] This expansion of ART coverage has dramatically improved survival among people living with HIV (PLHIV), resulting in an increase in the number of PLHIV

The findings and conclusions in this article are those of the author(s) and do not necessarily represent the official position of the U.S. Department of Health and Human Services, Public Health Service, or Centers for Disease Control and Prevention.
The authors have nothing to disclose.
[a] Epidemiology and Strategic Information Branch, Division of Global HIV/AIDS, Center for Global Health, Centers for Disease Control and Prevention (CDC), 1600 Clifton Road, Northeast, MS E-30, Atlanta, GA 30333, USA; [b] HIV Care and Treatment Branch, Division of Global HIV/AIDS, Center for Global Health, Centers for Disease Control and Prevention (CDC), 1600 Clifton Road, Northeast, MS E-04, Atlanta, GA 30333, USA
* Corresponding author.
E-mail address: jxk2@cdc.gov

Infect Dis Clin N Am 28 (2014) 323–337
http://dx.doi.org/10.1016/j.idc.2014.05.001
0891-5520/14/$ – see front matter Published by Elsevier Inc.

id.theclinics.com

to an estimated all-time high of 35.3 million in 2012 (**Table 1**).[3] Increased access to ART has averted an estimated 5.2 million AIDS-related deaths in low- and middle-income countries from 1995 to 2010, with a 28% reduction in deaths from 2006 to 2012 (**Table 2**).[1,4] Even as PLHIV live longer, the incidence of new infections continues

Table 1
Estimated adults and children living with HIV, by region

	2000	2003	2006	2009	2012
Sub-Saharan Africa					
Adults & Children	20,800,000	22,800,000	23,500,000	24,200,000	25,000,000
Adults	18,800,000	20,200,000	20,500,000	21,100,000	22,100,000
Women 15+ y of age	10,700,000	11,600,000	11,800,000	12,200,000	12,900,000
Children	2,100,000	2,600,000	3,000,000	3,100,000	2,900,000
Asia					
Adults & Children	3,820,000	4,380,000	4,550,000	4,580,000	4,780,000
Adults	3,820,000	4,280,000	4,340,000	4,470,000	4,580,000
Women 15+ y of age	1,187,000	1,430,000	1,480,000	1,620,000	1,650,000
Children	94,300	143,600	185,300	206,900	208,200
North Africa and Middle East					
Adults & Children	130,000	170,000	200,000	230,000	260,000
Adults 15+ y of age	120,000	150,000	180,000	210,000	250,000
Women 15+ y of age	59,000	69,000	77,000	86,000	100,000
Children	9300	13,000	16,000	18,000	20,000
Latin America and the Caribbean					
Adults & Children	1,580,000	1,570,000	1,560,000	1,650,000	1,750,000
Adults 15+ y of age	1,550,000	1,550,000	1,530,000	1,530,000	1,630,000
Women 15+ y of age	500,000	520,000	520,000	530,000	560,000
Children	65,000	72,000	73,000	67,000	56,000
North America, Western Europe, and Oceania					
Adults & Children	1,544,000	1,682,000	1,866,000	2,049,000	2,211,000
Adults 15+ y of age	1,543,000	1,679,000	1,863,000	2,046,000	2,208,000
Women 15+ y of age	323,000	366,000	408,000	448,000	488,000
Children	6600	6600	6300	6200	6100
Eastern Europe and Central Asia					
Adults & Children	760,000	1,000,000	1,100,000	1,200,000	1,300,000
Adults 15+ y of age	750,000	990,000	1,100,000	1,200,000	1,300,000
Women 15+ y of age	300,000	430,000	460,000	440,000	430,000
Children	8700	16,000	19,000	19,000	19,000
Global					
Adults & Children	28,700,000	31,700,000	32,800,000	34,000,000	35,300,000
Adults 15+ y of age	26,500,000	28,800,000	29,500,000	30,500,000	32,100,000
Women 15+ y of age	13,100,000	14,400,000	14,800,000	15,300,000	16,100,000
Children	2,300,000	2,900,000	3,300,000	3,400,000	3,300,000

From Global report: UNAIDS report on the global AIDS epidemic 2013. Available at: http://www.unaids.org/en/media/unaids/contentassets/documents/epidemiology/2013/gr2013/UNAIDS_Global_Report_2013_en.pdf. Accessed May 9, 2014; with permission.

Table 2
AIDS-related deaths in adults and children, by region

	2000	2003	2006	2009	2012
Sub-Saharan Africa	1,400,000	1,700,000	1,700,000	1,500,000	1,200,000
Asia	205,000	303,000	322,000	300,000	261,000
North Africa and Middle East	7300	10,000	13,000	15,000	17,000
Latin America and the Caribbean	100,000	104,000	92,000	80,000	63,000
North America, Western Europe, and Oceania	28,500	29,000	29,000	27,500	28,800
Eastern Europe and Central Asia	24,000	59,000	83,000	82,000	91,000
Global	1,700,000	2,200,000	2,300,000	2,000,000	1,600,000

From Global report: UNAIDS report on the global AIDS epidemic 2013. Available at: http://www.unaids.org/en/media/unaids/contentassets/documents/epidemiology/2013/gr2013/UNAIDS_Global_Report_2013_en.pdf. Accessed May 9, 2014; with permission.

to decline. An estimated 2.3 million new HIV infections occurred in 2012, which is a 34% decrease from 2000 (**Table 3**).[2] Overall incidence rate for adults 15 to 49 years of age reached a peak of 0.11% in 1997 and decreased to 0.05% in 2012 (**Fig. 1**).[1] The greatest decrease in HIV incidence is among children, which has been reduced by 52% in 10 years.[2] Many reasons exist for this decrease in incidence, including reduced infectiousness of PLHIV on ART, expansion of programs for prevention of mother-to-child transmission (PMTCT) of HIV, and introduction of harm-reduction programs focusing on safer sex and outreach to high-risk populations.[4]

The World Health Organization (WHO) defines key populations as those who are vulnerable to and most-at-risk for HIV.[5] The guidelines define most-at-risk populations as "men who have sex with men, transgender people, people who inject drugs and sex workers. Most-at-risk populations are disproportionately affected by HIV in most, if not all, epidemic contexts."[5] Vulnerable populations can be identified by focusing on the specific social and demographic characteristics of a region, and may vary depending on specific situations and contexts.[5] The concept of key populations relates to the epidemic terminology as defined by the Joint United Nations Programme on HIV/AIDS (UNAIDS), which defines a "concentrated epidemic" as one in which HIV

Table 3
Adults and children newly infected with HIV, by region

	2000	2003	2006	2009	2012
Sub-Saharan Africa	2,600,000	2,400,000	2,100,000	1,900,000	1,600,000
Asia	488,000	422,000	374,000	341,000	351,000
North Africa and Middle East	20,000	23,000	25,000	26,000	32,000
Latin America and the Caribbean	126,000	114,000	107,000	105,000	98,000
North America, Western Europe and Oceania	84,200	81,200	84,200	81,200	79,100
Eastern Europe and Central Asia	140,000	130,000	120,000	120,000	130,000
Global	3,500,000	3,100,000	2,800,000	2,600,000	2,300,000

From Global report: UNAIDS report on the global AIDS epidemic 2013. Available at: http://www.unaids.org/en/media/unaids/contentassets/documents/epidemiology/2013/gr2013/UNAIDS_Global_Report_2013_en.pdf. Accessed May 9, 2014; with permission.

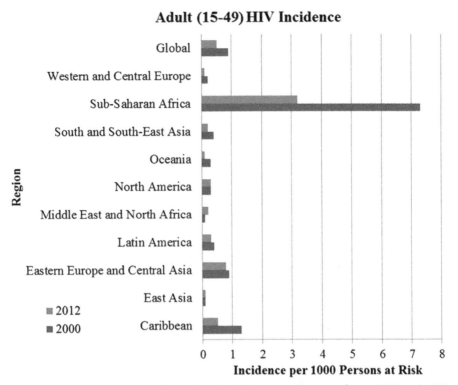

Fig. 1. Estimated HIV incidence by region in adults 15 to 49 years of age, 2000 and 2012. (*Data from* UNAIDS report on the global AIDS epidemic 2013. UNAIDS 2013. Available at: http://www.unaids.org/en/media/unaids/contentassets/documents/epidemiology/2013/gr 2013/UNAIDS_Global_Report_2013_en.pdf. Accessed May 9, 2014.)

has spread rapidly in one or more populations (usually >5% prevalence) but is not well established in the general population (usually <1% prevalence).[6] A "generalized epidemic" is an epidemic that is self-sustaining in the general population through heterosexual transmission.[6]

The purpose of this paper is to provide an overview of the diversity of the global HIV epidemic by region, including the impact of HIV treatment and prevention programs on epidemiologic trends, over the past decade.

SUB-SAHARAN AFRICA

HIV prevalence and incidence estimates in many developing countries, including those in sub-Saharan Africa, are derived using statistical models based primarily on either sentinel surveys among pregnant women or household surveys. Overall trends in HIV epidemiology show fewer new infections and decreased AIDS-related mortality in sub-Saharan Africa.[1] From 2000 to 2012, HIV incidence among adults in sub-Saharan Africa decreased by more than half, corresponding to an estimated 1 million fewer new HIV infections in 2012 compared with 2000.[1] The concurrent increase in estimated number of PLHIV, from 20.8 million in 2000 to 25 million in 2012, is largely from improved survival because of ART; AIDS-related deaths have decreased from approximately 1.4 million in 2000 to 1.2 million in 2012.[1] Evidence suggests that access to ART has reduced mortality rates and contributed to lower infection rates, resulting in slowly increasing HIV prevalence in most countries, with the notable exception of Angola, where new infections and AIDS-related deaths continue to increase.[1,3,4]

The main mode of transmission contributing to the HIV epidemic in sub-Saharan Africa is unprotected heterosexual intercourse.[1] Risk is increased with multiple sex partners and concurrent sexually transmitted infection, particularly herpes simplex type 2 (HSV-2).[7] A large proportion of new HIV infections may be attributable to long-term heterosexual relationships. Among sub-Saharan African couples in which at least one person is infected with HIV, at least two-thirds are in discordant relationships.[8] In Rwanda and Zambia, up to 95% of new infections occur in individuals who are living with their sex partners.[8] To what extent new infections are introduced into long-term relationships from other sex partners is unknown.

Among HIV-discordant couples in Africa, the man has traditionally been viewed as the infected partner, and most education and prevention programs have focused on reducing risks for male-to-female transmission. However, a meta-analysis by Eyawo and colleagues[8] showed that in approximately 47% of stable, heterosexual, HIV-discordant relationships, the infected partner was the woman. Globally, 50% of PLHIV are women, but this proportion is 59% in sub-Saharan Africa.[1]

Men at risk for HIV through heterosexual intercourse can reduce HIV risk by approximately 50% to 60% through undergoing voluntary medical male circumcision (VMMC).[9–11] A concerted effort has been endorsed by the WHO and UNAIDS since 2007 to prioritize VMMC for HIV prevention in 14 priority countries (Botswana, Ethiopia, Kenya, Lesotho, Malawi, Mozambique, Namibia, Rwanda, South Africa, Swaziland, Tanzania, Uganda, Zambia, and Zimbabwe).[12] The number of VMMCs has increased every year during the scale-up, reaching more than 500,000 in 2012.[12] This prevention approach is unique to this region and is specific to countries with low circumcision rates.

Another risk factor for HIV infection in sub-Saharan Africa is mother-to-child transmission of HIV. Although the use of ART in pregnancy can reduce the mother-to-child transmission rate to less than 1%, access to ART, HIV testing, and other PMTCT services remains incomplete.[1,13] In 2011, PMTCT services reached 59% of HIV-positive women in sub-Saharan Africa.[14] The estimated number of children infected each year has decreased from a high of 510,000 in 2002 to 2003 to 230,000 in 2012[1]; more than 350,000 children worldwide avoided acquiring HIV infection from 1995 to 2010, with approximately 86% of these children living in sub-Saharan Africa.[4] In addition, the estimated number of children who avoided infection doubled between 2008 and 2010 because access to ART increased dramatically during this period.[4]

The global trends in mother-to-child transmission of HIV have led to a disproportionate number of children living with HIV in sub-Saharan Africa; approximately 88% of all children younger than 15 years infected with HIV live in this region.[1] Approximately 55% fewer children were infected with HIV in 2012 than in 2003. However, access to ART is lower in children than in adults, and only 28% of children eligible for ART in sub-Saharan Africa are receiving treatment.[15] Frequently delays occur in the diagnosis of infant and pediatric HIV because of limited access to infant diagnostic tests, and the median survival of an untreated child in sub-Saharan Africa is only 12.4 months.[16] Environmental factors, such as greater exposure to infectious agents, reduced rates of vaccinations, and higher rates of malnutrition, cause untreated infants to have much lower rates of survival in sub-Saharan Africa than in industrialized countries.[16]

Although limited data exist on the role of MSM in the HIV epidemic in Africa, some studies have shown HIV prevalence among MSM populations in sub-Saharan Africa to be significantly higher than that of men in the general population.[17] HIV prevalence among MSM in surveyed populations has ranged from approximately 14% in Kampala, Uganda to 17% in surveyed populations in Botswana, Malawi, Namibia, and Nigeria, and up to 50% of MSM in Johannesburg, South Africa.[4] Sex between men remains highly stigmatized in sub-Saharan Africa, and many MSM also maintain sexual relationships with women.[18] To what extent HIV infection among MSM remains behaviorally segregated remains unclear, but viral genotype data from African MSM show the same circulating strains as in the general population, suggesting that overlap exists between MSM-acquired infection and HIV infection acquired through heterosexual transmission.[18] Stigmatization and criminalization of MSM in sub-Saharan Africa have limited the amount of reliable data on HIV prevalence, and few prevention or treatment programs target this key at-risk population.[18]

In addition to MSM, two key populations at risk for HIV infection are female sex workers (FSW) and individuals who pay for sex. An approximately linear relationship exists between HIV risk and number of sex partners for both men and women.[7] HIV prevalence among FSW, on average, is significantly higher (28%) than among women with no history of paid sex (17%).[7] HIV prevalence was also higher among men who reported sex with an FSW than among men who did not report this risk.[7] Research focusing on traditional high-risk groups in Africa, including FSW and MSM, has shown that these groups remain at higher risk for HIV infection than the general population, even in the setting of a generalized epidemic.[7] Injection drug use (IDU) is associated with a small proportion of HIV infections in sub-Saharan Africa, although its importance is increasing in Kenya, South Africa, Mauritius, and the United Republic of Tanzania.[19]

Considerable regional differences exist in the HIV epidemiology within the sub-Saharan Africa region; therefore, although all subregions share many of the epidemiologic characteristics discussed previously to varying degrees, some subregional differences are apparent. The subregion of Southern Africa is composed of countries with the highest estimated HIV prevalence in the world, including Swaziland (26.5%), Lesotho (23.1%), Botswana (23.0%), and South Africa (17.9%).[1] The severe epidemics in this subregion have no single cause. The combination of high rates of HSV-2, low rates of male circumcision, and sexual risk factors, including multiple partners and intergenerational sex, and large migrant populations, may all contribute to the high HIV burden.[20] However, new infections have continued to decline throughout the subregion. For example, approximately 300,000 fewer new HIV infections occurred in South Africa in 2012 than in 2000.[1]

The HIV prevalence is lower in the Eastern Africa region than in Southern Africa, ranging from approximately 2.9% in Rwanda to 7.2% in Uganda.[1] Incidence and AIDS-related deaths are also declining in this region, with the exception of Uganda, where HIV incidence increased throughout the late 2000s.[1] Lower rates of male circumcision, leading to higher risk for both HIV and ulcerative sexually transmitted infection; younger age at marriage; and younger age at sexual debut in Eastern Africa compared with Western Africa led to a more severe HIV epidemic in Eastern Africa.[20] In Western Africa, the HIV prevalence ranges from approximately 1.3% in Gambia to 3.2% in Cote d'Ivoire.[1] The largest estimated number of PLHIV in West Africa live in Nigeria (3.4 million), where there is an HIV prevalence of 3.1% and deaths caused by AIDS continue to increase.[1] The Central African region has an HIV prevalence between that of Eastern and Western Africa, which ranges from approximately 1.1% in the Democratic Republic of the Congo to 4.5% in Cameroon.[1] New infections and AIDS mortality have generally stabilized throughout the Central African subregion.[1]

ASIA

Asia has the second largest HIV burden after Africa. As in sub-Saharan Africa, the incidence of HIV is declining in Asia; however, these areas have important epidemiologic differences, mainly that HIV is concentrated among key populations. Despite reduced rates of HIV transmission, the number of PLHIV has increased to an estimated 4.8 million in 2012 from 3.8 million in 2000, largely because of improved survival.[1] AIDS-related deaths among adults and children in Asia have slowly declined during the 2000s to reach approximately 260,000 in 2012 from a high of 330,000 in 2005.[1] Although access to ART has improved, PMTCT services remain limited, with fewer than 20% of pregnant women receiving ART.[1] In addition, fewer than 60% of eligible persons were receiving ART in Asia in 2012.[1] Overall, new infections among children in Asia are decreasing.[1] The modes of transmission of HIV in Asia are primarily IDU, paid sex, and MSM, with considerable variations within and between countries.[4]

China and India have the highest burden of HIV in Asia.[1] The major mode of HIV transmission in China is heterosexual transmission; approximately 46.5% of the estimated 780,000 PLHIV in 2011 were estimated to have been infected with HIV through heterosexual transmission.[21] Injection drug use is also an important risk factor for HIV in China and accounts for approximately 28.4% of infections.[21] Among key populations at high risk, there was an HIV prevalence of approximately 0.3% among sex workers and 6.3% among MSM in 2011.[21] A subepidemic unique to China occurred among former plasma donors, which had spread through contaminated equipment during the 1990s.[22]

With 2.1 million PLHIV, India has the largest number of PLHIV in Asia. The overall estimated prevalence of 0.3% among adults aged 15 to 49 is lower than some countries in the region, including Cambodia (0.8%), Myanmar (0.6%), Vietnam (0.4%) and Malaysia (0.4%).[1] Other countries including Laos (0.3%), Nepal (0.3%), Philippines (<0.1%), and Pakistan (<0.1%) have similar or lower estimated adult HIV prevalence than India.[1] Within India, prevalence varies considerably by region, with HIV prevalence approximately 5 times as high in the Southern states of India as in the Northern states.[1,23] A high HIV prevalence exists among sex workers in India and HIV seems to be spreading from sex workers to their clients and to the clients' other sex partners.[23] Studies in India indicate that one-half to two-thirds of male clients of sex workers are either married or in a relationship with a woman.[23] An exception to this general pattern is in the Northeast region where IDU is the main risk factor.[23] As in China, overlapping epidemics exist between people who inject drugs (PWID) and sex workers, with many PWID buying and selling sex. The MSM population in India is not well characterized because sex between men is both stigmatized and illegal. However, limited studies indicate that HIV prevalence among MSM is significantly higher than in the general population (from 2%–19%) and that most MSM have female sex partners.[23]

Thailand, the only country in Asia with a generalized epidemic, had the highest estimated HIV prevalence in Asia, at 1.1% in 2012, although incidence and prevalence have been steadily declining.[1] Approximately 8800 new infections were reported in 2012, down from a high of 150,000 new infections in 1991.[1] Injection drug use is an important risk factor for HIV infection, particularly among women. Women who inject drugs have higher estimated HIV prevalence (30.8%) than men (24.2%), probably because of the overlap between drug use and sex work.[24] Men who have sex with men accounted for approximately 41% of new HIV infections in Thailand in 2010.[24]

NORTH AFRICA AND THE MIDDLE EAST

Unlike the HIV epidemics in sub-Saharan Africa and Asia, the North Africa and Middle East region has ongoing, steady increases in new infections and AIDS-related mortality.[4] From 2000 to 2012, the estimated number of PLHIV increased from 130,000 to 260,000, the estimated number of AIDS-related deaths increased from 7300 to 17,000, and the estimated new infections per year increased from 20,000 to 32,000.[1] Infections and deaths from AIDS among children have also increased.[1,4] Overall, the HIV prevalence is lower in North Africa and the Middle East compared with sub-Saharan Africa.[1] Near-universal male circumcision in the North Africa and Middle East region and lower rates of sexual risk behavior likely contribute to the low HIV prevalence.[25]

The epidemiology of HIV in North Africa and the Middle East has been difficult to track because of limited data, but surveillance is improving. Most countries in North Africa and the Middle East have concentrated epidemics among key populations. Current research indicates that the most important modes of HIV transmission in the region are IDU and unprotected intercourse, including among MSM.[4] Although MSM are stigmatized and precise numbers are difficult to track, research has shown that HIV infection rates among MSM are higher than in the general population.[25] Estimates for 2011 in Sudan indicate an HIV prevalence of 0.53% among adults and 3.64% among MSM.[26] As with MSM, the prevalence of HIV is higher among FSW than among the general population. The generalized HIV epidemics in Djibouti, Somalia, and South Sudan are suspected to be driven by commercial sex networks, but data on sex behavior are limited.[25]

Injection drug use is a significant mode of transmission throughout the region, including Pakistan, Afghanistan, Iran, Tunisia, Libya, Bahrain, Kuwait, and Oman.[25] HIV prevalence among PWID is highest in the Islamic Republic of Iran, where approximately 15% of PWID are HIV-positive.[27] People who inject drugs account for 67% of HIV cases in Iran and as much as 90% in Libya.[25] Levels of heroin and opium use are higher in North Africa and the Middle East than in other areas of the world.[25] The region is a drug route for heroin originating in Afghanistan, where more than 90% of the world's heroin is produced. Injection drug use remains stigmatized and illegal, despite its high prevalence, leading to limited knowledge of the precise prevalence of the risk behavior and the demographic characteristics of PWID.[25]

Despite the generally low prevalence, the increasing incidence of AIDS-related mortality indicates an inadequate response to HIV in North Africa and the Middle East. Only half of the countries in the region have PMTCT programs in place, and ART coverage is among the lowest in the world; only 11% of people in need of ART were on treatment in 2012.[28] The gap is even worse among children in need of ART, of which only 6% are on treatment. This treatment gap may be attributed to the low number of people who know their HIV status and the poor access to ART.[25] Overall, the epidemic is showing evidence of accelerating in this region.[1]

LATIN AMERICA AND THE CARIBBEAN

The HIV epidemic in Latin America (including South America, Central America, and Mexico) has stayed mostly stable over the past decade, with slowly declining HIV incidence and AIDS-related deaths resulting in a slightly increased number of PLHIV; the estimated number of PLHIV increased from 1.60 million in 2000 to 1.75 million in 2012.[1] When compared with South America, where no countries have a generalized epidemic, estimated adult HIV prevalence is higher in the Caribbean and Central America and exceeds 1% in the Bahamas, Belize, Guyana, Haiti, Jamaica, and

Suriname.[29] Females constitute a higher proportion of PLHIV (60%) in Latin America and the Caribbean than in any other region of the world. Despite the high burden of HIV in several countries of the Caribbean, however, new infections have decreased by more than 50% over the past decade.[2]

The highest HIV prevalence in Latin America is among MSM; 9 of 14 countries in the region have prevalence rates exceeding 10% among MSM.[4] Some parts of Colombia, Uruguay, and Bolivia have an HIV prevalence among MSM of approximately 20%, and one study showed that MSM in 15 countries in South and Central America are 33 times as likely to be infected with HIV as men in the general population.[4] The highest HIV prevalence among MSM in the world is in the Caribbean region, where approximately 25% of MSM are infected with HIV.[17] Transgender women (TGW) are also at very high risk for HIV infection. The highest HIV prevalence among TGW in Latin America is thought to be in Peru, where approximately 30.0% of TGW are infected with HIV.[29] Female sex workers are another high-risk population in the region, where approximately 6.1% of FSW are HIV-positive.[29]

Injection drug use contributes substantially to HIV transmission in Mexico and the southern areas of South America. In particular, Mexico seems to be experiencing an overlapping epidemic among PWID and FSW. Female sex workers who injected drugs in Ciudad Juarez and Tijuana had an HIV prevalence of 12% in one survey.[30]

Antiretroviral therapy coverage has increased substantially throughout Latin America and the Caribbean. In the Caribbean, approximately 79% of pregnant women with HIV received combined ART therapy, and AIDS-related deaths in the general population have decreased dramatically.[29] The ART coverage in Latin America is even higher, with more than 80% of persons in need receiving treatment.[1]

NORTH AMERICA, WESTERN EUROPE, AND OCEANIA

The epidemiologic methods for HIV surveillance are different in the higher-income countries of North America, Western Europe, and Oceania versus other regions of the world. Countries with fewer resources usually use health survey or sentinel surveillance data to estimate HIV prevalence, incidence, and mortality. In contrast, high-income countries have case-based surveillance systems to describe HIV epidemiology.[31] Overall trends in HIV prevalence are similar among the high-income countries of North America, Western Europe, and Oceania. The estimated number of PLHIV in North America has increased from 940,000 in 2000 to 1.3 million in 2012, but the prevalence among adults has stayed the same, approximately 0.5%, over the same period.[1] The estimated number of adult PLHIV in Western Europe increased to 860,000 in 2012 from 570,000 in 2000; in Oceania, adult PLHIV increased to 51,000 in 2012 from 34,000 in 2000.[1] In Western Europe, as in Oceania, estimated HIV prevalence among adults has stayed constant at 0.2%.[1] AIDS-related mortality has decreased over the past decade in all 3 regions.[1] Access to ART is high throughout these regions; 89% of HIV-positive persons receiving medical care in the United States underwent ART in 2010.[32]

All countries in North America, Western Europe, and Oceania have had steady or increasing numbers of PLHIV from 2006 to 2011.[1] All countries had more men infected with HIV, with approximately 2.5 men infected with HIV for every woman infected with HIV. The highest disparity was in Germany, where there are 5.6 infected men for every 1.0 infected woman.[31] HIV risk factors vary across the regions but, in general, most high-income countries report MSM as a major key population at risk. Countries in which MSM account for most PLHIV include the United States, Canada,

Spain, the Netherlands, Austria, Czech Republic, Australia, and New Zealand.[31] The incidence of HIV among MSM continues to increase in many countries, including the United States, United Kingdom, Switzerland, Spain, Greece, and France, among others.[31] In the United States, HIV prevalence among MSM has been increasing by approximately 8% per year since 2001.[17] The estimated HIV prevalence among MSM in North America (15%) is higher than in Western Europe (6%) and Oceania (4%).[17] Some counties have a primarily heterosexual epidemic, including Portugal, Norway, Sweden, Switzerland, Finland, and Latvia, although some of these risk categories may have been misclassified.[31] The only 2 countries in Western Europe, North America, and Oceania in which IDU is the most important risk factor for HIV are Estonia and Lithuania.[31]

A unique feature of the HIV epidemic in Western Europe is that approximately 35% of AIDS cases reported through 2006 were among migrants, with most from sub-Saharan Africa.[33] Across high-income nations, a racial and ethnic disparity exists in HIV prevalence, with ethnic minority groups having a higher HIV prevalence compared with the general population. In the United States, African Americans account for a disproportionate number of new HIV and AIDS diagnoses, and the same is true of Aboriginal persons in Canada.[34] Although case surveillance data provide accurate information about reported cases, information on "hidden" populations, such as sex workers and transgender individuals, is limited, because these classifications may not be captured on case report forms.[31]

EASTERN EUROPE AND CENTRAL ASIA

The Eastern Europe and Central Asia (EECA) region has a growing HIV epidemic, resulting in increasing numbers of PLHIV, AIDS deaths, and new infections among children, although overall incidence in the region is decreasing.[4] Approximately 760,000 adults and children were living with HIV in EECA in 2000, and this number increased to 1.3 million in 2012.[1] AIDS-related deaths have increased from approximately 24,000 to 91,000, and new infections have fluctuated over the same period.[1] This region is unusual in that new HIV infections continue to increase notably in Russia, Ukraine, Kazakhstan, and Kyrgyzstan.[1,35] In fact, in 4 countries in EECA (Kazakhstan, Kyrgyzstan, Georgia, Republic of Moldova), HIV incidence increased more than 25% from 2001 to 2011.[36] The highest estimated HIV prevalence in EECA is in Ukraine (0.9%).[1]

The predominant mode of HIV transmission in EECA is IDU. An estimated 3.1 million PWID live in EECA, and approximately 1 million of these individuals are infected with HIV.[37] Most (approximately 80%) HIV infections in Russia are among PWID.[36] The HIV incidence among PWID in Russia doubled from 2004 to 2009, and many HIV-infected PWID in the EECA region remain undiagnosed.[4] Similar to data on the epidemic in Asia, evidence shows significant overlap between sex work and IDU, which leads to amplified infection risk.[4] Men who have sex with men are thought to constitute less than 1% of the people newly diagnosed with HIV in EECA, but official estimates may underestimate the contribution of this high-risk group.[4] The estimated HIV prevalence among MSM in EECA is approximately 6.6%, which is considerably higher than among the general population.[17]

HIV data in EECA may be incomplete and underestimate the extent of HIV infections in the region because of low access to and uptake of HIV testing.[37] Few targeted approaches to prevention or treatment of HIV have been attempted among PWID in the region, despite the high prevalence of HIV in this subpopulation. Opiate substitution therapy is not available in Russia, Armenia, Tajikistan, Turkmenistan, or Uzbekistan.[36]

Needle and syringe exchange programs are available in all countries except Turkmenistan and Kosovo, but evidence from the International Harm Reduction Association indicates that the programs are limited in coverage.[38] In addition, ART coverage among PWID in EECA is low. Data are limited, but estimates show that less than 1% of HIV-positive PWID receive ART in Russia and Uzbekistan, and 5% to 12% in Estonia.[36,39]

Discussion and Program Implications

Most of the regions of the world have increasing HIV prevalence in the context of decreasing new infections and AIDS-related mortality, primarily reflecting the scale-up of ART programs in most regions. Worldwide increase in ART availability increases survival among PLHIV, leading to increased prevalence even as it decreases the likelihood of viral transmission from individuals adherent to ART. This finding was illustrated in the high-prevalence province of KwaZulu-Natal, South Africa, where increasing HIV prevalence in the province was almost completely explained by declining mortality among HIV-positive men and women aged 25 to 49 years as they gained access to ART.[40] This epidemiologic pattern will likely continue in KwaZulu-Natal and elsewhere as more persons are able to access ART. This represents an important change in the global epidemiology of HIV; it is now important to differentiate between persons living with long-term HIV infection and those newly infected. Consequently, the surveillance focus should shift to using HIV incidence to monitor prevention efforts.

In addition to a change in surveillance methodology to prioritize the identification of new infections, the massive HIV treatment scale-up that allowed 1.6 million more people access to ART in 2012 than in 2011 must continue. The number of people on ART in low- and middle-income countries has tripled from 2007 to 2012, but 9.7 million people are currently on treatment and 26.0 million are in need of ART (based on 2013 WHO eligibility guidelines).[41] Continued efforts to expand access to ART require identification of infected persons and linkage into HIV care. These programs could have increased impact if they more effectively identify key populations of HIV infected individuals and ensure high-quality care, treatment, and supportive services for those in need. Globally, men are less likely to receive ART than women, and PWID, MSM, and transgender individuals are underrepresented in access to HIV treatment relative to their burden of disease.[41] In addition, only 34% of children with HIV receive ART. Addressing this disparity, particularly in sub-Saharan Africa, should remain a high priority.[41]

The increased access to and effective use of ART may contribute to "treatment as prevention," meaning that treatment of HIV-infected individuals will function as a preventive measure by reducing transmission. Mathematical models have shown that 28% of all HIV infections would be prevented if 80% of PLHIV were given ART treatment.[42] Another study in South Africa showed that an individual living in an area with 30% to 40% ART coverage had a 34% decrease in risk of HIV infection compared with an individual living in an area with less than 10% ART coverage.[43] Updated WHO guidelines recommend ART for persons with CD4 counts less than 500 cells/μL. Global adaptation of these guidelines will further increase the number of persons on ART.[44] Another important component of treatment as prevention is provision of ART to HIV-infected pregnant women. Although PMTCT services have expanded dramatically, only 62% of pregnant women had access to PMTCT services in 2012, and only 30% of those who were eligible for treatment began ART.[1,2,4] To eliminate vertical transmission of HIV, PMTCT coverage must be increased. Since 2010, the WHO has recommended starting all HIV-infected pregnant women on lifelong HIV treatment at diagnosis ("Option B+").[45] This approach simplifies the medication regimen, decreases the likelihood of transmission through breastfeeding, decreases horizontal transmission to uninfected partners, and increases the likelihood of treatment during subsequent pregnancies.[46]

Despite the geographic heterogeneity of the HIV epidemic, increased ART coverage will reduce incidence in all regions. Increased access to ART combined with specific prevention interventions relevant to local populations and contexts may decrease incidence further.[47] In Africa, focus on PMTCT services and reduction in heterosexual risk, including VMMC and sexual risk-reduction strategies, should remain a high priority. Increasing HIV testing services and access to HIV care and treatment is important throughout North Africa and the Middle East. In countries where MSM remain at high risk, it is important to increase access to health care services, including testing and treatment. For countries in which PWID are at highest risk for infection, prevention strategies should focus on this high-risk group. Public health organizations should continue to focus on outreach to identify HIV-positive persons, link these persons to comprehensive care, increase quality of care, and retain these persons in treatment, and to provide ongoing education and prevention messages relevant to local communities. Great strides have been made in reducing HIV morbidity and mortality through the first decade of the 2000s, and continued focus on access to HIV treatment in addition to focused, region-appropriate prevention, care, and treatment will continue to reduce the burden of HIV disease going forward.

REFERENCES

1. Global report 2013: UNAIDS report on the global AIDS epidemic 2013. UNAIDS Web site. Available at: http://www.unaids.org/en/media/unaids/contentassets/documents/epidemiology/2013/gr2013/UNAIDS_Global_Report_2013_en.pdf. Accessed May 9, 2014.
2. AIDS by the numbers. UNAIDS Web site. Available at: http://www.unaids.org/en/media/unaids/contentassets/documents/unaidspublication/2013/JC2571_AIDS_by_the_numbers_en.pdf. Accessed January 3, 2014.
3. Ambrosioni J, Calmy A, Hirschel B. HIV treatment for prevention. J Int AIDS Soc 2011;14:28. http://dx.doi.org/10.1186/1758-2652-14-28.
4. Global HIV/AIDS response: epidemic update and health sector progress towards universal access. Progress report 2011. Available at: http://www.unaids.org/en/media/unaids/contentassets/documents/unaidspublication/2011/20111130_ua_report_en.pdf. Accessed January 3, 2014.
5. HIV/AIDS. Definition of key terms. World Health Organization Web site. Available at: http://www.who.int/hiv/pub/guidelines/arv2013/intro/keyterms/en/. Accessed April 7, 2014.
6. UNAIDS. UNAIDS terminology guidelines (October 2011). Available at: http://www.unaids.org/en/media/unaids/contentassets/documents/document/2011/20111009_UNAIDS_Terminology_Guidelines_MidtermAdditions_en.pdf. Accessed April 9, 2014.
7. Chen L, Jha P, Stirling B, et al. Sexual risk factors for HIV infection in early and advanced HIV epidemics in sub-Saharan Africa: systematic overview of 68 epidemiological studies. PLoS One 2007;2(10):e1001. http://dx.doi.org/10.1371/journal.pone.0001001.
8. Eyawo O, de Walque D, Ford N, et al. HIV status in discordant couples in sub-Saharan Africa: a systematic review and meta-analysis. Lancet Infect Dis 2010;10(11):770–7. http://dx.doi.org/10.1016/S1473-3099(10)70189-4.

9. Auvert B, Taljaard D, Lagarde E, et al. Randomized, controlled intervention trial of male circumcision for reduction of HIV infection risk: the ANRS 1265 trial. PLoS Med 2005;2(11):e298. http://dx.doi.org/10.1371/journal.pmed.0020298.

10. Bailey RC, Moses S, Parker CB, et al. Male circumcision for HIV prevention in young men in Kisumu, Kenya: a randomised controlled trial. Lancet 2007; 369(9562):643–56. http://dx.doi.org/10.1016/S0140-6736(07)60312-2.

11. Gray RH, Kigozi G, Serwadda D, et al. Male circumcision for HIV prevention in men in Rakai, Uganda: a randomised trial. Lancet 2007;369(9562):657–66. http://dx.doi.org/10.1016/S0140-6736(07)60313-4.

12. Centers for Disease Control and Prevention (CDC). Voluntary medical male circumcision - southern and eastern Africa, 2010-2012. MMWR Morb Mortal Wkly Rep 2013;62(47):953–7.

13. Cooper ER, Charurat M, Mofenson L, et al. Combination antiretroviral strategies for the treatment of pregnant HIV-1-infected women and prevention of perinatal HIV-1 transmission. J Acquir Immune Defic Syndr 2002;29(5):484–94.

14. UNAIDS. Regional fact sheet 2012. Sub-Saharan Africa. Available at: http://www.unaids.org/en/media/unaids/contentassets/documents/epidemiology/2012/gr2012/2012_FS_regional_ssa_en.pdf. Accessed April 3, 2014.

15. 2013 progress report on the global plan towards the elimination of new HIV infections among children by 2015 and keeping their mothers alive. Available at: http://www.unaids.org/en/media/unaids/contentassets/documents/unaidspublication/2013/20130625_progress_global_plan_en.pdf. Accessed January 17, 2014.

16. De Baets AJ, Ramet J, Msellati P, et al. The unique features of pediatric HIV-1 in sub-Saharan Africa. Curr HIV Res 2008;6(4):351–62.

17. Beyrer C, Baral SD, van Griensven F, et al. Global epidemiology of HIV infection in men who have sex with men. Lancet 2012;380(9839):367–77. http://dx.doi.org/10.1016/S0140-6736(12)60821-6.

18. Smith AD, Tapsoba P, Peshu N, et al. Men who have sex with men and HIV/AIDS in sub-Saharan Africa. Lancet 2009;374(9687):416–22. http://dx.doi.org/10.1016/S0140-6736(09)61118-1.

19. Sub-Saharan Africa: AIDS epidemic update regional summary. Available at: http://data.unaids.org/pub/Report/2008/JC1526_epibriefs_subsaharanafrica_en.pdf. Accessed January 3, 2014.

20. Orroth KK, Freeman EE, Bakker R, et al. Understanding the differences between contrasting HIV epidemics in east and west Africa: results from a simulation model of the Four Cities Study. Sex Transm Infect 2007;83(Suppl 1):i5–16. http://dx.doi.org/10.1136/sti.2006.023531.

21. Ministry of Health of the People's Republic of China. 2012 China AIDS response progress report. UNAIDS Web site. Available at: http://www.unaids.org/en/dataanalysis/knowyourresponse/countryprogressreports/2012countries/ce_CN_Narrative_Report%5B1%5D.pdf. Accessed April 28, 2014.

22. Wang L. Overview of the HIV/AIDS epidemic, scientific research and government responses in China. AIDS 2007;21(Suppl 8):S3–7. http://dx.doi.org/10.1097/01.aids.0000304690.24390.c2.

23. Asia: AIDS epidemic update: regional summary. Available at: http://data.unaids.org/pub/report/2008/jc1527_epibriefs_asia_en.pdf. Accessed April 28, 2014.

24. Thailand AIDS response progress report 2012. Available at: http://www.unaids.org/en/dataanalysis/knowyourresponse/countryprogressreports/2012countries/ce_th_narrative_report.pdf. Accessed April 28, 2014.

25. Abu-Raddad LJ, Ayodeji Akala F, Semini I. Characterizing the HIV/AIDS epidemic in the Middle East and North Africa. Time for strategic action. Washington, DC: The

International Bank for Reconstruction and Development/The World Bank; 2010. Available at: http://www-wds.worldbank.org/external/default/WDSContentServer/ WDSP/IB/2010/06/04/000333038_20100604011533/Rendered/PDF/548890PUB 0EPI11C10Dislosed061312010.pdf. Accessed January 22, 2014.

26. 2012 global AIDS report: Sudan. Available at: http://www.unaids.org/en/ dataanalysis/knowyourresponse/countryprogressreports/2012countries/ce_SD_ Narrative_Report%5B1%5D.pdf. Accessed April 28, 2014.

27. Islamic Republic of Iran AIDS progress report. Available at: http://www.unaids. org/en/dataanalysis/knowyourresponse/countryprogressreports/2012countries/ IRIran%20AIDS%20Progress%20Report%202012%20English%20final1_1.pdf. Accessed April 28, 2014.

28. Middle East and North Africa regional report on AIDS 2011. Available at: http:// www.unaids.org/en/media/unaids/contentassets/documents/unaidspublication/ 2011/JC2257_UNAIDS-MENA-report-2011_en.pdf. Accessed January 22, 2014.

29. De Boni R, Veloso VG, Grinsztejn B. Epidemiology of HIV in Latin America and the Caribbean. Curr Opin HIV AIDS 2014;9(2):192–8. http://dx.doi.org/10.1097/COH. 0000000000000031.

30. Stockman JK, Morris MD, Martinez G, et al. Prevalence and correlates of female condom use and interest among injection drug-using female sex workers in two Mexico-US border cities. AIDS Behav 2012;16(7):1877–86. http://dx.doi.org/10. 1007/s10461-012-0235-9.

31. Sullivan PS, Jones JS, Baral SD. The global north: HIV epidemiology in high-income countries. Curr Opin HIV AIDS 2014;9(2):199–205. http://dx.doi.org/10. 1097/COH.0000000000000039.

32. Vital signs: HIV prevention through care and treatment — United States. Centers for Disease Control and Prevention Web site. Available at: http://www.cdc.gov/ mmwr/preview/mmwrhtml/mm6047a4.htm?s_cid=mm6047a4_w#tab. Accessed March 25, 2014.

33. Del Amo J, Likatavičius G, Pérez-Cachafeiro S, et al. The epidemiology of HIV and AIDS reports in migrants in the 27 European Union countries, Norway and Iceland: 1999-2006. Eur J Public Health 2011;21(5):620–6. http://dx.doi.org/10. 1093/eurpub/ckq150.

34. North America, Western and Central Europe: AIDS epidemic update regional summary. Available at: http://data.unaids.org/pub/Report/2008/jc1532_epibriefs_ namerica_europe_en.pdf. Accessed February 9, 2014.

35. Beyrer C, Abdool Karim Q. The changing epidemiology of HIV in 2013. Curr Opin HIV AIDS 2013;8(4):306–10. http://dx.doi.org/10.1097/COH.0b013e328361f53a.

36. Wu Z, Shi CX, Detels R. Addressing injecting drug use in Asia and Eastern Europe. Curr HIV/AIDS Rep 2013;10(2):187–93. http://dx.doi.org/10.1007/ s11904-013-0153-0.

37. Jolley E, Rhodes T, Platt L, et al. HIV among people who inject drugs in Central and Eastern Europe and Central Asia: a systematic review with implications for policy. BMJ Open 2012;2(5). http://dx.doi.org/10.1136/bmjopen-2012-001465.

38. International Harm Reduction Association. Global state of harm reduction 2008: mapping the response to drug-related HIV and hepatitis C epidemics. Available at: http://www.ihra.net/files/2010/06/16/GSHRFullReport1.pdf. Accessed February 27, 2014.

39. Mathers BM, Degenhardt L, Ali H, et al. HIV prevention, treatment, and care services for people who inject drugs: a systematic review of global, regional, and national coverage. Lancet 2010;375(9719):1014–28. http://dx.doi.org/10.1016/ S0140-6736(10)60232-2.

40. Zaidi J, Grapsa E, Tanser F, et al. Dramatic increase in HIV prevalence after scale-up of antiretroviral treatment. AIDS 2013;27(14):2301–5. http://dx.doi.org/10.1097/QAD.0b013e328362e832.
41. Global update on HIV treatment 2013: results, impact and opportunities. WHO report in partnership with UNICEF and UNAIDS. June 2013. World Health Organization. Available at: http://www.unaids.org/en/media/unaids/contentassets/documents/unaidspublication/2013/20130630_treatment_report_en.pdf. Accessed February 19, 2014.
42. Abbas UL, Glaubius R, Mubayi A, et al. Antiretroviral therapy and pre-exposure prophylaxis: combined impact on HIV transmission and drug resistance in South Africa. J Infect Dis 2013;208(2):224–34. http://dx.doi.org/10.1093/infdis/jit150.
43. Tanser F, Bärnighausen T, Grapsa E, et al. High coverage of ART associated with decline in risk of HIV acquisition in rural KwaZulu-Natal, South Africa. Science 2013;339(6122):966–71. http://dx.doi.org/10.1126/science.1228160.
44. World Health Organization. Consolidated guidelines on the use of antiretroviral drugs for treating and preventing HIV infection: recommendations for a public health approach. June 2013. Available at: http://www.who.int/hiv/pub/guidelines/arv2013/download/en/. Accessed February 19, 2014.
45. World Health Organization. Antiretroviral drugs for treating pregnant women and preventing HIV infections in infants: recommendations for a public health approach. 2010 version. Available at: http://whqlibdoc.who.int/publications/2010/9789241599818_eng.pdf. Accessed January 17, 2014.
46. Chi BH, Stringer JSA, Moodley D. Antiretroviral drug regimens to prevent mother-to-child transmission of HIV: a review of scientific, program, and policy advances for sub-Saharan Africa. Curr HIV/AIDS Rep 2013;10(2):124–33. http://dx.doi.org/10.1007/s11904-013-0154-z.
47. Vermund SH, Hayes RJ. Combination prevention: new hope for stopping the epidemic. Curr HIV/AIDS Rep 2013;10(2):169–86. http://dx.doi.org/10.1007/s11904-013-0155-y.

HIV Testing, Staging, and Evaluation

Carla V. Rodriguez, PhD, MPH[a],*, Michael A. Horberg, MD, MAS[b]

KEYWORDS

- HIV epidemiology • HIV surveillance

KEY POINTS

- Overall HIV incidence has been stable over the last decade, although HIV prevalence has increased. HIV incidence in young MSM has been increasing over the last few years.
- Fourth-generation enzyme immunoassays (IAs) are recommended as part of the updated Centers for Disease Control and Prevention (CDC) and the Association of Public Health Laboratories diagnostic criteria for HIV infection. Fourth-generation IAs are able to detect p24 antigen and HIV-1/2 IgG and IgM antibodies as early as 2 weeks after infection.
- All HIV-infected persons, regardless of CD4 count, should initiate ART.
- On diagnosis with HIV, referral to infectious diseases or HIV specialist and a multidisciplinary care team is desirable to ensure best management of the patient and a comprehensive approach to care.

INTRODUCTION

The human immunodeficiency virus (HIV) that causes AIDS was first described in 1983. HIV-1 and HIV-2 are the two known distinct virus types and originate from different primate species.[1] HIV-1 is far more prevalent than HIV-2, which is only endemic in West Africa, with growing incidence in India.[2] HIV-1 and HIV-2 have similar transmission routes and can lead to the development of AIDS. However, persons infected with HIV-1 tend to have higher viral loads compared with those infected with HIV-2, which contributes to greater virulence and transmission, accelerated progression to AIDS, and higher risk of death compared with HIV-2.[2] HIV-1 is further classified into one of three phylogenetic groups: M (main), O (outlier), and N (non-M/non-O). The M group, which accounts for about 90% of HIV-1 infections, is further broken into 10 subtypes or clades: A-K, with E being the only nonrecombinant,

Disclosures: The authors have no professional or financial affiliations for themselves or their spouse/partner.
[a] Mid-Atlantic Permanente Research Institute, Kaiser Permanente, 2101 East Jefferson Street, 6 West, Rockville, MD 20852, USA; [b] HIV/AIDS, Mid-Atlantic Permanente Research Institute, Kaiser Permanente, 2101 East Jefferson Street, 6 West, Rockville, MD 20852, USA
* Corresponding author.
E-mail address: carla.v.rodriguez@kp.org

Infect Dis Clin N Am 28 (2014) 339–353
http://dx.doi.org/10.1016/j.idc.2014.06.002
id.theclinics.com

recombining only with subtype A.[3] Currently available combination antiretroviral therapy (ART) is active on all HIV-1 clades, with the exception of O subtypes, which are resistant to nonnucleoside reverse transcription inhibitors.[3] Subtype B is predominant in the Americas, Western and Central Europe, Australia, Thailand, North Africa, and the Middle East. Subtype C (sub-Saharan Africa, India, Brazil) accounts for 50% of all HIV-1 infections.

Worldwide there are now more than 35 million people living with HIV/AIDS. More than two-thirds of those infected live in sub-Saharan Africa, including 88% of the world's HIV-infected children.[4] The Asia-Pacific region, with 5 million infected persons, represents the area with the next highest prevalence of HIV/AIDS in the world. In 2012, an estimated 2.3 million people worldwide were newly infected with HIV and 1.6 million people died of AIDS. Approximately 10% of new infections and deaths were in children younger than 15 years.

In the United States, the peak of the epidemic in 1984 to 1985 saw approximately 130,000 new infections per year.[5] By 1991, new infections dropped to 49,000 per year. Since then, the incidence of HIV infections increased to 58,000 infections per year in 1997 and then declined to 50,000 infections per year in 2000, where it has since plateaued. A stable incidence rate comes despite a modest increase in the HIV testing rate. Estimates based on the National Health Interview Survey data suggest a rise in testing from 36.6% in 2000 to 45% in 2010. However, data from the National Health and Nutrition Examination Survey (NHANES) suggested no overall significant change.[6] In Canada, there were more than 3000 new infections in 2011.[7]

More effective ART has increased the number of people living with HIV to more than 1.1 million persons in the United States and 71,000 in Canada in 2011.[7,8] With higher prevalence come more opportunities for transmission if viral replication is not well controlled.[9] In addition, increased testing may create an inflated incidence rate that is simply an artifact of testing.[10] Despite increased testing and prevalence, the number of new infections per year has not increased over the last decade, suggesting that HIV testing, prevention, and treatment programs are working to reduce overall transmission. However, too often diagnosis comes too late, or not at all for too many Americans. In 2011, approximately one-third of all newly diagnosed HIV infections progressed to stage 3 (AIDS) within 12 months of diagnosis and an estimated 190,000 (16%) of people living with HIV were undiagnosed.[6] In Canada, approximately one-fourth of people living with HIV were unaware of their infection.[11] The epidemiology of HIV in key populations reflects the success of targeted interventions and informs areas for future work.

Race and Ethnicity

In the United States, blacks and African-Americans, Latinos, and men who have sex with men (MSM) continue to be disproportionately affected by HIV. Blacks/African-Americans bear the greatest burden. In 2010, the prevalence and incidence of HIV was 1650.8 and 68.9 per 100,000 persons, respectively.[12,13] These estimates are greater than seven times the HIV prevalence and incidence among whites. Latinos also continue to be disproportionately affected by HIV, with prevalence and incidence of 579.3 and 25.7 per 100,000, respectively, in 2010.

Through the Expanded Testing Initiative launched by the Centers for Disease Control and Prevention (CDC) in 2007, HIV screening and linkage to care programs targeted populations disproportionately affected by HIV: blacks, Latinos, and MSM.[6] Great gains have been achieved in the black population with regard to increased testing and reduced incidence. HIV testing among black non-Hispanics increased by 23% from 2000 to 2010, the only significant increase by race according to NHANES data.[6] Meanwhile, the annual HIV diagnosis rate among blacks decreased from 2008 to 2011.[8] In 2011, the percentage with AIDS at the time of HIV diagnosis was lowest among blacks (25.8%). Declines in diagnosis rates were also seen among Hispanics and persons of multiple races. Rates for American Indians/Alaska Natives and whites were stable. Although diagnosis rates increased among Asians, they maintained among the lowest overall incidence and prevalence rates, 8.4 and 121 per 100,000, respectively, in 2010.[12,13]

In Canada, Aboriginal people represent the ethnicity most disproportionately affected by HIV. In 2011, the HIV prevalence in this population was 544.0 per 100,000 and incidence rates were 3.5 times higher than among non-Aboriginal people.[7,11] The primary route of infection among Aboriginal people was injection drug use (IDU; 58%), followed by heterosexual sex (30%), MSM (9%), and MSM-IDU (3%).

The high proportion of undiagnosed HIV infection remains a public health challenge in North America. In the United States, HIV-infected blacks had the lowest proportion of undiagnosed infection in 2010. However, there were still approximately 85,000 (17%) black persons infected with HIV who did not know their serostatus.[12] HIV-infected Asians and Native Hawaiian/Other Pacific Islanders had the highest estimates of undiagnosed infection, 23% and 27%, respectively. Diagnosis of HIV at stage 3 (AIDS) was also highest among infected Hawaiians/Other Pacific Islanders (35.3%).[12]

MSM

Currently, about half of all people living with HIV in the United States and Canada are MSM.[7,12] New HIV infections among MSM peaked in the mid-1980s at more than 75,000 new infections per year. By the early 1990s, the incidence among MSM dropped to less than 18,000 per year. Unfortunately, after years of steady progress, new infections began to rise among MSM throughout the 1990s and into the 2000s.[5] This rise was likely associated with many factors, including "condom fatigue," a younger at-risk age demographic among MSM, and effective therapies lessening the fear of mortality. Additionally, this same time period also was associated with great use of erectile dysfunction medications and other sexually transmitted infections (STI), such as syphilis. Although in recent years prevention efforts may have helped stabilize infections (HIV testing increased by 22% from 2000 to 2010 in the 45 to 64 age group[6]), the incidence of HIV is again on the rise among MSM. In 2011 there were an estimated 31,000 new diagnoses.[8] Increasing incidence among MSM has recently been driven by those in the 13 to 24 age group, in whom new infections increased from 7200 in 2008 (27% of all MSM with new diagnoses) to 8800 (30%) in 2010.[13] Moreover, more than a quarter of MSMs who are HIV-infected were unaware of their status.[12] This underscores the need to sustain and reinvigorate prevention efforts for gay and bisexual men of all races and to ensure that each generation is effectively reached. Meanwhile, the number of new diagnoses attributed to MSM and IDU and heterosexual contact decreased.[8] As of 2011, most (75.9%) HIV-infected persons in the Unites States were male, and 68.7% were MSM. The lowest percentages of persons with AIDS at the time of HIV diagnosis was among MSM and heterosexual females, both 25.6%.[14]

In Canada, the proportion of new infections among MSM increased from 44% in 2008 to 47% in 2011.[7] However, the largest estimated prevalence of undiagnosed HIV infection in 2011 was among persons engaged in heterosexual sex (34% among persons born in countries where HIV is endemic and nonendemic, combined).[7] Among MSM and IDU, the estimated proportion living with undiagnosed HIV was 20% and 24%, respectively.

Pregnant Women and Perinatally Acquired HIV

The decline in perinatally acquired HIV has been a public health success story. Since the peak in the early 1990s to 2010, annual perinatal transmission (mother to child) has declined from an estimated 1650 to 212 cases (86% decline).[12,15] This decline is largely attributed to effective screening and treatment among pregnant women. From 2008 to 2010, perinatally acquired HIV decreased from 6.8 to 5.7 per 100,000 live births. These tremendous declines since the early days of the epidemic are because of successful perinatal prophylaxis, successful antiretroviral treatment of the mother, and recommendations against breastfeeding by HIV-infected mothers in the United States. Declines were greatest among children born to black women, although their rates were almost four times higher than the general population.[12] However, in every year since 2000, only 60% of pregnant women were tested for HIV in the last 12 months, although testing with each pregnancy is recommended.[16,17] Opportunities to strengthen prevention campaigns targeting adolescents abound as those who were infected perinatally age and begin navigating their own sexuality and issues related to family planning, prevention of STI, stigma, combination ART adherence, and associated economic burdens. In addition, long-term exposure to ART initiated perinatally and continued throughout adulthood during key developmental stages is not well understood.[16]

Youth

Programs geared toward all adolescents, not just those infected, are very much needed to stem transmission. In the United States, HIV incidence among adolescents and young adults has been relatively stable from 2007 to 2010.[13] In 2010, HIV incidence was 23.7 and 34.9 per 100,000 persons among persons 13 to 24 years and 25 to 34 years, respectively.[13] However, among young MSM aged 13 to 24, the incidence rose from 23% in 2007 to 30% in 2010.[13] Furthermore, the CDC estimated that in 2010 58% of HIV infections among persons aged 13 to 24 were undiagnosed. Additionally, almost half of US high school students in 2011 had engaged in sexual intercourse and one-third were sexually active.

STAGING

The viral kinetics of HIV is illustrated in **Fig. 1**. Plasma HIV RNA levels are typically not detectable until approximately 10 days after HIV infection. The p24 antigen becomes detectable after about 17 days, and its rise parallels the initial increase in viral load, both peaking at about 3 to 6 weeks postinfection. As the viral load declines, levels of HIV antibodies begin to increase.[18] The virus reaches a plateau, or "viral set point," at which point CD4 counts begin to rise, but usually not to a level before infection. Stages have been assigned to represent key phases in the continuum of HIV to AIDS: acute HIV infection, chronic HIV infection, and AIDS. In addition, the CDC has defined three stages of severity for the purposes of surveillance: (1) stage 1, CD4 count greater than or equal to 500 cells/UL (or CD4% $\geq$29) and no AIDS-definition condition (**Box 1**); (2) stage 2, CD4 count of 200 to 499 cells/UL (or CD4% 14–28) and no AIDS-definition condition; and (3) stage 3, CD4 count less than 200 cells/UL (or CD4% <14) or documentation of an AIDS-definition condition. Although CD4 counts define HIV stages of disease, they are not used to diagnose infection. Current treatment guidelines include offering ART to all patients regardless of CD4 count.[19]

Acute HIV Infection

Acute HIV infection has been defined as a transient nonspecific clinical syndrome corresponding with high viral load (typically within 2–6 weeks of transmission) and

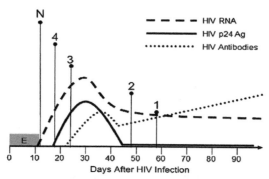

Fig. 1. Diagnostic markers of HIV infection. Time to reliable positivity of first (1), second (2), third (3), and fourth (4) generation and nucleic acid amplification test (N). HIV diagnostic assays superimposed on a graphic depiction of the kinetics of circulating HIV RNA, p24 antigen, and HIV antibodies. (*From* Cornett JK, Kirn TJ. Laboratory diagnosis of HIV in adults: a review of current methods. Clin Infect Dis 2013;57:712–8; with permission.)

Box 1
Opportunistic infections considered an AIDS-definition condition

- Candidiasis of bronchi, trachea, esophagus, or lungs
- Invasive cervical cancer
- Coccidioidomycosis
- Cryptococcosis
- Cryptosporidiosis, chronic intestinal (>1 month duration)
- Cytomegalovirus disease (particularly cytomegalovirus retinitis)
- Encephalopathy, HIV-related
- Herpes simplex: chronic ulcers (>1 month duration); or bronchitis, pneumonitis, or esophagitis
- Histoplasmosis
- Isosporiasis, chronic intestinal (>1 month duration)
- Kaposi sarcoma
- Lymphoma, multiple forms
- *Mycobacterium avium* complex
- Tuberculosis
- *Pneumocystis carinii* pneumonia
- Pneumonia, recurrent
- Progressive multifocal leukoencephalopathy
- *Salmonella* septicemia, recurrent
- Toxoplasmosis of brain
- Wasting syndrome caused by HIV

Data from AIDS.gov. Opportunistic infections. Available at: http://www.aids.gov/hiv-aids-basics/staying-healthy-with-hiv-aids/potential-related-health-problems/opportunistic-infections/.

as the phase between detectable p24 or HIV RNA and detectable antibodies. However, quantitative viral load tests are not currently approved in the United States for diagnosing HIV because of high false-positive fractions at lower viral load levels. Ideally, all HIV-positive persons would be detected during the acute stage of infection. Studies have shown that the highest rates of transmission occur during the acute stage of infection, regardless of viral load.[18] Also, the longer a person is unaware of their diagnosis, the greater likelihood they have of passing the infection to others, especially during the acute infection phase with extremely high viral loads.[18] While the presence of a proper clinical situation (recent potential exposure with or without clinical symptoms consistent with acute mononucleosis-like syndrome) and a high and increasing viral load often carries a diagnosis of acute HIV infection, acute HIV infection diagnosis is missed 80% of the time.[18] The HIV antibody test is often negative because symptoms present before HIV antibody seroconversion.

Chronic HIV Infection

The next phase of infection is called clinical latency or chronic HIV infection. The median time from HIV infection to AIDS has been estimated at 10 years, depending on age at infection.[20] Most of this period is characterized as chronic infection. Clinicians should suspect chronic HIV infection, if previous testing was negative, if the following signs or symptoms are present (although most often patients are asymptomatic): active or history of STI, opportunistic infection, tuberculosis, hepatitis B or C, cervical cancer, new severe psoriasis, new herpes zoster in someone younger than 50 years old; thrush; unexplained cachexia or weight loss, lymphadenopathy, thrombocytopenia, leukopenia, anemia; and prolonged unexplained illness with negative evaluation.[21]

HIV reproduces more slowly during this phase. Depending on the viral set point, patients may have lower levels of viremia and greater CD4 counts without the use of medication during the early years of this stage. Although the absolute CD4 count may be higher than those patients with more advanced HIV infection, the CD4% is likely abnormally lower. Although asymptomatic, untreated HIV infection leads to greater likelihood of transmission and ongoing immune system destruction. Present recommendations are for nearly all HIV-infected individuals to receive appropriate ART aiming for undetectable viral loads. Typically, viral load begins to rise, CD4 counts begins to drop, and patients can begin to develop constitutional symptoms of HIV, including fever, night sweats, fatigue, and weight loss during the middle and end of this period. Yet, most chronic HIV patients without AIDS-defining conditions are asymptomatic. Testing should be prompted by general recommendations for HIV testing or with higher risk for HIV infection (multiple sexual partners, intercourse without a condom, prior or present STI).

AIDS

The final stage of disease is defined as AIDS. Although the median time from HIV infection to AIDS is approximately 10 years, in 2011, one-third of all HIV infections in the United States progressed to AIDS within a year of diagnosis. This fact underscores the need to improve early diagnosis. AIDS is defined as having either CD4 count less than 200/μL or an AIDS-defining illness (see **Box 1**). All HIV-infected patients, regardless of their present CD4 count, are considered AIDS cases if they ever met either of these criteria. Furthermore, all HIV-infected patients meeting AIDS criteria should receive ART, regardless of their viral load.

TESTING
Screening Recommendations

Diagnosis is a key component to limiting the spread of HIV and mitigating the impact of the epidemic. Yet, approximately 17% of all HIV infections are undiagnosed. Without diagnosis, patients cannot be linked or retained in care, prescribed ART, or suppress the virus; thus, there is an increase in the risk of transmitting it to others. Recognizing the need, the US Preventive Services Task Force (USPSTF) 2013 guidelines upgraded HIV screening to an "A" grade and recommends screening for HIV in all persons aged 15 to 65 years, including pregnant women with each pregnancy; and targeted screening in younger adolescents and older adults for those at increased or ongoing risk.[16] The USPSTF 2013 guidelines also recommend annual screening in uninfected persons who are MSM and active injection drug users; and repeat testing (every 3–5 years) for those at "increased risk" of transmission, including those (1) who have acquired or request testing for other STIs; (2) who engage in unprotected vaginal or anal intercourse and are not in exclusive monogamous relationships with an uninfected partner; (3) with sexual partners who are HIV-infected, bisexual, or injection drug users; (4) who exchange sex for drugs or money; or (5) who live or receive medical care in a high-prevalence setting.[16] In practice, many clinicians (including the author MAH) would test those at increased risk annually. The USPSTF defines a "high-prevalence setting" as one with an HIV prevalence greater than or equal to 1%, including STI clinics, correctional facilities, homeless shelters, tuberculosis clinics, clinics serving MSM, and adolescent health clinics with a high prevalence of sexually transmitted diseases. To support screening and reduce barriers related to diagnosis, the Patient Protection and Affordable Care Act (ACA) eliminates exclusions for preexisting conditions, prohibits insurance from rescinding coverage, puts an end to lifetime and annual coverage limits, and extends eligibility for dependent coverage to up to 26 years. Additionally, the ACA requires that all new health plans provide certain services, including those rated A or B by the USPSTF, at no added cost to the patient. Medicare and Medicaid, in states that opt for the Medicaid expansion, must also provide such services at no cost.[22]

Diagnostic Tools

The tools needed to screen and the additional laboratory diagnostics that support ongoing testing and treatment management in HIV-infected populations have improved greatly since the start of the epidemic. The first enzyme immunoassay (IA) to detect HIV antibodies was introduced in 1985 and could detect positive specimens no earlier than 6 weeks after infection (see **Fig. 1**). Unlike current tests, early diagnostics, including Western blot and immunofluorescence assay, were designed for IgG detection, were unable to differentiate between HIV-1 clades, and lacked the sensitivity and specificity of current diagnostics.[18] Today's fourth-generation IAs became available in the United States in 2010 and are recommended as part of the updated CDC and the Association of Public Health Laboratories diagnostic criteria for HIV infection. These IAs are able to reliably detect p24 antigen and HIV-1/2 IgG and IgM antibodies as early as 2 weeks after infection, thus being able to diagnose even acute cases with great sensitivity. **Fig. 1** illustrates the temporal ability for first- to fourth-generation IAs to detect HIV infection.

Point-of-care rapid HIV tests, approved by the US Food and Drug Administration (FDA) in 2002, changed the landscape for HIV testing in acute care settings. Rapid tests detect anti-HIV IgG and IgM in sputum, whole blood, plasma, or serum.[18] Results are available within 30 minutes and thus have an opportunity to influence medical decision making, obviate the need to track patients down to report results, and facilitates engagement in care where appropriate. The reported accuracy of rapid tests has been mixed, with later studies showing accuracy comparable with third- and fourth-generation IAs.[18] A study of the OraQuick Rapid HIV-1 Antibody Test (OraSure Technologies, Inc. Bethlehem, PA, USA) in 3238 patients seeking emergency department care demonstrated 100% sensitivity and 99.94% specificity compared with enzyme IA and confirmatory Western blot.[23] HIV home self-tests, approved by the FDA in 2013, allow patients further anonymity and have been shown to be highly acceptable, preferred, and more likely to result in partner self-testing.[24] However, subsequent linkage to care among persons who self-test has not been fully evaluated and confirmatory testing is recommended.

Current CDC recommendations, as presented at the 2012 HIV Diagnostics Conference Feedback Session (December 2012) are illustrated in **Fig. 2**. Recommended HIV laboratory diagnostic testing algorithm for serum or plasma specimens (excerpted from draft recommendations) is as follows[25]:

1. An FDA-approved fourth-generation HIV-1/2 IA should be used to screen for acute HIV-1 infection and for established infections with HIV-1 or HIV-2.
2. Specimens with a reactive fourth-generation IA (or repeatedly reactive, if repeat testing is recommended by the manufacturer) should be tested with an FDA-approved second-generation antibody IA that differentiates HIV-1 antibodies from HIV-2 antibodies.
3. Positive results on the initial IA and HIV-1/HIV-2 antibody differentiation IA should be considered positive for HIV-1 or HIV-2 antibodies and should initiate medical care that includes laboratory tests (such as viral load, CD4 count, and antiretroviral resistance assays—see below) to confirm the presence of HIV infection, stage HIV disease, and assist in the selection of an initial antiretroviral drug regimen.
4. Specimens that are reactive on the initial assay and negative on the HIV-1/HIV-2 antibody differentiation IA should be tested with an FDA-approved nucleic acid test (NAT) for HIV-1 RNA (many providers commonly use an HIV-1 RNA viral load assay if NAT is not available). Under these circumstances, a reactive NAT result indicates the presence of acute HIV-1 infection. A negative result indicates the

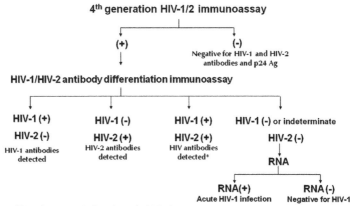

Fig. 2. Recommended HIV laboratory diagnostic testing algorithm for serum or plasma specimens. (*From* US Centers for Disease Control, Draft laboratory testing guidance, 2012. Available at: http://www.cdc.gov/hiv/pdf/policies_Draft_HIV_Testing_Alg_Rec_508.2.pdf. Accessed January 10, 2014.)

absence of HIV-1 infection, either a false-positive result on the initial IA or rarely, recent HIV-2 infection. If HIV-2 infection is a possibility, a NAT for HIV-2 DNA can be considered. However, HIV-2 infection is rare in the United States, and there is no FDA-approved NAT for HIV-2.

5. This testing algorithm, beginning with a fourth-generation IA, should be followed for specimens from persons with a preliminary positive rapid HIV test result.

Alternatives for use with other FDA-approved HIV tests are as follows:

1. Third-generation HIV-1/2 IA used as the initial test: Perform subsequent testing as specified in the recommended algorithm. This alternative misses some acute HIV infections in antibody-negative persons.
2. Alternative FDA-approved supplemental antibody test (eg, HIV-1 Western blot or indirect immunofluorescence assay) used as the second test instead of an HIV-1/HIV-2 antibody differentiation IA: If negative or indeterminate, perform HIV-1 NAT; if HIV-1 NAT is negative, perform HIV-2 antibody IA. This alternative might misclassify HIV-2 infections as HIV-1, and incur additional costs, and increases turnaround time for test results.
3. HIV-1 NAT as second test instead of the HIV-1/HIV-2 antibody differentiation IA: If HIV-1 NAT result is negative, perform an HIV-1/HIV-2 antibody differentiation IA or other FDA-approved supplemental antibody test. If result of this antibody test is negative or indeterminate, perform an HIV-2 antibody test. This alternative fails to distinguish acute HIV infection from established infection, increases turnaround time for test results, and incurs additional costs.

Quantitative viral load and CD4 testing are not recommended for diagnosis of HIV, although their use in monitoring of HIV disease is discussed later.

INITIAL EVALUATION AND CARE
Initial Evaluation

On diagnosis with HIV, referral to infectious diseases or HIV specialist is desirable to ensure best management of the patient. Care is often provided by a multidisciplinary care team, which could include (1) the HIV specialist; (2) nurse case manager; (3) clinical pharmacist to help with maximal ART adherence, adverse medication effects management, and complex drug-drug interactions, social worker for case management, and health educator. Other members of the care team could include other specialists, mental health experts, and transportation and housing specialists. The initial evaluation of an HIV-infected patient needs to be thorough and fairly exhaustive. A comprehensive present and past medical history (with special attention to HIV-related information), physical examination, and medication history should be obtained for all patients on initiation of care (**Box 2**). In addition, a complete review of systems and physical examination is essential. The suggested review of systems and physical examination are listed in **Box 3**.

Clinical Testing and Case Management

The initial laboratory examination for a patient newly diagnosed with HIV infection needs to be fairly exhaustive (**Box 4**). Parameters of the stage of infection, comorbidities, and other health parameters (including renal and hepatic function) must be established before further therapy.

Once patients are identified as HIV-positive, regular testing is recommended to monitor therapeutic response and sustained viral suppression. HIV-1 RNA levels (viral load) should be assessed before treatment initiation and every 2 to 4 weeks (but not

Box 2
Initial assessment: history, review of systems, and physical examination

Initial history

- HIV diagnosis: How, where, and when the diagnosis was made

- History compatible with an acute retroviral illness (or prior negative test)

- Infections potentially related to HIV (eg, thrush, oral hairy cell leukoplakia, recurrent vaginitis, varicella zoster virus, cervical cancer or dysplasia, *Pneumocystis carinii* pneumonia, or other opportunistic infections)

- HIV medications: Prior use of antiretroviral therapy or preexposure/postexposure prophylaxis, including specific drugs, duration of therapy, complications or side effects, drug resistance, and adherence

- Comorbidities: History of and risk factors for coronary heart disease, dyslipidemia, diabetes mellitus, and osteoporosis

- Psychiatric history: Treatment of symptoms of depression, anxiety, suicidal ideation or posttraumatic stress disorder, psychiatric hospitalizations

- Sexually transmitted diseases: Gonorrhea, chlamydia, chancroid, syphilis, herpes simplex virus, viral hepatitis, human papilloma virus, and trichomoniasis, including treatment history and outcome

- Women: Gynecologic and obstetric history, plans for future pregnancy, birth control practices, abnormal Pap smears, menstrual history, mammogram (if applicable)

- Pediatric: Maternal obstetric and birth history, exposure to perinatal antiretrovirals, exposure to infectious diseases, growth and development

- Any prior malignancies

- Hematologic complications: Idiopathic thrombocytopenic purpura, neutropenia, or anemia

- Inquire about dates of
  - Last PAP smear
  - Exposure to tuberculosis: Last screening test for tuberculosis (If positive, was patient treated with isoniazid? Establish duration of therapy and document date of last negative purified protein derivative)
  - Immunization history: Hepatitis A and B vaccine, TDAP vaccine, pneumococcal vaccine, influenza vaccine
  - Last dental visit
  - Family history: Significant familial medical conditions

Allergies

- Dates and types of reactions

Social history

- Demographics: Sexual orientation, sexual identity, race/ethnicity

- Health-related behaviors: Tobacco, alcohol, and drugs

- Patient birthplace and residence history

- Travel history: Establish risk for reactivation of geographically endemic infections, such as histoplasmosis and coccidiodomycosis

- History of donated blood, organs, or semen

- Employment history

- Establish mode of infection and sexual history
  - Have your sexual partners been women, men, or both?

- ○ To what extent have you had unprotected sexual contact, regardless of the gender or number of partners?
- ○ Do you have a history of injection drug use?
- ○ Have you shared needles for injection drug use?
- ○ Have you had a transfusion or received blood products, especially between 1975 and 1985?
- ○ Have you been the recipient of artificial insemination by an unidentified donor?
- Review specific sexual practices and discuss safer sex techniques
- Document patient's statement regarding marital and relationship status; partner's health and HIV status and his or her access to health care, including HIV testing; and whether the spouse or partner is aware of patient's seropositive status
- Disclosure: Determine who knows about the patient's HIV status/diagnosis
- Determine participation in any HIV support groups
- Review diet and unusual dietary habits; review good nutrition and foods to be avoided
- Inquire about exercise and pets (including cats and birds)

Medications

- Current medications, including over-the-counter medications
- Prior experience with HIV therapy: Specific drugs, duration of therapy, complications or side effects from therapy
- Any use of alternative agents (nutritional, psychological, herbal, acupuncture)

Adapted from Aberg JA, Gallant JE, Ghanem KG, et al. Primary care guidelines for the management of persons infected with HIV: 2013 update by the HIV Medicine Association of the Infectious Diseases Society of America. Clin Infect Dis 2014;58(1):e1–34; with permission.

more than 8 weeks) after initiation or change in ART until viral load becomes suppressed (depending on assay used; <50 copies/mL). Monitoring viral load every 3 to 4 months in untreated patients and patients on stable ART is recommended. Patients who have suppressed viral load for more than 2 to 3 years and are adherent to therapy may be monitored every 6 months.[17]

CD4 cell counts should be monitored to assess the urgency for initiating ART and its efficacy and to determine the need for prophylaxis against opportunistic infections. The Infectious Disease Society of America recommends monitoring CD4 at entry into care and, if therapy is delayed, annually to determine if immune function is stable or declining and before initiation of ART. Follow-up tests should be conducted every 3 to 4 months, and 6 to 12 months in patients on suppressive ART regimens whose CD4 counts are well above the threshold for opportunistic infections. Other baseline tests that should be assessed before the initiation of treatment are listed in **Box 4**. Special considerations must be made for pregnant women, infants, and children infected with HIV.[17] These considerations include the following:

1. All pregnant women should be treated for HIV infection, regardless of immunologic or virologic status, to prevent transmission to fetus. Infants exposed to HIV in utero should undergo HIV diagnostic testing at 13 to 21 days of life and again at 1 to 2 months and 4 to 6 months of age.
2. HIV-infected infants should undergo HIV resistance testing and initiate therapy in the first year of life, regardless of immunologic, virologic, or clinical status.
3. CD4 cell counts and viral loads in children born to HIV-infected mothers should be monitored every 3 to 4 months until 18 months when it is hoped the child is

Box 3
Review of systems and physical examinations

Initial Assessment: Review of Signs and Symptoms	Initial Assessment: Physical Examination
A complete review of systems with special attention to the following areas: • General: unexplained weight loss, night sweats, fever, body fat changes • Skin: skin discoloration, seborrheic dermatitis, psoriasis, new pigmented lesions, folliculitis, pruritis, vesicular lesions, nodules, hair changes, onychomycosis • Lymph nodes: localized or generalized enlargement of lymph nodes, a recent decrease in size of previously enlarged nodes • Eyes: vision change or loss • Mouth: gum disease, aphthous ulcers, thrush, oral hairy leukoplakia • Gastrointestinal: diarrhea, nausea, stomach cramps • Endocrinology: diabetes mellitus, hypogonadism • Neurologic and psychiatric: persistent and severe headaches, memory loss, loss of concentration, depression, apathy, paresthesias, paralysis or weakness, cognitive difficulties, seizures and sleep disorders, mood swings • Genitourinary: recurrent candidal vaginitis, anal lesions • Orthopedic: hip pain, nontraumatic or compressions fractures, diagnosis of or risk factors for osteopenia/osteoporosis	A complete physical examination should be performed on all patients. It is common in the asymptomatic patient to have a normal physical examination. Special attention should be paid to the following areas: • Vital signs: including height and weight • General including body habitus, evidence of obesity, wasting, lipodystrophy, assessment of frailty and ambulatory ability • Skin: seborrheic dermatitis, ecchymoses, purpura, petechiae, Kaposi sarcoma, herpes simplex or zoster, psoriasis, molluscum contagiosum, onychomycosis, folliculitis, condylomata, cutaneous fungal infections • Lymph nodes: generalized or localized lymphadenopathy • Eye: retinal exudates or cotton wool spots, hemorrhages, pallor, icterus; dilated fundoscopic examination, especially if $CD4^+$ are <100/μL • Oropharynx: oral hairy leukoplakia, candidiasis (thrush, palatal erythema, angular cheilosis), aphthous ulcers, gingivitis, periodontal disease, Kaposi sarcoma, tonsillar or parotid gland enlargement • Cardiovascular: heart examination, peripheral pulses, presence/absence of edema • Chest: lung examination • Breast: nodules, nipple discharge • Abdomen: hepatomegaly, splenomegaly, masses, tenderness • Genitourinary: ulcers, warts, chancres, rashes, abnormal gynecologic examination, discharge • Anorectal: ulcers, warts, fissures, internal or external hemorrhoids, masses, Kaposi sarcoma • Neuropsychiatric: depression, mania, anxiety, signs of personality disorder, difficulties in concentration, attention, and memory, signs of dementia, speech problems, gait abnormalities, focal deficits (motor or sensory), lower extremity vibratory sensation (distal sensory neuropathy, abnormal reflexes)

Box 4
Initial evaluation: baseline laboratory tests

Recommended	Consider
Patients who have been diagnosed with HIV outside of your care system should have a confirmatory antibody test done unless medical documentation of previous positive antibody test or HIV RNA level above limits of quantification is available	• *Toxoplasma gondii* IgG (to identify patients at risk for reactivation)
• Complete blood count with differential and platelets	• Cytomegalovirus IgG: especially for patients at low risk for prior exposure (women and transfusion recipients)
• CD4$^+$ cell count and %, CD8$^+$ cell count and %, and CD4/CD8 ratio	• G6PD level: before considering primaquine, dapsone or pyrimethamine use in patients with genetic risk for enzyme deficiency (Mediterranean, Asian, African descent)
• HIV RNA level	• Coreceptor tropism assay (if CCR5 antagonist being considered)
• Liver enzymes: alanine aminotransferase, aspartate aminotransferase, total bilirubin, alkaline phosphatase	• HLA B*5701 for increased hypersensitivity reaction to abacavir (if never screened and not presently taking this medication)
• Serum creatinine and glomerular filtration rate estimate	• Baseline chest radiograph: if prior pulmonary disease
• Electrolytes including serum phosphorous	• PAP smear of anus
• HIV viral genotypic analysis (assuming patient not on antiretroviral medications)	• Serum testosterone level (in males with fatigue, weight loss, loss of libido, erectile dysfunction, or depression or who have evidence of reduced bone mineral density; morning free testosterone preferred)
• Urinalysis	
• Gonorrhea/chlamydia chlamydia nucleic acid amplification test testing at appropriate sites (consider pharynx, rectum, and cervical and urethral/urine)	
• Syphilis screening	
• Hepatitis: hepatitis A IgG; hepatitis B core antibody, hepatitis B surface antigen; hepatitis C antibody (Confirm a negative hepatitis C antibody with hepatitis C RNA if clinical suspicion for hepatitis C is high. All positive hepatitis C virus antibodies should be evaluated with a quantitative hepatitis C virus RNA assay and hepatitis C virus genotype)	
• Tuberculosis screening (tuberculin skin test or interferon-γ releasing assay. Interferon-γ releasing assay preferred if history of bacille Calmette-Guérin vaccination)	
• PAP smear of cervix and cervical human papilloma virus screening if appropriate	
• Fasting lipid panel	
• Fasting serum blood sugar	
• Trichomoniasis testing in all HIV-positive women	

Adapted from Aberg JA, Gallant JE, Ghanem KG, et al. Primary care guidelines for the management of persons infected with HIV: 2013 update by the HIV Medicine Association of the Infectious Diseases Society of America. Clin Infect Dis 2014;58(1):e1–34; with permission.

HIV-uninfected (assuming appropriate perinatal treatment to mother and baby). If the child is born HIV-infected or later acquires HIV infection, monitoring is similar to adult HIV-infected patients. However, it is critical the HIV-infected infant, child, or adolescent be cared for longitudinally by a pediatric infectious disease specialist well versed in HIV disease care and treatment.

SUMMARY

The overall HIV picture is one where testing and incidence have been stable for over a decade. Worrying trends for certain populations sound the call for reinvigorating primary prevention efforts to target people of color, MSM, adolescents and young adults, and pregnant women. Fortunately, science and policy have come a long way to improve the accuracy, speed, privacy, and affordability of HIV testing. Similarly, more potent and much better tolerated HIV treatments and a multidisciplinary care approach have increased adherence and viral suppression. Furthermore, the ACA facilitates increased affordability and access of improved HIV diagnostics and treatment in the United States. ACA changes include expanding HIV testing among Americans aged 15 to 65 without copay; greater access to insurance and health care; and expansion of Medicaid in many states, the largest provider of HIV "insurance" in the United States. Continued challenges are to improve long-term outcomes in people on lifetime regimens; reduce comorbidities associated with those regimens; and prevent further transmission, particularly in those communities disproportionately affected. That we talk of an HIV cure today is remarkable in and of itself.

REFERENCES

1. Hahn BH, Shaw GM, De Cock KM, et al. AIDS as a zoonosis: scientific and public health implications. Science 2000;287:607–14.
2. Gottlieb GS, Eholie SP, Nkengasong JN, et al. A call for randomized controlled trials of antiretroviral therapy for HIV-2 infection in West Africa. AIDS 2008;22:2069–72 [discussion: 2073–4].
3. Buonaguro L, Tornesello ML, Buonaguro FM. Human immunodeficiency virus type 1 subtype distribution in the worldwide epidemic: pathogenetic and therapeutic implications. J Virol 2007;81:10209–19.
4. UNAIDS. Global report: UNAIDS report on the global AIDS epidemic 2013. Geneva (Switzerland): Joint United Nations Programme on HIV/AIDS; 2013.
5. Hall HI, Song R, Rhodes P, et al. Estimation of HIV incidence in the United States. JAMA 2008;300:520–9.
6. Centers for Disease Control and Prevention. HIV testing trends in the United States, 2000–2011. Atlanta (GA): U.S Department of Health and Human Services, Centers for Disease Control and Prevention; 2013.
7. Public Health Agency of Canada. Summary: estimates of HIV prevalence and incidence in Canada, 2011. Ottawa (Canada): Her Majesty the Queen in Right of Canada; 2012.
8. Centers for Disease Control and Prevention. HIV surveillance report, 2011. Atlanta (GA): Division of HIV/AIDS Prevention, National Center for HIV/AIDS, Viral Hepatitis, STD and TB Prevention, Centers for Disease Control and Prevention (CDC), US Department of Health and Human Services; 2013. p. 1–35.
9. Cohen MS, Chen YQ, McCauley M, et al. Prevention of HIV-1 infection with early antiretroviral therapy. N Engl J Med 2011;365:493–505.
10. Koepsell T, Weiss N. Epidemiologic methods: studying the occurrence of illness. 1st edition. New York: Oxford University Press; 2003.

11. Public Health Agency of Canada. HIV/AIDS epidemic update: HIV testing and surveillance systems in Canada. Ottawa (Canada): Her Majesty the Queen in Right of Canada; 2010.
12. Centers for Disease Control and Prevention. Monitoring selected national HIV prevention and care objectives by using HIV surveillance data—United States and 6 dependent areas—2011. HIV Surveillance Supplemental Report 2013. 2013;18.
13. Centers for Disease Control and Prevention. Estimated HIV Incidence in the United States, 2007–2010. HIV Surveillance Report. 2012;17.
14. Centers for Disease Control and Prevention. Monitoring selected national HIV prevention and care objectives by using HIV surveillance data—United States and 6 U.S. dependent areas—2010. HIV Surveillance Supplemental Report. 2012;17.
15. Centers for Disease Control and Prevention. Achievements in public health: reduction in perinatal transmission of HIV infection—United States, 1985–2005. MMWR Morb Mortal Wkly Rep 2006;55(21):592–7.
16. Moyer VA. Screening for HIV: U.S. preventive services task force recommendation statement. Ann Intern Med 2013;159:51–60.
17. Aberg JA, Gallant JE, Ghanem KG, et al. Primary care guidelines for the management of persons infected with HIV: 2013 update by the HIV Medicine Association of the Infectious Diseases Society of America. Clin Infect Dis 2014;58:e1–34.
18. Cornett JK, Kirn TJ. Laboratory diagnosis of HIV in adults: a review of current methods. Clin Infect Dis 2013;57:712–8.
19. Thompson MA, Aberg JA, Hoy JF, et al. Antiretroviral treatment of adult HIV infection: 2012 recommendations of the International Antiviral Society-USA panel. JAMA 2012;308:387–402.
20. Bacchetti P, Moss AR. Incubation period of AIDS in San Francisco. Nature 1989; 338:251–3.
21. Burgess JK, Kasten MJ. Human immunodeficiency virus: what primary care clinicians need to know. Mayo Clin Proc 2013;88:1468–74.
22. Kates J. Implications of the Affordable Care Act for people with HIV infection and the Ryan White HIV/AIDS Program: what does the future hold? Top Antivir Med 2013;21:138–42.
23. Lyss SB, Branson BM, Kroc KA, et al. Detecting unsuspected HIV infection with a rapid whole-blood HIV test in an urban emergency department. J Acquir Immune Defic Syndr 2007;44:435–42.
24. Pant Pai N, Sharma J, Shivkumar S, et al. Supervised and unsupervised self-testing for HIV in high- and low-risk populations: a systematic review. PLoS Med 2013;10:e1001414.
25. Centers for Disease Control and Prevention. Draft laboratory testing guidance. Atlanta (GA): National Center for HIV/AIDS, Viral Hepatitis and TB Prevention, Centers for Disease Control, US Health and Human Services; 2012.

Engagement in Human Immunodeficiency Virus Care

Linkage, Retention, and Antiretroviral Therapy Adherence

Ellen F. Eaton, MD[a,*], Michael S. Saag, MD[a],
Michael Mugavero, MD[b]

KEYWORDS

- Human immunodeficiency virus retention • Linkage to care • Adherence monitoring

KEY POINTS

- Early entry into and subsequent retention in care improves human immunodeficiency virus outcomes.
- Early initiation of and adherence to antiretroviral therapy (ART) improves outcomes.
- Monitoring and measuring care engagement and ART adherence are foundational.
- Monitoring missed visits and ART adherence self-report is readily achievable in clinical settings.
- A range of evidence-based interventions are available that can optimize adherence to care and ART and be implemented in clinical settings.

INTRODUCTION

Successful diagnosis, treatment, and retention in care for patients infected with the human immunodeficiency virus (HIV) have been shown to correlate with clinical outcomes and reduction in HIV transmission. In the modern antiretroviral therapy (ART)

Disclosure Statement: The authors certify that they have no affiliations with or involvement in any organization or entity with any financial interest (eg, honoraria; educational grants; participation in speakers' bureaus; membership, employment, consultancies, stock ownership, or other equity interest; and expert testimony or patent-licensing arrangements) or nonfinancial interest (eg, personal or professional relationships, affiliations, knowledge, or beliefs) in the subject matter or materials discussed in this article.
[a] Division of Infectious Disease, University of Alabama, Birmingham, 229 Tinsley Harrison Tower, 1900 University Boulevard, Birmingham, AL 35223, USA; [b] Division of Infectious Disease, University of Alabama, Birmingham, BBRB 206H, 845 19th Street South, Birmingham, AL 35223, USA
* Corresponding author.
E-mail address: eeaton@uab.edu

era, HIV has become a chronic illness that can be managed successfully with medication adherence and close monitoring. Patients infected with HIV develop significant morbidity and mortality despite pharmacologic advancements if they fall out of care or fail to take their ART regimen consistently. The finding that more than half of persons diagnosed with HIV infection in the United States are not engaged in regular medical care highlights the significance of retention in care in contemporary HIV management. In this article, best practices for HIV retention, including adherence and retention monitoring, treatment, and tools for optimizing care, are summarized.

IMPROVED HIV OUTCOMES WITH COMBINATION ART

Improved survival with ART has been appreciated since the late 1980s, when zidovudine monotherapy was used in patients with advanced HIV and AIDS. In the early 1990s, newer antiretrovirals such as zalcitabine and didanosine, and later, stavudine and lamivudine, began to show promise. These drugs were successfully used in combination regimens, and clinical trials confirmed the benefits of combination therapy over monotherapy. Clinical trials evaluating combinations of protease inhibitors and nonnucleoside reverse transcriptase inhibitors had more favorable results, ushering in the era of modern combination ART.[1] There are now multiple options for ART in newly diagnosed and treatment-experienced patients infected with HIV, which contributes to reduced morbidity and mortality. Survival continues to increase for those diagnosed with HIV and AIDS.[2] Despite excellent therapeutic options, some patients infected with HIV never achieve virologic suppression, because they cannot or do not remain linked to an HIV treatment program and adherent to ART. One of the greatest challenges in the fight against HIV remains patient retention, with implications for individual and population health outcomes.

Linkage and Retention in Care

Early entry into care

Timely diagnosis, linkage and retention in care, and early treatment of HIV have been shown to reduce complications and HIV transmissions. A South Carolina study[3] evaluated retention in care by studying clinic visit attendance over the first 2 years after HIV diagnosis. Those who attended 4 clinic visits (at least 1 per 6-month interval) over the first 24 months of care had a greater reduction in viral load, whereas those who attended sporadically or dropped out of care had higher mortality. Furthermore, early initiation of ART benefits patients, their partners, and their community's health. In a large study of 9 countries,[4] serodiscordant couples were assigned to early or later initiation of ART. The early ART group received therapy when CD4 counts were between 350 and 550, whereas the delayed group did not receive therapy until CD4 counts were less than 250, in accordance with local treatment recommendations at that time in participating countries. There was a 96% relative reduction in linked HIV-1 transmission events with early initiation of ART. In addition, early initiation of ART led to a 41% reduction in HIV-related clinical events compared with delayed therapy. Although many guidelines recommend earlier initiation of ART, the real world challenge of late diagnosis persists. Most newly diagnosed persons have initial CD4 counts lower than levels at which ART is recommended in all guidelines. Moreover, over the past 2 decades, there has been a modest increase in CD4 counts at diagnosis and care entry (1.6 cells/μL per year), highlighting the need for innovative testing strategies to facilitate more timely diagnosis and ART initiation.[5]

The HIV treatment cascade (**Fig. 1**A) shows an approximately 50% drop-off in patients between diagnoses with HIV to consistent engagement in care, with large,

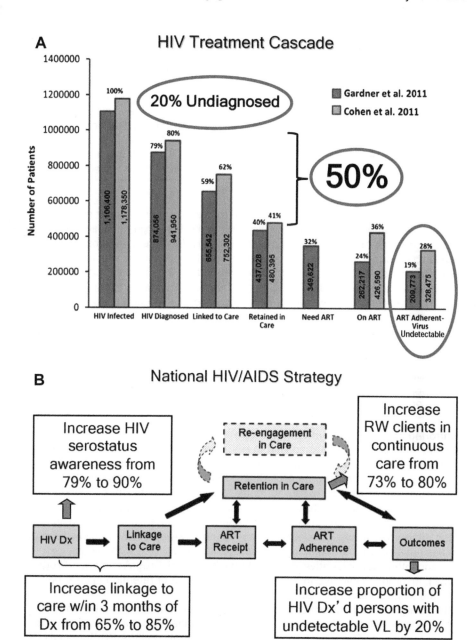

Fig. 1. (*A*) Treatment cascade: emphasis on importance of linkage and retention in care. (*B*) Goals of the US National HIV/AIDS strategy by 2015. (*Data from [A]* Gardner EM, McLees MP, Steiner JF. The spectrum of engagement in HIV care and its relevance to test-and-treat strategies for prevention of HIV infection. Clin Infect Dis 2011;52(6):796; Cohen SM, Van Handel MM, Branson BM, et al. Vital signs: HIV prevention through care and treatment—United States. MMWR Morb Mortal Wkly Rep 2011;60:1621; and *Adapted from [B]* Ulett KB, Willig JH, Lin HY, et al. The therapeutic implications of timely linkage and early retention in HIV care. AIDS Patient Care STDS 2009;23:42; and Mugavero MJ, Norton WE, Saag MS, et al. Health care system and policy factors influencing engagement in HIV medical care: piecing together the fragments of a fractured health care delivery system. Clin Infect Dis 2011;52(S2):239.)

incremental declines in initial linkage and subsequent retention in medical care. The US National AIDS Strategy (http://www.whitehouse.gov/administration/eop/onap/nhas/) is heavily grounded in addressing this gap, the closing of which has the most promise for increasing the number of patients with HIV in the United States attaining the goal of achieving and maintaining undetectable levels of HIV-1 RNA (viral load) in plasma. Those who sustain undetectable plasma HIV-1 RNA are predicted to live close to normal life spans and do not transmit HIV to others, therefore benefiting both themselves and the community.[6,7] As a result, the US National HIV/AIDS Strategy has set forth targeted goals for 2015, shown in **Fig. 1B**, which when achieved will markedly improve patient survival and reduce transmission in the United States.

Attendance to clinic visits

Retention in care is essential to effective HIV management and is best measured by assessment of attendance to clinic visits. One of the first large studies showing the importance of retention came from an analysis of HIV-infected veterans. In patients who were prescribed ART for 1 year, there was less CD4 count and viral load improvement in veterans with fewer attended clinic visits in the 12 months after ART initiation. Survival was also associated with frequency of kept clinic visits: an exposure response relationship was observed, with incremental increases in long-term mortality observed among patients attending fewer clinic visits (calculated based on attendance to ≥ 1 visit per 3-month interval) after ART initiation.[8] Missing clinic visits has also been associated with failure to receive ART, delays in viral suppression, and increased mortality.[9,10] One public HIV specialty clinic[11] evaluated commonalities in those who did not receive ART within 6 months of follow-up. In multivariate analysis, missed physician appointments, along with female sex and having a CD4 count greater than or equal to 200, was a predictor of not receiving ART.

Monitoring and measuring retention in care

Effective HIV care retention is so vital to HIV management that experts recommend monitoring entry into and retention in care.[12] One monitoring strategy being used increasingly is the measurement of CD4 count and viral load reported to public health surveillance as a surrogate for entry to care.[13,14] Serial HIV biomarker laboratory assessment reported to public health is used as a surrogate for HIV care visits and overcomes challenges of monitoring patients who move from 1 clinic to another, which might misclassify a patient as not retained if relying solely on clinic records. Studies have shown that combining public health surveillance with medical records data and other administrative data systems (eg, AIDS Drug Assistance Program (ADAP), insurance claims) can enhance the monitoring of retention in care beyond any data system used in isolation.[13]

Measuring retention in care is complex. Approaches that have been used to measure retention include missed visits, appointment adherence, visit constancy, gaps in care, the Human Resources and Services Administration HIV/AIDS Bureau (HRSA HAB) performance measure, and the Department of Health and Human Services (DHHS) Core Indicator for retention (**Table 1**). Although all have been used, there is no gold standard for measuring retention.[15] Missed visits may be a particularly useful retention indicator to HIV clinics and providers (**Fig. 2**). Unlike other retention measures, which require a year or longer of observation time for calculation, information on missed clinic visits is immediately available (see **Table 1**). Because studies have shown the strong prognostic value of missed visits for clinical events and mortality, interventions can be instituted in clinical settings in response to missed clinic visits. The ready availability of missed visits as a trigger for intervention is vital for clinical

Table 1
Approaches to measuring retention in care

Retention Measure	Missed Visit Data Needed?	Ease of Calculating	Follow-up Time
Missed visit	Yes	Easy	~1 d
Appointment adherence	Yes	Moderate	~1 y
No-show rate	Yes	Moderate	~1 y
Visit constancy (persistence): visit per 3-mo, 4-mo or 6-mo intervals	No	Moderate	≥1 y
Gaps	No	Easy	~1 y
HRSA/HAB	No	Moderate to difficult	1 y
DHHS	No	Moderate to difficult	2 y

Adapted from Giordano TP. Measuring retention in HIV care. Medscape 2012. Available at: http://www.medscape.com. Accessed June 3, 2014.

intervention, because by the time 1 to 2 years has elapsed to determine that a patient is not retained by other measures, locator information is often inaccurate, and it becomes increasingly challenging to engage patients. Although other retention measures have clear value and roles, missed visits represent a unique tool for immediate measurement and action. As noted earlier, it is advised that community clinics and public health providers develop systematic monitoring of patients' attendance to clinic visits, capitalizing on the unique strengths of public health surveillance and clinic medical records data. Such integrated approaches hold promise to improve

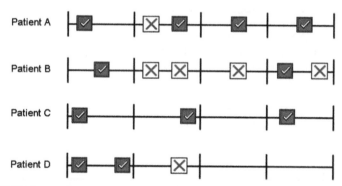

	Missed Visits	Appt. Adherence	Visit Constancy	Gap in Care	HRSA HAB Measure
Patient A	Yes; 1	80%	100%	No	Yes
Patient B	Yes; 4	33%	50%	Yes	Yes
Patient C	No; 0	100%	75%	No	Yes
Patient D	Yes; 1	67%	25%	Yes	No

Fig. 2. Examples of approaches to measure missed visits. (*From* Mugavero MJ, Davila JA, Nevin CR, et al. From access to engagement: measuring retention in outpatient HIV clinical care. AIDS Patient Care STDS 2010;24:609; with permission.)

both individual patient and community health, by informing targeted approaches for engagement and retention in care, focusing on those in greatest need.[14]

Interventions to improve entry and retention in care

Linkage case management and outreach are beneficial for those newly diagnosed with HIV. The Antiretroviral Treatment Access Study[16] evaluated the effect of strengths-based case management on linkage to care. The linkage case management arm of the study allowed up to 5 sessions with a trained professional within 90 days, focusing on patients' individual strengths and assets to foster linkage to care. The patients were significantly more likely to attend clinic visits at 6 months (18% increase) and at 12 months (15% increase) when case managed relative to the standard of care control group. Intensive outreach has also been shown to increase clinic attendance and lead to favorable viral load suppression. The US Special Projects of National Significance Outreach Initiative[17] included an outreach study that led to undetectable viral load rates of 45%, from a baseline of 14%, over 12 months. Patient navigation has also been shown to increase clinic visits and improve biomarkers. The US Special Projects of National Significance Outreach Initiative also studied patient navigators for patients infected with HIV inconsistently engaged in care in 4 studies; at baseline, 64% had attended 2 visits in the previous 6 months. The intervention increased attendance at clinic visits by 87% at 6 months and 79% at 12 months, and also increased those with undetectable HIV-1 RNA by 50% at 12 months.[18]

Two clinic-based approaches to improving retention in care were identified in the Centers for Disease Control and Prevention (CDC)-sponsored and HRSA-sponsored Retention in Care (RiC) Project (ClinicalTrials.gov: CDCHRSA9272007). Using a preintervention versus postintervention design, a modest 3% relative improvement in clinic-wide visit adherence was observed with a low-cost, low-effort intervention, including posters and brochures emphasizing a theme of *Stay Connected for your Health*, in addition to brief messages regarding retention in care from all clinic staff.[19] Important subgroups, including new patients and those with low CD4 counts and detectable HIV-1 RNA levels, reported greater improvements in visit adherence. The second intervention approach tested in the RiC study included personal reminder calls at 7 and 2 days before visits, as well as within 24 to 48 hours of missed clinic visits. Statistically significant increases in visit adherence (5%) and visit constancy (10%) were observed in the intervention arm relative to the standard of care control group.[20] The intervention was particular efficacious among disproportionately affected groups, including African Americans/blacks, women, and those lacking private health insurance.

Adherence to ART

Monitoring ART adherence

Adherence to ART is critical to HIV control and transmission reduction. Like retention, it is essential to monitor adherence to ART to optimize care. Because adherence behavior may change over time, routine adherence assessment longitudinally is vital. Many options exist for adherence monitoring: self-reports, pharmacy refill data, pill counts, electronic drug monitors (EDMs), and drug concentrations from biological samples (**Table 2**). Some studies have looked at combining these measures, but no method or combination seems superior based on current data. Experts recommend routine monitoring by patient self-report and pharmacy refill data if medications are not automatically refilled. Numerous methods for obtaining patient self-report are available. Furthermore, serum drug concentrations, EDM, and pill box counts are not routinely recommended for adherence monitoring in routine

Table 2	
Recommendations for measuring ART adherence in routine HIV care settings	
ART Adherence Approach	**Strength/Quality**
Self-reported adherence	IIA
Pharmacy refill data (MPR)	IIB
Not drug concentrations	IIIC
Not pill counts	IIIC
Not electronic devices (microelectromechanical systems)	IC

Data from Thompson MA, Mugavero MJ, Amico KR, et al. Guidelines for improving entry into and retention in care and antiretroviral adherence for persons with HIV: evidence-based recommendations from an International Association of Physicians in AIDS Care panel. Ann Intern Med 2012;156(11):817–33, W-284–94. http://dx.doi.org/10.7326/0003-4819-156-11-201206050-00419.

clinical care settings.[18] Similarly, plasma HIV-1 RNA (viral load) is not recommended as a screening tool for ART adherence. Once the viral load is detectable, the patient has already been nonadherent. Rather than waiting for an increasing viral load, the biological correlate of nonadherence, adherence should be measured directly by self-report or pharmacy refill (Medication Possession Ratio) in an attempt to identify and improve ART nonadherence.

Improving adherence

Adherence has been associated with many factors: pill count, dosing schedule/frequency, side effects, meal requirements, and drug interactions.[21] Advances in pharmacology have improved many of these limitations, and there are several once-daily combination pills available to patients infected with HIV. Still, resistance, treatment experience, medical and psychological comorbidities, and cost may preclude the use of these newer, convenient formulations. When possible, a once-daily regimen should be prescribed, and there is evidence that once-daily regimens are noninferior to more frequent dosing. Furthermore, there is improved adherence with once-daily dosing.[21–23] For patients whose HIV RNA is suppressed on a complex ART regimen, research[12] suggests they can successfully switch to a once-daily regimen, contingent on similar efficacy and treatment history. There is also benefit of fixed-dose combination pills. These formulations reduce the pill burden, leading to improved adherence.[12] Fixed-dose combinations reduce the likelihood of taking an incomplete regimen or confusion with the dosing schedules of various pills within the regimen. This strategy reduces concerns for resistance, which may occur in the setting of differential ART adherence with multiple pill regimens.[24]

Adherence reminders

Several tools are available for patient use to improve adherence (**Table 3**). Pill boxes, reminders, and calendars have all been used and studied observationally.[12] Petersen and colleagues[25] studied pill box organizers and found them to increase adherence and virologic suppression. In addition, pill boxes are inexpensive and user friendly. However, there is a lack of comparative data on adherence tools, and no single aid is recommended over others. Newer technology, such as pagers and cellular phones with SMS (short message service) and texting capabilities, allows for electronic reminders and is most effective when it includes an interactive component with patient response. Such interactive technology reminders can improve adherence and viral load even in resource-limited environments. One study of Kenyan patients infected

Table 3
Evidence-based ART adherence approaches

ART Adherence Approach	Strength/Quality
Reminder devices and interactive communication technologies	IB
Education and counseling using adherence-related tools	IA
Various individual, group, and peer education and counseling	IIA–IIIC
Case management services (eg, food/housing)	IIIB
Integration of medical management into pharmacy systems	IIIC

Data from Thompson MA, Mugavero MJ, Amico KR, et al. Guidelines for improving entry into and retention in care and antiretroviral adherence for persons with HIV: evidence-based recommendations from an International Association of Physicians in AIDS Care panel. Ann Intern Med 2012;156(11):817–33, W-284–94. http://dx.doi.org/10.7326/0003-4819-156-11-201206050-00419.

with HIV[26] evaluated the use of cellular phones with SMS messaging. Those who received SMS reminders were 13% to 16% more likely to have 90% adherence to highly active ART (HAART) than those who did not receive SMS reminders. These reminders also reduced treatment interruptions. Reminder tools are usually more effective when combined with counseling on adherence. One study[27] evaluated the effects of electronic monitoring-based counseling and showed a significant increase in adherence and reduction in viral load with this intervention approach. Similarly, a study in China[28] assessed EDM combined with feedback and found that the combination increased adherence and CD4 counts. Rates of adherence and mean CD4 counts in the intervention arm increased from 87% to 97% and 90 cells/μL, respectively, at 12 months. Routine adherence monitoring and counseling are important to successful HIV care.

Behavioral interventions

A wide range of educational and behavioral interventions are recommended for HIV-infected individuals (see **Table 3**).[12] Counseling has consistently been shown to increase adherence, and there are data suggesting an improvement in HIV viral load. One study[29] looked at the benefits of psychoeducative intervention in patients starting first-line or second-line ART and found that those in the intervention arm were more likely to have greater than 95% adherence (94% vs 69%) and more likely to have HIV viral load less than 400 copies/mL (89% vs 66%). Based on this and other supportive evidence, one-on-one ART education and adherence counseling is recommended for all patients infected with HIV.[12] Multiple studies have evaluated individual adherence counseling, most with positive results. Telephone counseling seems to be successful as well. One study of serial telephone calls[30] improved adherence but had no effect on viral load. A multisite, randomized controlled trial (RCT) of patients enrolled in the AIDS Clinical Trial Group showed that those receiving structured telephone calls had improved adherence and clinical outcomes. The telephone intervention arm also had a 32% lower risk of virologic failure.[31] There are limited data supporting home visits. One study[32] showed that home visits from a nurse and social worker allowed more patients infected with HIV to achieve greater than 90% adherence. Involving partners and caregivers is also less well characterized. Incorporating seronegative partners in counseling has a positive effect on adherence, but involving caregivers has not been consistently shown to improve adherence or HIV biological markers.[12]

Group education and multidisciplinary counseling are recommended for HIV-infected individuals based on mostly favorable research on adherence and HIV-1

RNA. The evidence base includes multiple group strategies and diverse patient populations, making it difficult to identify which strategy is optimal. In addition, several studies included an additional adherence tool, such as education by a pharmacist, which may improve outcomes.[33] Multidisciplinary education, whereby team members with distinct roles lend expertise to patients, has been shown to improve clinical outcomes. This strategy allows nutritionists, pharmacists, social workers, and case managers to educate via a team approach. One multidisciplinary intervention[34] focused on identifying and correcting adherence barriers led to significant improvements of HIV-1 RNA viral load and increased the duration of ART therapy. Another multidisciplinary intervention, when combined with reminder tools, highlighted the importance of reducing perceived barriers to adherence and developing strategies to overcome them. This intervention, studied by Levy and colleagues,[35] focused on many factors from nutrition to life skills and significantly reduced the number of missed doses in a month. Peer support has less consistently improved outcomes, but several studies combining peer support with other adherence interventions have shown improvement in adherence or biological outcomes. What remains unknown is the specific benefit from peer support versus coadministered treatment interventions.[12]

Additional Interventions

Case management, supportive services (housing, food, transportation), and pharmacy support

Access to housing, food, transportation, and pharmacy support are beneficial to patients infected with HIV and are often obtained with the assistance of a medical case manager or social worker. A randomized study of homeless patients infected with HIV assigned to Housing Opportunities for People with AIDS rental assistance or usual care[36] showed improvements in housing status and health in housed participants. At 18 months, the housed individuals had reductions in health care utilization and improved physical and mental health per self-report. The treatment group also had improvements in depression and stress. Likewise, addressing food insecurity has important benefits for patients infected with HIV. Research in Nigeria and Zambia[12] on food supplementation for food-insecure patients showed improvements in clinical outcomes as well as adherence and retention. Lack of transportation is also a prominent barrier to retention, especially for women, substance abusers, and those with mental illness. Andersen and colleagues[37] studied the effects of transportation on women with HIV and difficulty with clinic attendance. Those provided with transportation significantly decreased the number of missed appointments. Pharmacy interventions such as side effect and adherence monitoring may be beneficial, but directly administered ART (DAART) is not routinely recommended. DAART requires that a specialist observes the patient taking their medication. Weekend doses are generally provided on Fridays, and extra doses are provided if a patient misses the scheduled, observed administration. A pilot pharmacy medication management program evaluating Medi-Cal patients[38] found that assessing for side effects and adherence and adjusting medications to patient-specific needs increased adherence and led to fewer contraindicated ART regimens than those receiving usual care.

Nursing-based and community-based counselor care

In resource-limited settings, scarce access to physicians and clinics can limit retention, adherence, and HIV-related health outcomes. Nontraditional models in which nurse or community counselors home deliver services have similar results to doctor-based or clinic-based care in these settings.[12] Studies in both Uganda and

South Africa[12] using nurses rather than physicians to deliver care showed that adherence and biological markers, respectively, were not inferior to results obtained from traditional physician-delivered care.

Priority Populations

Most of the guidance outlined earlier comes from routine clinic populations, but there are additional considerations for special circumstances, including pregnancy, substance abuse, mental illness, incarceration, and children living with HIV.

Pregnancy

Care of the HIV-infected pregnant patient focuses on the health of the patient and child in addition to prevention of mother to child transmission. This subject is particularly important, given that more than 50% of HIV-infected individuals worldwide are women. With improved ART regimens that are safe in pregnancy and provide prevention of mother to child transmission, the US Preventive Services Task Force recommends universal screening of all pregnant women, regardless of risk.[39]

In settings with high HIV prevalence, HIV testing and targeting ART therapy for HIV-infected pregnant women is recommended over universal treatment.[12] A Zambian study[40] evaluated universal single-dose nevirapine for all pregnant women versus targeted nevirapine for only HIV-infected pregnant woman and found that uptake was higher in the universal treatment group. However, adherence was lower for those unaware of their HIV status and those who were illiterate. Labor ward interventions have also improved ART coverage and adherence. A cluster RCT in Zambia[41] found that universal HIV testing, counseling, and targeted ART initiation improved ART coverage of HIV-infected pregnant women. With universal HIV testing of pregnant women and targeted ART and counseling, rates of mother to child transmission should decline.

Substance use disorders

Active substance use is consistently associated with poor adherence, and HIV-infected substance users have higher morbidity and mortality than age-matched patients infected with HIV without substance use.[42] Treating substance use with methadone and buprenorphine maintenance, and integrating DAART into these programs, improves adherence and virologic control.[12] Retention in care and ART prescriptions were increased in 1 RCT when buprenorphine treatment was used in HIV clinics. Clinic-based buprenorphine treatment was compared with case management and referral to an external opioid program, and the clinic-based treatment resulted in fewer positive opioid and cocaine drug tests and fewer missed clinic visits.[43] In addition to offering opioid dependence treatment, providing DAART to substance users is beneficial.[44] Several studies have shown improvements in viral load and CD4 count with DAART compared with usual self-administered therapy for substance users.[12] One study of a methadone maintenance program showed that DAART, when compared with usual care, significantly improved ART adherence and viral suppression, and these results were maintained over 24 weeks. Several prospective studies had similar findings, when DAART was administered as part of a methadone treatment program.[45]

Mental illness

Mental illness such as depression has also been linked to poor engagement in care and ART nonadherence. The association between depressive symptoms and nonadherence has also been shown for subclinical depression.[46] This relationship makes screening for and treatment of depression critical to HIV management. Several randomized, controlled studies[12] have proved that cognitive-behavioral therapy (CBT) for depression in combination with adherence counseling improves adherence and reduces depressive symptoms. The gains in adherence were maintained for up to 12 months.[47] In contrast, an RCT[48] of CBT for stress management alone without adherence counseling failed to improve adherence or treatment outcomes. These results point to the need for coadministered therapy, CBT plus adherence counseling, as the most effect intervention for improving adherence and mental health outcomes in patients infected with HIV with concurrent mental illness.

Incarceration, homelessness, and marginally housed individuals

Institutionalization and lack of secure housing present unique challenges to ART adherence and retention. Incarceration provides an opportunity to improve ART adherence, and the prevalence of HIV is higher among incarcerated individuals regardless of low-resource or high-resource setting. However, barriers still exist, including protecting confidentiality, stigma, and transitions from institutions to the community. Several international studies have shown that administering DAART to incarcerated HIV-infected persons increases adherence and viral suppression when compared with self-administration.[12] Homeless and marginally housed individuals often have complex challenges to adherence, including unstable housing, inconsistent medication storage, food insecurity, mental illness, and substance use. Mistrust of medications, mistrust of the health care system, and poor relationships with providers have also been associated with poor adherence.[49] Nonetheless, adherence levels consistent with other HIV-infected populations can be achieved in homeless patients. For example, a study of homeless individuals in San Francisco[50] evaluated use of ART over a 12-month period. Average adherence in those continuing HAART over the study period was 74%, and more than half of these had undetectable viral loads at the study conclusion.

Case management is recommend for all homeless patients and includes referrals for substance use treatment, mental health services, and housing provisions. Another study of homeless and marginally housed patients in San Francisco[51] found that adherence and CD4 counts were improved with case management but viral suppression was not. Pillbox organizers are recommended for homeless patients with HIV, because pillbox use in this population is associated with improvements in adherence and viral suppression.[16]

Children, adolescents, and young adults

For infants and young children perinatally infected with HIV, adherence to ART is dependent on their caregivers. Barriers to adherence in this population include medication taste and difficulty with pills.[52] Behavioral interventions have been used with mixed results. One study used multisystemic therapy, a form of home-based family therapy, which led to improvement in viral suppression at 3 months but no change in caregiver-reported adherence. Pill swallowing training may also improve outcomes.[53] Garvie and colleagues[54] studied pill swallowing training in 23 pediatric patients and found significant improvements in ART adherence, CD4, and viral suppression. Like other priority populations, pediatric and adolescent patients benefit from DAART with short-term biomarker improvements, but this benefit is not sustained after DAART is discontinued. In Cambodia, DAART for orphaned children cost $60 per child annually and improved immunologic outcomes, making it a cost-effective strategy for young patients.[55]

There is also a decline in adherence in many HIV-infected adolescents. Adolescents and young adults have lower rates of retention in care and viral suppression and higher rates of viral rebound when compared with older patients. One study[56] proved that with intensive case management, newly infected and poorly adherent gay young men improved their clinic attendance and, at 6 months, had increased likelihood of ART prescription. Based on this and similar results in youth, experts recommend intensive age-appropriate case management through young adulthood to improve entry and retention in care.[12]

Future Research

Long-term studies on durable interventions that optimize care engagement and ART adherence to achieve and sustain viral suppression are needed. Novel technologies offer promise in terms of patient adherence and retention and may be particularly suited for younger patients. More research on cost-effectiveness of adherence tools is needed to inform policy at a national and international level. In the era of ART, many patients die with chronic illness, often accelerated by HIV. More research is needed on the effects of varying ART regimens on comorbidities such as coronary artery disease, chronic renal disease, and diabetes. There is also limited evidence on multimorbidity in HIV and the interactions between multiple medications and differential adherence to medications taken for comorbid conditions (eg, hypertension, hypercholesterolemia). Issues such as dosing frequency, pill burden, and drug interactions of non-HIV medications are also relevant in patients with multiple chronic medical conditions. As numerous generic ARTs become available, balancing factors such as pill counts with costs will become an increasingly complex challenge. Advancing our understanding of these issues through rigorous scientific endeavors will improve the overall care of patients infected with HIV. Because HIV care engagement and ART adherence are the prominent barriers to reducing individual and community viral load, with implications for health outcomes and new HIV infections, it is imperative that we accelerate the pace of scientific discovery and rapidly disseminate and implement effective strategies in communities and clinics.

REFERENCES

1. Hogg RS, Heath KV, Yip B, et al. Improved survival among HIV-infected individuals following initiation of antiretroviral therapy. JAMA 1998;279(6):450–4. PubMed PMID: 9466638.
2. Centers for Disease Control and Prevention. HIV surveillance report, 2009, vol. 21. 2011. Available at: http://www.cdc.gov/hiv/surveillance/resources/reports/2009report. Accessed December 21, 2011.
3. Tripathi A, Youmans E, Gibson JJ, et al. The impact of retention in early HIV medical care on viro-immunological parameters and survival: a statewide study. AIDS Res Hum Retroviruses 2011;27:751–8.
4. Cohen MS, Chen YQ, McCauley M, et al, HPTN 052 Study Team. Prevention of HIV-1 infection with early antiretroviral therapy. N Engl J Med 2011;365:493–505.
5. Lesko CR, Cole SR, Poole C, et al. A systematic review and meta-regression of temporal trends in adult CD4+ cell count at presentation to HIV care, 1992-2011. Clin Infect Dis 2013;57(7):1027–37.
6. McManus H, O'Connor CC, Boyd M, et al, Australian HIV Observational Database. Long-term survival in HIV positive patients with up to 15 years of antiretroviral therapy. PLoS One 2012;7(11):e48839. http://dx.doi.org/10.1371/journal.pone.0048839.
7. Quinn TC, Wawer MJ, Sewankambo N, et al. Viral load and heterosexual transmission of human immunodeficiency virus type 1. Rakai Project Study Group. N Engl J Med 2000;342(13):921–9.

8. Giordano TP, Gifford AL, White AC Jr, et al. Retention in care: a challenge to survival with HIV infection. Clin Infect Dis 2007;44(11):1493–9.

9. Mugavero MJ, Amico KR, Westfall AO, et al. Early retention in care and viral load suppression: implications for a test and treat approach to HIV prevention. J Acquir Immune Defic Syndr 2012;58:86–93.

10. Mugavero MJ, Lin HY, Willig JW, et al. Missed visits and mortality in patients establishing initial outpatient HIV treatment. Clin Infect Dis 2009;48:248–56.

11. Giordano TP, White AC Jr, Sajja P, et al. Factors associated with the use of highly active antiretroviral therapy in patients newly entering care in an urban clinic. J Acquir Immune Defic Syndr 2003;32:399–405.

12. Thompson MA, Mugavero MJ, Amico KR, et al. Guidelines for improving entry into and retention in care and antiretroviral adherence for persons with HIV: evidence-based recommendations from an International Association of Physicians in AIDS Care panel. Ann Intern Med 2012;156(11):817–33. http://dx.doi.org/10.7326/0003-4819-156-11-201206050-00419. W-284–94.

13. Zetola NM, Bernstein K, Ahrens K, et al. Using surveillance data to monitor entry into care of newly diagnosed HIV-infected persons: San Francisco, 2006-2007. BMC Public Health 2009;9:17.

14. Sweeney P, Gardner LI, Buchacz K, et al. Shifting the paradigm: using HIV surveillance data as a foundation for improving HIV care and preventing HIV infection. Milbank Q 2013;91(3):558–603.

15. Mugavero MJ, Davila JA, Nevin CR, et al. From access to engagement: measuring retention in outpatient HIV clinical care. AIDS Patient Care STDS 2010;24:607–13.

16. Gardner LI, Metsch LR, Anderson-Mahoney P, et al, Antiretroviral Treatment and Access Study Group. Efficacy of a brief case management intervention to link recently diagnosed HIV-infected persons to care. AIDS 2005;19:423–31.

17. Naar-King S, Bradford J, Coleman S, et al. Retention in care of persons newly diagnosed with HIV: outcomes of the outreach initiative. AIDS Patient Care STDS 2007;21(Suppl 1):S40–8.

18. Bradford JB, Coleman S, Cunningham W. HIV system navigation: an emerging model to improve HIV care access. AIDS Patient Care STDS 2007;21(Suppl 1):S49–58.

19. Gardner L, Marks G, Craw J, et al. A low-effort clinic-wide intervention improves attendance for HIV primary care. Clin Infect Dis 2012;55:1124–34.

20. Gardner LI, Giordano TP, Marks G, et al, For the Retention in Care Study Group. Enhanced personal contact with HIV patients improves retention in primary care: a randomized trial in six US HIV clinics. Clin Infect Dis 2014. [Epub ahead of print].

21. Nachega JB, Parienti JJ, Uthman OA, et al. Lower pill burden and once-daily antiretroviral treatment regimens for HIV infection: a meta-analysis of randomized controlled trials. Clin Infect Dis 2014;58:1297–307.

22. Flexner C, Tierney C, Gross R, et al, ACTG A5073 Study Team. Comparison of once-daily versus twice-daily combination antiretroviral therapy in treatment-naive patients: results of AIDS clinical trials group (ACTG) A5073, a 48-week randomized controlled trial. Clin Infect Dis 2010;50:1041–52.

23. Molina JM, Podsadecki TJ, Johnson MA, et al. A lopinavir/ritonavir-based once-daily regimen results in better compliance and is non-inferior to a twice-daily regimen through 96 weeks. AIDS Res Hum Retroviruses 2007;23:1505–14.

24. Gardner EM, Sharma S, Peng G, et al. Differential adherence to combination antiretroviral therapy is associated with virological failure with resistance. AIDS 2008;22(1):75–82.

25. Petersen ML, Wang Y, van der Laan MJ, et al. Pillbox organizers are associated with improved adherence to HIV antiretroviral therapy and viral suppression: a marginal structural model analysis. Clin Infect Dis 2007;45:908–15.

26. Pop-Eleches C, Thirumurthy H, Habyarimana JP, et al. Mobile phone technologies improve adherence to antiretroviral treatment in a resource-limited setting: a randomized controlled trial of text message reminders. AIDS 2011;25:825–34.

27. de Bruin M, Hospers HJ, van Breukelen GJ, et al. Electronic monitoring-based counseling to enhance adherence among HIV-infected patients: a randomized controlled trial. Health Psychol 2010;29:421–8.

28. Sabin LL, DeSilva MB, Hamer DH, et al. Using electronic drug monitor feedback to improve adherence to antiretroviral therapy among HIV-positive patients in China. AIDS Behav 2010;14:580–9.

29. Tuldrà A, Fumaz CR, Ferrer MJ, et al. Prospective randomized two-arm controlled study to determine the efficacy of a specific intervention to improve long-term adherence to highly active antiretroviral therapy. J Acquir Immune Defic Syndr 2000;25:221–8.

30. Collier AC, Ribaudo H, Mukherjee AL, et al. Adult AIDS Clinical Trials Group 746 Substudy Team. A randomized study of serial telephone call support to increase adherence and thereby improve virologic outcome in persons initiating antiretroviral therapy. J Infect Dis 2005;192:1398–406.

31. Reynolds NR, Testa MA, Su M, et al, AIDS Clinical Trials Group 731 and 384 Teams. Telephone support to improve antiretroviral medication adherence: a multisite, randomized controlled trial. J Acquir Immune Defic Syndr 2008;47:62–8.

32. Williams AB, Fennie KP, Bova CA, et al. Home visits to improve adherence to highly active antiretroviral therapy: a randomized controlled trial. J Acquir Immune Defic Syndr 2006;42:314–21.

33. Antoni MH, Carrico AW, Durán RE, et al. Randomized clinical trial of cognitive behavioral stress management on human immunodeficiency virus viral load in gay men treated with highly active antiretroviral therapy. Psychosom Med 2006;68:143–51.

34. Frick P, Tapia K, Grant P, et al. The effect of a multidisciplinary program on HAART adherence. AIDS Patient Care STDS 2006;20:511–24.

35. Levy RW, Rayner CR, Fairley CK, et al, Melbourne Adherence Group. Multidisciplinary HIV adherence intervention: a randomized study. AIDS Patient Care STDS 2004;18:728–35.

36. Wolitski RJ, Kidder DP, Pals SL, et al, Housing and Health Study Team. Randomized trial of the effects of housing assistance on the health and risk behaviors of homeless and unstably housed people living with HIV. AIDS Behav 2010;14:493–503.

37. Andersen M, Hockman E, Smereck G, et al. Retaining women in HIV medical care. J Assoc Nurses AIDS Care 2007;18:33–41.

38. Hirsch JD, Rosenquist A, Best BM, et al. Evaluation of the first year of a pilot program in community pharmacy: HIV/AIDS medication therapy management for Medi-Cal beneficiaries. J Manag Care Pharm 2009;15:32–41.

39. Branson BM, Handsfield HH, Lampe MA, et al, Centers for Disease Control and Prevention (CDC). Revised recommendations for HIV testing of adults, adolescents, and pregnant women in health-care settings. MMWR Recomm Rep 2006; 55(RR–14):1–17.

40. Stringer JS, Sinkala M, Stout JP, et al. Comparison of two strategies for administering nevirapine to prevent perinatal HIV transmission in high-prevalence, resource-poor settings. J Acquir Immune Defic Syndr 2003;32:506–13.

41. Megazzini KM, Sinkala M, Vermund SH, et al. A cluster-randomized trial of enhanced labor ward-based PMTCT services to increase nevirapine coverage in Lusaka, Zambia. AIDS 2010;24:447–55.
42. Altice FL, Kamarulzaman A, Soriano VV, et al. Treatment of medical, psychiatric, and substance-use comorbidities in people infected with HIV who use drugs. Lancet 2010;376:367–87.
43. Lucas GM, Chaudhry A, Hsu J, et al. Clinic-based treatment of opioid-dependent HIV-infected patients versus referral to an opioid treatment program: a randomized trial. Ann Intern Med 2010;152:704–11.
44. Berg KM, Litwin A, Li X, et al. Directly observed antiretroviral therapy improves adherence and viral load in drug users attending methadone maintenance clinics: a randomized controlled trial. Drug Alcohol Depend 2011;113:192–9.
45. Conway B, Prasad J, Reynolds R, et al. Directly observed therapy for the management of HIV-infected patients in a methadone program. Clin Infect Dis 2004; 38(Suppl 5):S402–8.
46. Gonzalez JS, Batchelder AW, Psaros C, et al. Depression and HIV/AIDS treatment nonadherence: a review and meta-analysis. J Acquir Immune Defic Syndr 2011;58:181–7.
47. Safren SA, O'Cleirigh C, Tan JY, et al. A randomized controlled trial of cognitive behavioral therapy for adherence and depression (CBT-AD) in HIV-infected individuals. Health Psychol 2009;28:1–10.
48. Berger S, Schad T, von Wyl V, et al. Effects of cognitive behavioral stress management on HIV-1 RNA, CD4 cell counts and psychosocial parameters of HIV-infected persons. AIDS 2008;22:767–75.
49. Mostashari F, Riley E, Selwyn PA, et al. Acceptance and adherence with antiretroviral therapy among HIV-infected women in a correctional facility. J Acquir Immune Defic Syndr Hum Retrovirol 1998;18:341–8.
50. Moss AR, Hahn JA, Perry S, et al. Adherence to highly active antiretroviral therapy in the homeless population in San Francisco: a prospective study. Clin Infect Dis 2004;39:1190–8.
51. Kushel MB, Colfax G, Ragland K, et al. Case management is associated with improved antiretroviral adherence and CD4+ cell counts in homeless and marginally housed individuals with HIV infection. Clin Infect Dis 2006;43:234–42.
52. Ryscavage P, Anderson EJ, Sutton SH, et al. Clinical outcomes of adolescents and young adults in adult HIV care. J Acquir Immune Defic Syndr 2011;58: 193–7.
53. Ellis DA, Naar-King S, Cunningham PB, et al. Use of multisystemic therapy to improve antiretroviral adherence and health outcomes in HIV-infected pediatric patients: evaluation of a pilot program. AIDS Patient Care STDS 2006;20: 112–21.
54. Garvie PA, Lensing S, Rai SN. Efficacy of a pill-swallowing training intervention to improve antiretroviral medication adherence in pediatric patients with HIV/AIDS. Pediatrics 2007;119:893–9.
55. Myung P, Pugatch D, Brady MF, et al. Directly observed highly active antiretroviral therapy for HIV-infected children in Cambodia. Am J Public Health 2007;97: 974–7.
56. Wohl AR, Garland WH, Wu J, et al. A youth-focused case management intervention to engage and retain young gay men of color in HIV care. AIDS Care 2011; 23:988–97.

Antiretroviral Therapy
Current Drugs

Alice K. Pau, PharmD[a],*, Jomy M. George, PharmD[b]

KEYWORDS

- HIV • Antiretroviral therapy • Nucleoside/nucleotide reverse transcriptase inhibitors
- Non-nucleoside reverse transcriptase inhibitors • Protease inhibitors
- Integrase strand transfer inhibitors • Fusion inhibitor • CCR5 antagonist

KEY POINTS

- To date, 28 antiretroviral drugs have been approved by the Food and Drug Administration.
- Effective combination antiretroviral therapy can durably suppress human immunodeficiency virus (HIV) viremia and has dramatically improved HIV-associated morbidity and mortality.
- For antiretroviral treatment-naïve patients, a combination regimen typically consists of 2 nucleoside reverse transcriptase inhibitors plus a third drug.
- Because of the increased number of options, the selection of an antiretroviral therapy regimen can be individualized, based on efficacy, adverse effects, comorbidity, dosing frequency, pill burden, potential for drug interactions, or drug resistance.
- Success and durable combination require strict adherence to long-term therapy.
- This article reviews the clinical pharmacology of the antiretroviral drugs commonly used in the United States.

INTRODUCTION

The 1980s saw the devastation of the newly emerging and deadly disease of acquired immunodeficiency syndrome (AIDS). The identification of the retrovirus, now known as human immunodeficiency virus (HIV), as the causative pathogen in the mid-1980s was the key milestone in the control of this disease. The discovery of the multistep replicative life cycle of HIV in human CD4+ T cells led to the identification of potential drug targets to halt or slow the replicative process (**Fig. 1**). This

Financial Disclosure: None.

Jomy M. George is now with Virology US Medical Strategy, US Pharmaceuticals Medical Affairs, Bristol-Myers Squibb, 777 Scudders Mill Road, Plainsboro Township, NJ 08536, USA.

[a] Division of Clinical Research, National Institute of Allergy and Infectious Diseases, National Institutes of Health, Building 10, Room 11C103 (MSC 1880), Bethesda, MD 20892, USA; [b] Department of Pharmacy Practice and Administration, Philadelphia College of Pharmacy, University of the Sciences in Philadelphia, 600 South 43rd Street, GH-108K, Philadelphia, PA 19104, USA

* Corresponding author.

E-mail address: apau@niaid.nih.gov

Infect Dis Clin N Am 28 (2014) 371–402

http://dx.doi.org/10.1016/j.idc.2014.06.001

0891-5520/14/$ – see front matter Published by Elsevier Inc.

id.theclinics.com

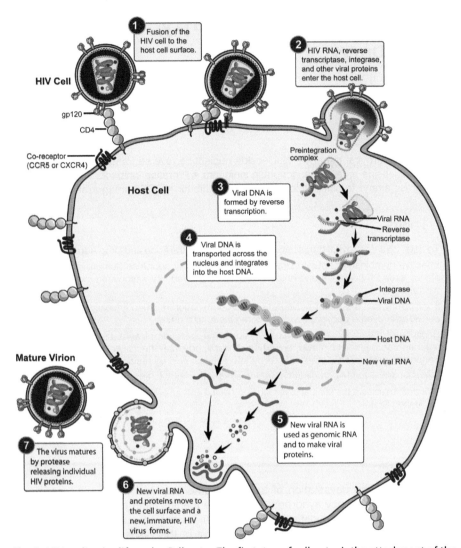

Fig. 1. HIV replicative life cycle. *Cell entry*: The first step of cell entry is the attachment of the HIV envelope glycoprotein gp120 onto human chemokine receptors (CCR5 or CXCR4) on the CD4 cell surface. After the initial attachment, the next step requires fusion of the viral and cell membranes, allowing the viral proteins to enter into the cytoplasm. *Reverse transcription*: After cell entry, as HIV is a retrovirus, the virus's RNA template transcribes into a double-stranded viral DNA in the presence of the enzyme reverse transcriptase. *Integration*: The viral double-stranded DNA produced after reverse transcription is then transported into the cellular nucleus. In the presence of the integrase enzyme, a multistep process allows the integration of viral DNA into host genome and ultimately formation of proviruses. *Formation of infectious virions by HIV proteases*: After successful integration of viral DNA into the host genome and formation of proviral proteins, the next step of the HIV-1 life cycle is the cleavage of these polyproteins and formation of infectious virions. The viral enzyme protease is the key element for this process. (*Adapted from* National Institutes of Allergy and Infectious Diseases. Available at: http://www.niaid.nih.gov/topics/HIVAIDS/Understanding/Biology/pages/hivreplicationcycle.aspx. Accessed March 12, 2014; with permission.)

identification resulted in unprecedented scientific progress in the drug discovery and drug development process.

Zidovudine, a nucleoside reverse transcriptase inhibitor (NRTI), was the first approved antiretroviral agent for use in 1987 after it had shown to provide a dramatic survival benefit when compared with placebo in patients with advanced AIDS.[1] Although NRTI monotherapy showed a reduction in viral load, delayed disease progression, and prolonged survival, the use of a single agent did not provide sustained viral suppression. Furthermore, it rarely reversed immune function. The approval of 3 HIV protease inhibitors (PI) in the mid-1990s dramatically changed the course of the HIV epidemic. The use of combination therapy consisting of a PI with 2-NRTI resulted in the rapid reduction of HIV RNA; improved immune function[2]; regression of difficult-to-treat opportunistic infections, such as Kaposi sarcoma[3] and progressive multifocal leukoencephalopathy[4]; and reduced mortality.[5] Since then, combination antiretroviral therapy became the mainstay of treatment. **Table 1** provides a glimpse of the advances in antiretroviral therapy over the years.

As of early 2014, 28 antiretroviral drugs belonging to 6 different mechanistic classes have been approved for use in the United States. Several of the older agents are no longer used in clinical practice, as they are replaced by newer drugs that are more potent and less toxic, have less dosing frequency, and with lower pill burden. This large armamentarium of drugs provides clinicians with ample options to individualize therapy. Despite the potency of current antiretroviral regimens, residual HIV remains in different sanctuary reservoirs. As a result, even temporary discontinuation of treatment results in viral rebound in almost all patients[6]; thus, in order to maintain viral suppression with current treatment, therapy needs to be continued indefinitely. Maintaining strict adherence to long-term antiretroviral therapy is a challenge for many asymptomatic HIV-infected patients. Intermittent adherence may lead to selection of drug resistance mutations, limiting future options. This article provides an overview of the goals and principles of antiretroviral treatment and factors to consider when selecting a regimen for an individual patient, with a main focus on the pharmacology of commonly used antiretroviral drugs in 2014.

GOALS AND PRINCIPLES OF ANTIRETROVIRAL THERAPY

The key goals of antiretroviral therapy are to

- Achieve and maintain suppression of plasma viremia to less than the current assays' level of detection
- Improve overall immune function as demonstrated by increases in CD4+ T-cell count
- Prolong survival
- Reduce HIV-associated morbidity
- Improve overall quality of life
- Reduce risk of transmission of HIV to others

In order to achieve these goals, the clinicians and patients must recognize several key principles:

- Current antiretroviral regimens do not eradicate HIV; viral rebound occurs rapidly after treatment discontinuation, followed by CD4 decline, with potential for disease progression
- Strict adherence to the prescribed regimen is essential in order to avoid viral rebound and the potential for selection of drug resistance mutations.

Table 1
A short history of advances in antiretroviral therapy (1987–2014)

Years	Advances in Antiretroviral Therapy	Comments
1987–1993	NRTI monotherapy (zidovudine or didanosine)	Improved patient survival and slow disease progression, but it does not halt CD4 decline.
1993–1996	Dual NRTI therapy	It has greater viral suppression than monotherapy and slow disease progression, with greater toxicities.
1994	PMTCT: with zidovudine monotherapy	The PACTG 074 trial showed dramatic reduction of PMTCT when zidovudine was given orally during pregnancy, with IV zidovudine given during labor and delivery, and oral zidovudine given to the newborn.
1996	PI + 2-NRTI regimens: highly active antiretroviral therapy or HAART	PI + 2-NRTI was the first regimen shown to suppress HIV RNA to less than the lower limit of detection and improve CD4 cell count and survival.
1998	NNRTI + 2-NRTI regimens	Efavirenz + 2-NRTI was found to be as potent as contemporary PI-based regimens. The NNRTI-based regimen became a new HAART regimen option.
1998	3-NRTI regimen	Approval of abacavir led to the hope of PI-sparing regimens (abacavir/zidovudine/lamivudine) to reduce PI-associated toxicities. However, this regimen was found to be less potent than PI or NNRTI-based regimens.
Late 1990s–early 2000s	Ritonavir-boosted PI	Ritonavir is commonly used as a pharmacokinetic enhancer (instead of an active HIV PI) to increase bioavailability of other PIs and to reduce the pill burden and dosing frequency.
2003–2008	Approval of second-generation antiretroviral agents of existing drug classes for drug-resistant HIV: tenofovir, tipranavir, darunavir, and etravirine	The increase in multiple drug class–resistant HIV led to the need of newer agents, resulting in the approval of newer-generation drugs from existing drug classes.
2003	First fusion inhibitor (enfuvirtide) approved for multidrug-resistant HIV	T-20 added to an optimized background regimen can significantly reduce HIV RNA in patients with multiple drug class resistance. The need for subcutaneous injection and resultant injection site reactions limit its use.
2006	Atripla: fixed-dose formulation of efavirenz, tenofovir, and emtricitabine approved	First fixed-dose combination, one-pill once-daily product approved, to reduce the pill burden and improve adherence.
2007	First CCR5 antagonist (maraviroc) approved for multidrug-resistant HIV	Use of maraviroc is limited by the need of performance of viral tropism testing before treatment. It was later approved for treatment-naïve patients.

(continued on next page)

Years	Advances in Antiretroviral Therapy	Comments
Table 1 *(continued)*		
2007	*First INSTI* (raltegravir) approved for multidrug-resistant HIV	It can significantly reduce HIV RNA in patients with multiple drug class resistance. It was later approved for treatment-naïve patients.
2011	*Antiretroviral use as prevention of transmission to uninfected partners*	In the HPTN 052 study, where HIV disconcordant couples were enrolled, the HIV-infected partners were randomized to receive antiretroviral therapy or no therapy, HIV transmission was significantly reduced when antiretroviral therapy was used.
2012	*Preexposure prophylaxis with tenofovir + emtricitabine*	There is FDA approval of tenofovir/emtricitabine for continuous preexposure prophylaxis for HIV-negative individuals who are at high risk of acquiring HIV infection. This approval marks the first approval of antiretroviral therapy for HIV-uninfected persons.

Abbreviations: FDA, Food and Drug Administration; HAART, highly active antiretroviral therapy; HPTN, HIV prevention trials network; INSTI, integrase strand transfer inhibitor; IV, intravenous; NNRTI, non-nucleoside reverse transcriptase inhibitor; PACTG, pediatric AIDS clinical trial group; PMTCT, prevention of mother to child HIV transmission.

- A combination regimen should consist of preferably 3 (but at least 2) active agents based on genotype resistance test results.

HIV LIFE CYCLE AND TARGETS OF ANTIRETROVIRAL DRUG THERAPY

Fig. 1 illustrates the different steps of the HIV life cycle and drug targets (adapted from http://www.niaid.nih.gov/topics/HIVAIDS/Understanding/Biology/pages/hivreplicationcycle.aspx).[7] HIV virions enter the CD4+ T cells and use the CD4 cells as the machinery for reproduction of new virions. The currently approved antiretroviral drugs aim at halting viral replication at 6 different stages of the HIV life cycle. **Table 2** lists the drugs approved by the Food and Drug Administration (FDA) within each drug class.

RATIONALE FOR COMBINATION ANTIRETROVIRAL THERAPY

As described earlier, HIV replication requires a multistep process. Using a combination of different agents targeting different steps within the HIV life cycle provides either a synergistic or additive antiviral effect, thus enhancing the efficiency in which viral replication is suppressed. Based on data from large randomized clinical trials, 4 different combinations are commonly prescribed to treatment-naïve patients. All these combinations include a backbone of 2-NRTIs, plus one of these classes of drugs: a PI (usually boosted with ritonavir), a non-nucleoside reverse transcriptase inhibitor (NNRTI), an integrase strand transfer inhibitor (INSTI), or the C-C chemokine receptor type 5 (CCR5) antagonist maraviroc (for more detailed description of different regimens, please refer to the article by Johnson and Sax elsewhere in this issue). Transmission of drug-resistant HIV may occur, thus a genotypic resistance testing is

Table 2
US FDA-approved antiretroviral agents (listed in chronologic order by year of drug approval) and their targets in the HIV life cycle

Drug Class	CCR5 Antagonist	Fusion Inhibitor	NRTI	NNRTI	INSTI	PI
FDA-Approved Drugs	Maraviroc	Enfuvirtide	Zidovudine Didanosine Zalcitabine Stavudine Lamivudine Abacavir Tenofovir Emtricitab-ine	Nevirapine Delavirdine Efavirenz Etravirine Rilpivirine	Raltegravir Elvitegravir[a] Dolutegravir	Saquinavir Indinavir Ritonavir Nelfinavir Amprenavir Lopinavir[b] Fosamprenavir Atazanavir Tipranavir Darunavir

Abbreviations: FDA, Food and Drug Administration; INSTI, integrase strand transfer inhibitor; NNRTI, non-nucleoside reverse transcriptase inhibitor; PI, protease inhibitor.
[a] Only approved as a fixed-dose combination product with cobicistat (a pharmacokinetic enhancer), tenofovir, and emtricitabine.
[b] Only approved as a fixed-dose combination product with low-dose ritonavir as a pharmacokinetic enhancer.

generally recommended before initiation of therapy in order to avoid prescription of suboptimal therapy.[8] Despite the efficacy of these antiretroviral regimens, some patients may experience treatment failure with HIV drug resistance. In these patients, therapy may be more complex and require the use of multiple drug classes, based on genotypic or phenotypic drug susceptibility testing (for more detailed discussion, please refer to the article by Daar and Calvo elsewhere in this issue).

Early generation antiretroviral agents have provided the evidence that viral suppression can be achieved. However, these earlier agents have largely fallen out of favor because of their large pill burden, frequent daily dosing, as well as intolerable side effects. Newer agents marketed in the past decade aim to provide some advantages, including new mechanisms of action; greater virologic potency, especially toward multidrug-resistant HIV; fewer toxicities; less drug-drug interactions; and lower pill burden or dosing frequency. The remainder of this article describes the different currently used agents in each drug class. The accompanying tables provide a comparison of the characteristics of drugs in each class to help the readers in selecting the most optimal drugs for each patient.

NRTIs

The NRTIs are the first class of antiretroviral drugs approved for use in the United States and remains as a key component of most combination regimens.[8] The NRTIs are phosphorylated intracellularly to their active diphosphate or triphosphate metabolites, which then inhibit the enzymatic action of the HIV reverse transcriptase by incorporating into the nucleotide analogue causing DNA chain termination or by competing with the natural substrate of the virus. This process in turn halts the conversion of viral RNA into double-stranded DNA. Zidovudine was first approved in 1987 for patients with advanced HIV (CD4 count <200 cells per cubic millimeter) or with AIDS-defining conditions,[1] followed by the approval of didanosine, zalcitabine, stavudine, and lamivudine. These drugs were initially prescribed as a monotherapy followed by the combination of 2-NRTI (such as zidovudine + didanosine, zidovudine +

zalcitabine, [zidovudine or stavudine] + lamivudine, or stavudine + didanosine). A combination antiretroviral regimen today typically consists of 2-NRTI as a backbone to be used in combination with a third or fourth drug, typically an NNRTI, a boosted-PI, an INSTI, or a CCR5 antagonist. The use of older NRTIs is limited by some serious toxicities, mostly related to their effects on human cellular mitochondrial DNA in different tissues.[9] Some of these include bone marrow toxicities and myopathy associated with zidovudine; peripheral neuropathy with stavudine, didanosine, and zalcitabine; and pancreatitis with didanosine and stavudine. These older NRTIs are also associated with serious and sometimes fatal toxicities, such as lactic acidosis and hepatic steatosis. Additionally, cosmetically disfiguring and mostly irreversible lipoatrophy has been associated with long-term use of the thymidine analogues stavudine and zidovudine. Newer NRTIs, such as abacavir, tenofovir, lamivudine and emtricitabine, seem to be weaker inhibitors of mitochondrial DNA polymerase gamma and associated with much less toxicities that are associated with mitochondrial injury.[10] NRTIs are not metabolized via the CYP450 enzyme system and, thus, have less potential for significant drug-drug interactions. Most NRTIs, except for abacavir, require dosage adjustment in patients with renal insufficiency. Dosing recommendations in patients with renal impairment can be found in the product labels and in the treatment guidelines.[8]

Today, the most commonly used NRTIs are tenofovir and abacavir, both used in combination with emtricitabine or lamivudine. These agents, along with zidovudine, are discussed later. A comparison of the characteristics of the different agents can be found in **Table 3**.

Abacavir

Abacavir is a carbocyclic nucleoside analogue that is converted to its active metabolite carbovir triphosphate, which in turn inhibits the effect of HIV reverse transcriptase.[11] It is readily and extensively absorbed orally. It is metabolized by alcohol dehydrogenase and glucuronyl transferase. No dosage adjustment is needed in patients with renal insufficiency. Abacavir is commonly used in combination with lamivudine as a 2-NRTI backbone, and it is available as a fixed-dose combination with lamivudine (Epzicom) or with zidovudine and lamivudine (Trizivir). Although a 3-NRTI combination of abacavir + zidovudine + lamivudine has been approved as an initial regimen for antiretroviral-naïve patients, it is generally not recommended[8] because of the inferior potency of this regimen.[12] Abacavir + lamivudine can be given once daily without regard to food. Abacavir use has been associated with an immunologically mediated systemic hypersensitivity reaction manifested by symptoms such as high fever, diffuse skin rash, flulike syndrome, gastrointestinal (GI) disturbances, and respiratory compromise.[13] These symptoms usually occur within the first few weeks of treatment initiation for which abacavir should be discontinued promptly. It is not recommended to rechallenge a patient who has experienced this hypersensitivity reaction, as reintroduction of abacavir can lead to the rapid onset of more severe symptoms, such as profound hypotension and vascular collapse.[13–15] This reaction has been found to be highly associated with the presence of the HLA-B*5701 allele.[16,17] Testing of HLA-B*5701 should be done before initiation of abacavir, and those who test positive should not be given this agent.[8] In some but not all prospective and retrospective studies, the current or recent use of abacavir was associated with cardiovascular events, such as acute myocardial infarction, especially in patients with significant history of cardiac diseases.[18,19] To date, this association remains controversial. Because of concerns of lower rates of virologic suppression associated with abacavir + lamivudine as an NRTI backbone compared with tenofovir + emtricitabine in

Table 3
Characteristics of selected nucleos(t)ide reverse transcriptase inhibitors

	Abacavir (Ziagen)	Emtricitabine (Emtriva)	Lamivudine (Epivir)	Tenofovir Disoproxil Fumarate (Viread)	Zidovudine (Retrovir)
Abbreviation	ABC	FTC	3TC	TDF	ZDV (or AZT)
US FDA approval year	1999	2003	2003	2001	1987
US FDA indications for HIV-1 infected adults	ART-naïve and ART-experienced patients	1. ART-naïve and ART-experienced patients 2. Preexposure prophylaxis (use with tenofovir)	1. ART-naïve and ART-experienced patients 2. Hepatitis B infection	1. ART-naïve and ART-experienced patients 2. Hepatitis B infection 3. Preexposure prophylaxis (when used with emtricitabine)	1. ART-naïve and ART-experienced patients 2. Prevention of perinatal HIV transmission
Approval for HIV-1 infected children	3 mo and older	Newborn and older	3 mo and older	2 y and older	Newborn and older
Generic formulation	Yes	No	Yes	No	Yes
Fixed-dose combination product marketed in the United States	Epzicom (+lamivudine) Trizivir (+lamivudine + zidovudine)	Truvada (+tenofovir) Atripla (+efavirenz + tenofovir) Complera (+rilpivirine + tenofovir) Stribild (+elvitegravir + cobicistat +tenofovir)	Epzicom (+abacavir) Combivir (+zidovudine) Trizivir (+abacavir + zidovudine)	Truvada (+emtricitabine) Atripla (+efavirenz + emtricitabine) Complera (+rilpivirine + emtricitabine) Stribild (+elvitegravir +cobicistat +emtricitabine)	Combivir (+lamivudine) Trizivir (+abacavir +lamivudine)
Usual dose (adult)	600 mg PO once daily or 300 mg PO twice daily	200 mg PO once daily Oral solution: 240 mg daily	300 mg PO once daily or 150 mg PO twice daily	300 mg PO once daily	300 mg PO twice daily
Adjust dose in renal insufficiency	No	Yes	Yes	Yes	Yes
Formulations (as individual drugs)	Oral tablet: 300 mg Oral solution: 20 mg/mL	Oral capsule: 200 mg Oral solution: 10 mg/mL	Oral tablets: 150 mg and 300 mg Oral solution: 10 mg/mL	Oral tablets: 150, 200, 250, and 300 mg Oral powder: 40 mg/g	Oral tablet and capsule: 500 mg

Significant and/or common adverse effects	Hypersensitivity reaction (primarily in patients with HLA-B*5701 allele); perform HLA-B*5701 testing before prescribing abacavir	Skin pigmentation	Generally well tolerated Rarely reported, peripheral neuropathy	Renal insufficiency (proximal renal tubulopathy, manifested as increase in serum creatinine, hypophosphatemia, glucosuria) Decrease in bone mineral density	Bone marrow suppression (macrocytic anemia, neutropenia) Nausea, vomiting, headache Nail pigmentation Lactic acidosis, hepatic steatosis Cardiomyopathy Lipoatrophy Myopathy
CYP3A4 interaction	None	None	None	None	None
Primary resistance mutations[61]	K65R, L74V, Y115F, M184V	K65R, M184V	K65R, M184V	K65R, K70E	M41L, D67N, K70R, L210W, T215Y/F, K219Q/E
Other considerations	HLA-B*5701 testing should be performed before initiating abacavir In some studies, lower virologic responses reported with pre-ART viral load >100,000 copies per milliliter Some observation studies reported an association of abacavir use and increased cardiovascular events	Symptomatic hepatic flare has been associated with initiation or discontinuation of emtricitabine in patients with hepatitis B coinfection	Symptomatic hepatic flare has been associated with initiation or discontinuation of lamivudine in patients with hepatitis B coinfection	Symptomatic hepatic flare has been associated with initiation or discontinuation of tenofovir in patients with hepatitis B coinfection	Mitochondrial toxicities (such as lactic acidosis, lipoatrophy, cardiomyopathy, myopathy) generally associated with long-term use

Abbreviations: ART, antiretroviral therapy; FDA, Food and Drug Administration.

treatment-naïve patients with a baseline viral load greater than 100,000 copies per milliliter, some experts suggest that, except when using with dolutegravir, abacavir + lamivudine use in patients with baseline HIV RNA greater than 100,000 copies per milliliter should be done with caution.[8]

Emtricitabine and Lamivudine

Emtricitabine and lamivudine share similar structure and activities. They possess similar HIV-1 resistance profiles whereby the most frequently selected resistance mutation is M184V. They are both active against hepatitis B virus (HBV) and should be used as part of a regimen in patients with hepatitis B coinfection. Exacerbation of hepatitis may occur after initiation[20] (as a form of immune reconstitution) or discontinuation[21] of these agents. These two agents are rapidly absorbed orally, with emtricitabine having a slightly longer intracellular half-life. They are both renally excreted, whereby dosage adjustment is necessary in patients with renal impairment. These drugs are generally very well tolerated, with skin discoloration being the most commonly reported side effect. Both agents are commonly used as part of a 2-NRTI backbone, together seen with emtricitabine abacavir, tenofovir, or zidovudine. They are both available in different fixed-dose combination products on the market (see **Table 3**). As they provide similar antiviral activities without additive effect, there is no benefit in using these two drugs in combination.

Tenofovir Disoproxil Fumarate (or Tenofovir)

Tenofovir disoproxil fumarate is a nucleotide analogue, which inhibits the reverse transcriptase of both HIV and HBV. It is approved for use as part of the treatment of HIV and HBV infection. Tenofovir with emtricitabine also has been approved for use as preexposure prophylaxis for individuals who are at high risk of acquisition of HIV.[22] Tenofovir is available as part of a fixed-dose combination product with various different antiretroviral drugs (see **Table 2**). It is rapidly absorbed orally and is eliminated renally by both glomerular filtration and active tubular secretion. It can be given as once daily therapy without regard to food. Dosage adjustment is necessary in patients with renal impairment. Use of tenofovir has been associated with new onset or worsening of renal dysfunction, primarily as a consequence of renal proximal tubulopathy (or Fanconi syndrome), which may manifest as increase in serum creatinine, glycosuria, proteinuria, or hypophosphatemia.[23] These effects on the kidneys may be increased when tenofovir is used with a boosted PI.[24,25] Renal function, electrolytes, and urinalysis should be monitored in patients receiving tenofovir and particularly in those who have preexisting renal dysfunction or who are receiving other nephrotoxic drugs. Tenofovir use has been associated with reduced bone mineral density and increases in biomarkers associated with bone metabolism, which may lead to an increase in fracture risk.[26,27] Osteomalacia and hypophosphatemia with symptomatic bone and muscular pain have been reported in patients that may have been a consequence of proximal renal tubulopathy.[28,29] Tenofovir use with emtricitabine or lamivudine and a third agent (either an NNRTI, a boosted PI, or an INSTI) have been found to result in a potent antiretroviral effect, leading to durable viral suppression in the clinical trial participants. Because of its potency and ease of use, tenofovir is part of most preferred combination antiretroviral regimens for treatment-naïve patients.

Zidovudine

Zidovudine is a thymidine analogue that is converted to its active triphosphate form intracellularly, which is then attached to the DNA polymerase of the reverse transcriptase leading to chain termination. It was the first NRTI approved, showing a survival benefit compared with placebo, in patients with advanced HIV.[1] In 1994, zidovudine monotherapy received FDA approval for pregnant women after 14-week gestation, which included intrapartum intravenous zidovudine; oral zidovudine was given to the newborn. This therapy resulted in a dramatic reduction in perinatal HIV transmission.[30] It is well absorbed orally and undergoes glucuronidation in the liver and eventually elimination by the kidneys. Zidovudine is dosed at twice daily without regard to food. It is commonly prescribed with lamivudine to form the 2-NRTI backbone of a combination regimen. It is available as coformulated products with lamivudine (Combivir) as well as with lamivudine and abacavir (Trizivir). The side effects of zidovudine have led to its limited utility in today's treatment armamentarium. Some common side effects include bone marrow suppression (primarily macrocytic anemia and neutropenia), nausea and vomiting, nail pigmentation, and headache. Serious but less common side effects have also been reported, which include myopathy, cardiomyopathy, and lactic acidosis (often with hepatic steatosis). Because of its long-term efficacy and safety data for pregnant women and the fetus, zidovudine remains as one of the recommended antiretroviral drugs to be given during pregnancy. For nonpregnant patients, the utility of zidovudine is more limited, primarily because of its toxicity profile and the need for twice-daily dosing.

NNRTIs

NNRTIs are different from NRTIs in that they do not require intracellular phosphorylation to exert their pharmacologic action. NNRTIs are noncompetitive inhibitors of reverse transcriptase, which results in a conformational change and, thus, decreases the action of this enzyme.

NNRTIs are potent agents for virologic suppression but are limited by drug interactions, selected side effects, and overall low threshold for the emergence of resistant mutants (exception is etravirine). All of the NNRTIs are highly metabolized by CYP450 and are particularly potent inducers with the exception of rilpivirine. Caution should be exercised when prescribing concomitant agents that are also highly metabolized by CYP450. Clinicians should consult the prescribing information or other guidelines for information on the management of drug interactions. The description of the US FDA indications in HIV-1 infected adults and children, usual dose, formulations, daily pill burden, significant and/or common adverse effects, major drug interactions, primary resistance mutations, and special considerations are summarized in **Table 4.**

Efavirenz

Efavirenz is rapidly absorbed orally, and the extent of absorption is increased in the setting of a high-fat meal. It is, therefore, recommended to take efavirenz on an empty stomach to avoid excessive adverse effects. It is more than 99% protein bound and is metabolized via oxidative metabolism primarily by CYP2B6 and CYP3A4. Efavirenz is a potent inducer of both of these enzymes and should be used with caution when given with drugs that are metabolized by CYP2B6 and 3A4. It has a long half-life (40–55 hours), which allows for once-daily dosing.[31]

Efavirenz is dosed at 600 mg orally once daily and should be given preferably at bedtime because of the central nervous system (CNS) side effects, which include vivid dreams, dizziness, and hallucinations. More than 50% of patients experienced a myriad of CNS side effects. Although less common, the use of efavirenz has also been associated with psychotic disturbances, such as depression, insomnia, mania,[31]

Table 4
Characteristics of NNRTIs

	Efavirenz (Sustiva)	Etravirine (Intelence)	Nevirapine (Viramune)	Rilpivirine (Edurant)
Abbreviation	EFV	ETR	NVP	RPV
US FDA approval year	1998	2008	1996	2011
US FDA indications for HIV-infected adults	ART-naïve and experienced patients	ART-experienced patients	ART-naïve and ART-experienced patients For ART-naïve patients; only recommended for women with CD4 count <250 cells per cubic millimeter and for men with CD4 count <400 cells per cubic millimeter	ART-naïve patients with baseline HIV RNA <100,000 copies/mL
US FDA indications for HIV-infected children	Infants 3 mo or older	6 y or older	Recommended in all ages	Not recommended for children
Generic formulation	No	No	Yes	No
Fixed-dose combination product marketed in the United States	Atripla (+emtricitabine +tenofovir)	None	None	Complera (+emtricitabine +tenofovir)
Usual dose (adult)	600 mg PO once daily (take on empty stomach, at bedtime)	200 mg PO twice daily	200 mg PO once daily × 14 d, then 200 mg PO BID or 400 mg (extended release) PO once daily	25 mg PO once daily (taken with a ~500-calorie meal)
Adjust dose in renal insufficiency	No	No	No	No
Formulations (as individual drugs)	Capsule: 50 mg, 200 mg Tablet: 600 mg	Tablet: 25 mg, 100 mg, 200 mg	Oral suspension: 50 mg/5 mL Tablet: 200 mg Extended-release tablet: 100 mg, 400 mg	Tablet: 25 mg

Daily pill burden	1	2	1–2	1
Significant and/or common adverse effects	Rash Hepatoxicity CNS disturbances: vivid dreams, hallucinations, depression, suicidality	Rash Elevations in hepatic transaminases	Rash (more frequent and more severe than other NNRTIs) Hepatotoxicity (can lead to fulminant hepatic failure)	Rash Elevations in hepatic transaminases CNS disturbances: depression
Major drug interactions[a]	Substrate of CYP3A4, 2B6: cautionary use with drugs that are strong CYP3A4 or 2B6 inhibitors or inducers Moderate induction of CYP3A4, 2B6: cautionary use with drugs that are major 3A4, 2B6 substrates	Substrate of CYP3A4, 2C19, 2C9: cautionary use with drugs that are strong inhibitors or inducers of these enzymes Moderate inhibition of 2C19, 2C9. P-glycoprotein: cautionary use with drugs that are major 2C19, 2C9 substrates Weak inducer of CYP3A4: cautionary use with drugs that are major CYP3A4 substrates	Substrate of CYP3A4: cautionary use with drugs that are strong CYP3A4 inhibitors or inducers Potent induction of CYP3A4, 2B6: cautionary use with drugs that are major substrates for 3A4, 2B6	Substrate of CYP3A4: cautionary use with drugs that are strong CYP3A4 inhibitors or inducers Should not be coadministered with proton pump inhibitors
Primary resistance mutations[61]	L100I, K101P, K103N, V106M, V108I, Y181C/I, Y188L, G190S/A, P225H, M230L	L100I, K101P, E138K, Y181C/I/V	L100I, K101P, K103N, V106M, V108I, Y181C/I, Y188L, G190A, M230L	K101E/P, E138K, V179L, Y181I/V Y188L, H221Y, F227C, M230I/L
Special considerations	Alternative agent should be used for women who desire to get pregnant or who are not using effective contraception	Not recommended to be used with ritonavir-boosted atazanavir, fosamprenavir, or tipranavir	Higher rate and more serious cutaneous events (including Stevens-Johnson syndrome and toxic epidermal necrolysis), reported with nevirapine use than with other NNRTI	Should be avoided in patients with a baseline viral load of ≤100,000 copies per milliliter and CD4 count <200 cells per cubic millimeter

Abbreviations: ART, antiretroviral therapy; CNS, central nervous system.

[a] Please refer to http://aidsinfo.nih.gov/guidelines/html/1/adult-and-adolescent-arv-guidelines/32/drug-interactions for a comprehensive list of drug-drug interactions.

and suicidality.[32] The incidence of these side effects is highest in the first 4 weeks of therapy and is known to resolve after this time period. Nevertheless, patients should be counseled on these potentially harmful side effects. Rash has been reported in approximately 26% of patients taking efavirenz in clinical trials and usually resolves within the first few weeks of therapy. Serious skin reactions, such as Stevens-Johnson syndrome, have been reported and should be promptly discontinued if suspected. Other reported side effects include hypercholesterolemia (up to 40%) and increase hepatic transaminases (up to 8%). It should be noted that efavirenz is a pregnancy category D whereby the use of this agent in the first trimester has been associated with neural tube defects in both primates and human.[31] It is generally recommended to avoid efavirenz in women of childbearing age if possible. However, it may be continued in pregnant women already on an efavirenz-containing regimen, which produces virologic suppression.[33] This exception was made because neural tube defects occur most likely in the first 5 to 6 weeks of pregnancy and that pregnancy is usually not detected before 6 weeks.

Efavirenz is a preferred NNRTI for treatment-naïve patients in the United States[8] and worldwide[34] and is a popular treatment option given that it is coformulated with the NRTIs emtricitabine and tenofovir (Atripla). The long half-life of efavirenz allows for this one pill once a day antiretroviral regimen. Although the long half-life clearly represents a pharmacokinetic advantage, it should also be noted that HIV can rapidly develop resistance to this agent because of the relative ease of single amino acid substitutions; thus, patient adherence is especially important.

Etravirine

Etravirine is a viable treatment option in patients who have developed resistance to both efavirenz and nevirapine. Its oral bioavailability is increased in the setting of food, and it is recommended to be taken with food. It is metabolized in the liver via CYP3A4, 2C9, and 2C19 to its metabolites and primarily excreted into feces as an unchanged drug (86%). Because its metabolism is mediated by multiple CYP450 enzymes for which it is a substrate, inducer, and inhibitor, caution should be exercised when giving this agent with drugs that are also highly metabolized via this enzyme system. Currently, etravirine is dosed at 200 mg orally twice daily. Unlike efavirenz, etravirine is not associated with CNS disturbances. Rash occurred in 15% of patients in clinical trials and usually resolved within the first few weeks of therapy. Hyperglycemia and hypercholesterolemia have also been reported. It is only approved for use in treatment-experienced patients. In patients who experienced virologic resistance to other NNRTIs, etravirine should not be used with a 2-NRTI backbone alone. Instead, other antiretroviral drugs, such as a ritonavir-boosted PI, an INSTI, or enfuvirtide, should be added to the regimen.[35] In patients who fail a rilpivirine-based regimen with the emergence of the E138K mutation, use of etravirine should be avoided, as this mutation also confers resistance to etravirine.[36]

Nevirapine

The use of nevirapine has been largely limited by the development of resistance to this agent and its CD4 count dependent incidence of serious side effects. It is highly orally bioavailable and moderately protein bound (60%). It is extensively metabolized by CYP3A4 and 2B6 and undergoes enterohepatic recirculation. It auto-induces its metabolism after the first 14 days of therapy for which a dosage adjustment from 200 mg once daily to 400 mg daily dosage (as 400 mg extended-release formulation once daily or 200 mg twice daily) is required. Approximately 80% of the drug is eliminated into the urine.[37]

Hepatotoxicity, often accompanied by systemic symptoms, including fulminant hepatic failure, has been reported in patients receiving nevirapine, with the highest incidence in women with a CD4 count of 250 or more cells per cubic millimeter and men with a CD4 count of 400 or more cells per cubic millimeter.[37] Rash has also been frequently reported with this agent in up to 13% of patients, often occurring within the first 6 weeks of therapy. Drug rash with eosinophilia and systemic symptoms syndrome, Stevens-Johnson syndrome, and toxic epidermal necrolysis have all been reported with nevirapine use. Nevirapine is no longer one of the recommended NNRTIs; however, it remains an option mainly in pregnant women who are HIV positive and for infant antiretroviral prophylaxis, especially in developing countries.[8,33,34]

Rilpivirine

Rilpivirine is the most recently approved of the NNRTIs on the market, which offers some distinct advantages over other agents in its class. Rilpivirine should be taken with food, as its absorption is markedly increased in its presence and depends on gastric pH. Acid-suppressing agents should be separated by at least 2 hours of rilpivirine administration, and proton pump inhibitors should be avoided entirely. It is highly bound to albumin (99%) and is metabolized by CYP3A4, for which it is only a substrate and not an inducer nor an inhibitor of this enzyme. This represents an advantage over other NNRTIs, as the drug interactions with this agent may be more predictable. Caution should be exercised when administering this agent with drugs that are potent inducers or inhibitors of CYP3A4, as these drugs may significantly alter the serum levels of rilpivirine. It has a long half-life of more than 50 hours, which allows for convenient once-a-day dosing. It is primarily excreted into feces.[38]

Rilpivirine is dosed 25 mg orally once daily in both treatment-naïve and experienced patients and is currently recommended as an alternative NNRTI in patients with a baseline viral load of 100,000 or less copies per milliliter.[8] Rilpivirine is not recommended in patients with a viral load greater than 100,000 copies per milliliter, as it was shown to have inferior rates of virologic suppression compared with efavirenz in treatment-naïve patients.[39] Rilpivirine is coformulated into a single-tablet, once-daily regimen (Complera) with emtricitabine and tenofovir.

Rilpivirine is generally well tolerated. Like all NNRTIs, rilpivirine use has also been associated with rash (3%), although to a much lesser extent compared with nevirapine and efavirenz. CNS side effects, including depression, were reported in about 9% of patients in the double-blinded clinical trials comparing rilpivirine with efavirenz.[39] Elevations in hepatic transaminases have also been reported and, therefore, should be used with caution in patients with liver dysfunction. Rilpivirine offers the advantage of a single-tablet regimen, potentially fewer drug interactions, and is generally well tolerated, including fewer CNS side effects. Its use may be limited by its inferior efficacy rates in patients with high baseline viral loads and drug interactions with acid-suppressing agents.

PI

PIs exhibit their pharmacologic action late in the HIV replication cycle by binding to HIV proteases, leading to blockage of the proteolytic activities of the enzyme, resulting in the inability to form mature, infectious virions. In combination with 2-NRTIs, certain ritonavir-boosted PI regimens are considered preferred therapies in treatment-naïve patients. PI plus NRTI combination regimens have shown to be effective not only in treatment-naïve patients but also with other antiretroviral therapy drug classes for patients who experience treatment failure.

Currently, 9 PIs are available on the US market. Of these 9, only 7 are discussed in this review: ritonavir, saquinavir, lopinavir, fosamprenavir, tipranavir, atazanavir, and darunavir. Indinavir and nelfinavir are not discussed, as their role in therapy has diminished because of the large pill burden and intolerable side effects. The PIs remain an important class of antiretroviral drugs mainly because of their high barrier to resistance. These agents generally require an accumulation of multiple resistance mutations for resistance to occur. Class-associated side effects include metabolic abnormalities including dyslipidemia (primarily triglycerides), insulin resistance, hyperglycemia, and lipodystrophy. The incidence of these side effects is augmented by the use of concomitant ritonavir, which is recommended to be given with most available PIs. Ritonavir, although it possesses anti-HIV activity, is not currently used as an active agent in the treatment of HIV in part because of the high pill burden required as an active PI and high rate of GI side effects and lipid abnormalities. Instead, its role is limited to boosting or enhancing the pharmacokinetic profile of other PIs. Being a potent CYP3A4 inhibitor (in both the liver and the gut lumen), low-dose ritonavir inhibits the metabolism of most PIs resulting in an overall increase in drug exposure and plasma half-life, allowing for use of the active PI in a lower dose and reduced dosing frequency. Currently, all PIs are given with ritonavir (100–400 mg daily) as the standard of therapy. The available PIs vary greatly in regard to their pharmacokinetics, dosing, virologic potency, pill burden, and side-effect profile. Prescribers should be aware of these differences to individualize therapy for patients according to their concomitant medications, comorbidities, and allergies/intolerances.

Virtually all of the available PIs are metabolized by CYP450. Caution should be exercised when prescribing concomitant agents that are also highly metabolized by CYP3A4. The description of the US FDA indications in HIV-1 infected adults and children, usual dose, formulations, daily pill burden, significant and/or common adverse effects, major drug interactions, primary resistance mutations, and special considerations are summarized in **Tables 5** and **6**.

Atazanavir

Atazanavir undergoes rapid oral absorption. When unboosted, the area under the concentration time curve (AUC) is increased by almost 70% when given with a light meal compared with approximately 35% with a high-fat meal. When given with ritonavir, the AUC of atazanavir is increased by almost 2.5-fold. Atazanavir requires an acidic gastric environment to be optimally absorbed. Concomitant use with acid suppressants, such as proton pump inhibitors and acid-reducing agents such as histamine-2-receptor antagonists (H2RAs) and antacids, significantly reduce atazanavir serum concentrations. The prescribing information provides recommendations on optimal dosage and/or timing adjustments for atazanavir when patients are also taking any acid-reducing agents.[40] Atazanavir is extensively metabolized by CYP3A4. Because its metabolism is primarily mediated by CYP3A4, the potential for significant drug interactions is high. In addition, atazanavir is a moderate inhibitor of UGT1A1, which may increase the AUC of agents that are metabolized by this enzyme (eg, certain integrase inhibitors). Despite this increase in concentration, dosage adjustments are not necessary, as this interaction has not amounted to adverse responses. Unboosted atazanavir (at 400 mg once-daily dosage) is only recommended for treatment-naïve patients who are not receiving tenofovir or a proton pump inhibitor. For most other patients, boosted atazanavir regimen of 300 mg/100 mg ritonavir orally daily is recommended.

Atazanavir is better tolerated when compared with patients treated with lopinavir, fosamprenavir, and efavirenz with lower rates of dyslipidemia and virtually no effect on glucose or insulin sensitivity.[40] The most common side effect is an increase in indirect bilirubin, which occurred in approximately 40% of patients in clinical trials. Although this indirect hyperbilirubinemia has not been correlated with hepatotoxicity, some patients may be adverse to this cosmetic side effect usually manifested by scleral icterus. Only 5% of patients in clinical trials experienced jaundice. Postmarketing surveillance reported cases of cholelithiasis[41] and nephrolithiasis,[42] which may be increased with cumulative exposure and in the presence of ritonavir boosting. Ritonavir boosting may also increase the overall incidence of dyslipidemia. Rash was also reported in about 20% of patients, with a median onset of 7 weeks. A less common but serious adverse reaction reported with atazanavir include PR interval prolongation which was largely limited to first-degree atrioventricular (AV) block; thus, atazanavir should be used with caution in patients with a preexisting cardiac conduction abnormality, especially in patients who are on concomitant medications that may also have PR prolongation effects. Boosted atazanavir is a preferred PI regimen primarily because of the overall lower pill burden (2 pills), its high barrier to drug resistance, and virologic potency demonstrated in treatment-naïve and experienced patients.

Darunavir

Darunavir is the most recently approved PI on the market. Unlike atazanavir and fosamprenavir, darunavir must be boosted with ritonavir in all patients. It undergoes rapid absorption after oral administration, and its AUC is significantly increased by up to 14-fold in the presence of ritonavir. Darunavir should also ideally be administered with food as the AUC is increased by 30%. It is highly protein bound (95%) to alpha$_1$-acid glycoprotein and is metabolized by CYP3A4. When used with ritonavir, it is a potent CYP3A4 inhibitor; thus, the potential for significant drug interactions is high. Its elimination half-life is approximately 15 hours when boosted with ritonavir.

Darunavir was initially FDA approved for treatment-experienced patients only, at a dosage of 600 mg with ritonavir 100 mg both given twice daily. It was later approved in treatment naïve-patients and treatment-experienced patients with no darunavir-associated mutations as a once-daily regimen of 800 mg/ritonavir 100 mg.[43] The most common GI side effects (nausea, vomiting, diarrhea) associated with darunavir are likely attributed to ritonavir. Darunavir contains a sulfonamide moiety and should be prescribed cautiously in patients with a known sulfa allergy. The overall incidence of rash was similar among patients with and without a reported history of sulfonamide allergy. Rash occurred in 10% of patients treated with darunavir and occurred within the first 4 weeks of therapy. Hepatotoxicity, namely, acute hepatitis, has also been associated with darunavir use in both clinical trials (0.5%) and in postmarketing reports. It should be used with caution in patients with underlying liver dysfunction. Like other PIs, darunavir is also associated with metabolic complications, which include dyslipidemia and hyperglycemia; however, a smaller percentage of patients experienced these side effects compared with lopinavir/ritonavir in a clinical trial.[44] It has the highest barrier to resistance of the available PIs, requiring multiple primary mutations. It has also demonstrated superior virologic efficacy compared with lopinavir/ritonavir.[44] Like atazanavir, boosted darunavir is a preferred PI because of its low pill burden and tolerability profile.[8]

Fosamprenavir

Fosamprenavir is the phosphorylated prodrug of amprenavir. The oral bioavailability of amprenavir is greatly increased by approximately 63% when given as the prodrug. It is highly bound to alpha$_1$-acid glycoprotein and primarily metabolized in the liver via CYP3A4, with a high potential for significant drug interactions. Even though fosamprenavir is approved to be used without ritonavir, it has less optimal virologic response;

Table 5
Characteristics of selected protease inhibitors

	Atazanavir (Reyataz)	Darunavir (Prezista)	Fosamprenavir (Lexiva)
Abbreviation	ATV	DRV	FPV
US FDA approval year	2003	2006	2003
US FDA indications for HIV-1 infected adults	ART-naïve and ART-experienced patients	ART-naïve and ART-experienced patients	ART-naïve and ART-experienced patients
US FDA indications for HIV-1 infected children	6–18 y of age	3 y and older	2–18 y of age
Generic formulation	No	No	No
Usual dose (adult)	*ART naïve*: 300 mg PO daily + ritonavir 100 mg PO daily or 400 mg PO daily *ART experienced*: 300 mg PO daily + ritonavir 100 mg PO daily	*ART naïve*: 800 mg PO daily + ritonavir 100 mg PO daily *ART experienced*: 600 mg PO BID + ritonavir 100 mg PO BID	*ART naïve*: 1400 mg + ritonavir (100–200) mg PO daily or 700 mg PO BID + ritonavir 100 mg PO BID *ART experienced*: 700 mg PO BID + ritonavir 100 mg PO BID
Adjust dose in renal dysfunction	No	No	No
Formulations	Oral capsules: 150 mg, 200 mg, 300 mg	Oral tablets: 75 mg, 150 mg, 600 mg, 800 mg Oral suspension: 100 mg/mL (200 mL)	Oral tablets: 700 mg Oral suspension: 50 mg/mL (225 mL)
Daily pill burden	2 pills, once daily administration	2–4 pills; once or twice daily administration depending on ART naïve or experienced	3–4 pills, once or twice daily administration depending on ART naïve or experienced

Significant and/or common adverse effects	Increased indirect bilirubin[a] Jaundice[a] Cholelithiasis[a] Rash Nephrolithiasis[a] Dyslipidemia[a,b] PR interval prolongation	Rash (contains sulfonamide moiety) Dyslipidemia[b] Elevation of hepatic transaminases	Rash (contains sulfonamide moiety) Dyslipidemia[b] Hyperglycemia Headache Nausea Diarrhea
Major drug interactions[c]	Potent CYP3A4 inhibition: cautionary use with drugs that are major CYP3A4 substrates Substrate of CYP3A4: cautionary use with drugs that are strong CYP3A4 inhibitor or inducer Atazanavir requires acidic gastric pH for optimal absorption: may be used with acid suppressive agents including antacids, H2RAs, and PPIs in some circumstances, and with dosage separation; refer to product label for recommendations	Potent CYP3A4 inhibition: cautionary use with drugs that are major CYP3A4 substrates Substrate of CYP3A4: cautionary use with drugs that are strong CYP3A4 inhibitor or inducer	Potent CYP3A4 inhibition: cautionary use with drugs that are major CYP3A4 substrates Substrate of CYP3A4: cautionary use with drugs that are strong CYP3A4 inhibitor or inducer
Primary resistance mutations[61]	I50L (most common), I84V, N88S	I47V, I50V, I54M/L, L76V, I84V	I50V, I84V

Abbreviations: ART, antiretroviral therapy; H2RAs, histamine-2 receptor antagonists; PPIs, proton pump inhibitor.
[a] Higher incidence observed with boosted ATV.
[b] Dyslipidemia is observed with all approved protease inhibitors, particularly hypertriglyceridemia: Boosted LPV = FPV > boosted ATV > DRV.
[c] Please refer to http://aidsinfo.nih.gov/guidelines/html/1/adult-and-adolescent-arv-guidelines/32/drug-interactions for a comprehensive list of drug-drug interactions.

Table 6
Characteristics of selected protease inhibitors

	Lopinavir/Ritonavir (Kaletra)	Saquinavir (Invirase)	Tipranavir (Aptivus)
Abbreviation	LPV/r	SQV	TPV
US FDA approval year	2000	1995	2005
US FDA indications for HIV-1 infected adults	ART-naïve and ART-experienced patients	ART-naïve and ART-experienced patients	ART-experienced patients
US FDA indications for HIV-1 infected children	14 d and older	Not approved for children	≥2 y of age
Generic formulation	No	No	No
Usual dose (adult)	*All patients:* 400 mg/100 mg PO BID Once-daily dosing (only in patients with <3 LPV-associated resistance mutations): 800 mg/200 mg PO daily	*All patients:* 1000 mg PO BID + ritonavir 100 mg PO BID	*All patients:* 500 mg PO BID + ritonavir 200 mg PO BID
Adjust dose in renal dysfunction	No	No	No
Formulations	Oral tablet: 100/25 mg, 200 mg/50 mg Oral solution: 80 mg/20 mg per 1 mL (160 mL)	Oral tablet and capsule: 500 mg tablet 200 mg capsule	Oral capsule: 250 mg Oral solution: 100 mg/mL
Daily pill burden	4 pills	6 pills	8 pills
Significant and/or common adverse effects	Rash Dyslipidemia[a] Diarrhea Elevations in transaminases Hyperglycemia/insulin resistance Pancreatitis PR & QT interval prolongation	Nausea, vomiting Dyslipidemia[a] Hyperglycemia PR & QT interval prolongation	Rash (contains sulfonamide moiety) Hepatitis Intracranial hemorrhage Headache Diarrhea
Major drug interactions[b]	Mediated by mainly CYP3A4 via Potent inhibition: cautionary use with drugs that are major CYP3A4 substrates	Mediated by mainly CYP3A4 via Potent inhibition: cautionary use with drugs that are major CYP3A4 substrates Substrate of CYP3A4: cautionary use with drugs that will strongly inhibit or induce CYP3A4 metabolism	Substrate of CYP3A4
Primary resistance mutations (generally requires multiple mutations to confer resistance)[61]	V32I, I47V/A, L76V, V82A/F/T/S	G48V, L90M	I47V, Q58E, T74P V82L/T, N83D, 84V

Abbreviation: ART, antiretroviral therapy.

[a] Dyslipidemia is observed with all boosted protease inhibitors, particularly hypertriglyceridemia: Boosted LPV = FPV > boosted ATV > DRV.

[b] Please refer to http://aidsinfo.nih.gov/guidelines/html/1/adult-and-adolescent-arv-guidelines/32/drug-interactions for a comprehensive list of drug-drug interactions.

thus, in general, ritonavir-boosting is recommended. When given with ritonavir, the fosamprenavir may be reduced from 1400 mg twice daily to fosamprenavir 1400 mg plus ritonavir 100 or 200 mg, both given once daily or fosamprenavir 700 mg plus ritonavir 100 mg, both given twice daily.[8]

The most common side effects associated with fosamprenavir include rash, nausea, vomiting, and diarrhea and metabolic abnormalities, including hypertriglyceridemia. Amprenavir contains a sulfonamide moiety, which may increase the risk of rash in some patients. The overall incidence of rash varied in clinical trials between those who had a previous sulfa allergy versus those who did not (12%–33%) and most often occurred within the first 2 weeks of therapy. The potential for cross reactivity to other sulfonamide drugs is unknown and should be used with caution. Fosamprenavir is less favored overall compared with other PI-based regimens because of the higher pill burden and modest virologic efficacy compared with other boosted PI regimens.[8]

Lopinavir

Lopinavir is the only PI that is coformulated with the ritonavir. The current formulation of lopinavir is absorbed rapidly when given via oral administration and is not affected significantly by the presence or absence of food. When given with ritonavir, the AUC is increased significantly potentiating a potent antiviral pharmacologic effect. It undergoes significant oxidative metabolism mediated by CYP3A4 and, along with ritonavir, is a potent CYP3A4 inhibitor and, thus, has the potential for significant drug interactions.

The typical dosage in treatment-naïve and experienced patients is lopinavir 400 mg/ritonavir 100 mg twice daily or lopinavir 800 mg/ritonavir 200 mg once daily. When given in combination with potent CYP3A4 inducers, such as efavirenz, nevirapine, and amprenavir, the dosage should be increased to lopinavir 500 mg/ritonavir 125 mg twice daily. It should be noted that the once-daily regimen should not be prescribed for pregnant women[33] and for treatment-experienced patients with evidence of 3 or more of certain lopinavir-associated mutations.[45]

Common adverse effects of lopinavir/ritonavir include metabolic abnormalities, such as hypercholesterolemia, hypertriglyceridemia, hyperglycemia, and insulin resistance. In comparison with other PI agents on the market, the incidence of hypercholesterolemia and hypertriglyceridemia occurs at higher rates with lopinavir/ritonavir, up to 39% and 36%, respectively. Pancreatitis has also been observed primarily in patients with marked elevations in triglycerides. GI side effects are also common, primarily nausea and diarrhea, and likely attributed to the 200 mg of concomitant ritonavir. Postmarketing cases of complete AV blockade and cardiomyopathy primarily in neonates receiving lopinavir solution, which contains approximately 42% volume/volume of ethanol and 15% weight/volume of propylene glycol, have been reported.[45] Furthermore, postmarketing cases of hepatotoxicity, PR and QT prolongation, and torsades de pointes have been reported with the use of lopinavir/ritonavir. It should be avoided in patients with congenital and structural heart diseases. Because of the higher pill burden, need for 200 mg of ritonavir, higher incidence of metabolic abnormalities, and lower tolerability rates when compared with the newer PI agents, lopinavir/ritonavir is no longer recommended as the preferred PI.[8]

Saquinavir

Saquinavir was the first approved PI. Oral bioavailability of saquinavir is poor, as it undergoes significant first pass metabolism but is increased with a high-fat meal.[46] Saquinavir should be given with a meal and always boosted with ritonavir. Common adverse effects include GI disorders, with nausea being the most commonly reported

(10%). Saquinavir was shown to cause PR interval and QT prolongation in a dose-dependent manner in a healthy volunteer study.[46,47] Cases of torsades de pointes have been reported. Patients with structural heart disease, preexisting conduction abnormalities, and ischemic heart disease are at an increased risk of cardiac conduction abnormalities. Baseline electrocardiogram is recommended before initiation of saquinavir. Saquinavir is contraindicated in patients with prolonged QTc, refractory hypokalemia or hypomagnesemia, and complete AV block.[46] Saquinavir is generally otherwise well tolerated, but its use has fallen largely out of favor because of its high daily pill burden, need for twice-daily dosing, and the potential cardiac toxicities.

Tipranavir

Tipranavir, at a dosage of 500 mg twice daily given with 200 mg twice daily of ritonavir, is a salvage option for treatment-experienced patients with documented resistance to one or more PIs. This dosage is a total daily pill burden of 8 pills. Tipranavir is the only PI that requires 400 mg of ritonavir daily to boost its concentrations[48] primarily because of its very low oral bioavailability. In pharmacokinetic studies, 400 mg daily of ritonavir boosted tipranavir trough concentrations by 29-fold compared with unboosted tipranavir. It is highly protein bound (99%) to both albumin and alpha$_1$-acid glycoprotein and metabolized via CYP450 via 3A4 (substrate) and 2D6 (potent inducer). Tipranavir is different from other PIs in that it also induces p-glycoprotein, a major drug transporter, which poses an additional risk for significant drug interactions. Coupled with the higher dose of ritonavir, which also poses its own drug interaction profile, this combination produces unpredictable drug interactions and should be used with caution when given concomitantly with other drugs.

Tipranavir is also associated with rare but serious life-threatening side effects. Cases of clinical hepatitis and fatal hepatic decompensation have been reported.[49] Therefore, extreme caution should be used in patients with hepatitis B or C coinfection. Furthermore, both fatal and nonfatal cases of intracranial hemorrhage have been reported with the use of tipranavir.[49] Caution should be taken when prescribing tipranavir to individuals with medical conditions that may predispose them to intracranial bleed. GI side effects include nausea, vomiting, diarrhea, and abdominal pain and are common, most likely because of the higher dosage of ritonavir used. Rash was also reported in up to 18% of patients in clinical trials accompanied by joint pain, fever, and myalgia. Tipranavir should be discontinued in the event of severe skin rash. Tipranavir contains a sulfonamide moiety; therefore, it should be used with caution in patients with a known sulfa allergy. Boosted tipranavir can be used in select patients, namely, treatment-experienced patients with documented PI resistance but with demonstrated susceptibility to tipranavir. However, the pill burden, tolerability, and toxicity profile preclude its widespread use.

INTEGRASE INHIBITORS

A decade after the introduction of then novel compounds, such as PI and NNRTI, raltegravir was introduced to the US market as the first INSTI with a novel mechanism of action (see **Fig. 1** step 4). Integrase inhibitors block the integrase enzyme from catalyzing the formation of covalent bonds between the host and viral DNA; this in turn prevents the incorporation of viral DNA into the host chromosome. Currently, there are 3 licensed INSTIs (raltegravir, elvitegravir, and dolutegravir) on the US market, each with its own unique characteristics. INSTIs are particularly potent and can rapidly decrease the HIV RNA.[50] INSTIs are generally well tolerated. An antiretroviral therapy regimen consisting of an INSTI + 2-NRTI is now recommended a preferred regimen in treatment naïve patients.[51] Among the INSTIs, only elvitegravir is primarily metabolized by the CYP3A4 system and has the potential for interacting with other drugs using the same metabolic pathway. All the INSTIs may bind to polyvalent cations and, thus, have the potential of interaction with products such as antacids containing magnesium, aluminum, and calcium; separating the dosage administration by several hours can reduce this interaction potential.[52–54] The description of the US FDA indications in HIV-1 infected adults and children, usual dose, formulations, daily pill burden, significant and/or common adverse effects, major drug interactions, primary resistance mutations, and special considerations are summarized in **Table 7**.

Dolutegravir

Dolutegravir is the most recently approved INSTI on the US market. It is recommended to be given at a dosage of 50 mg orally once daily in both treatment-naïve and experienced patients (who do not harbor certain integrase associated mutations).[52] It may be given without regard to meals, but its absorption is increased in the setting of a high-fat meal (area under the curve increased by 61%). It is more than 99% protein bound and primarily metabolized by UGT1A1 and minimally by CYP3A.

When given with drugs that are inducers of UGT1A and CYP3A, including efavirenz, rifampin, boosted fosamprenavir, and tipranavir, dolutegravir should be dosed at a higher dosage of 50 mg twice daily. The 50-mg twice-daily dosage is also recommended in patients with suspected INSTI resistance or with 2 or more of certain INSTI-associated resistance mutations.[52] Dolutegravir is active against some HIV-1 strains that are resistant to elvitegravir and raltegravir, and thus can be a viable option in patients with prior or current virologic failure with elvitegravir or raltegravir containing regimens.[55]

Dolutegravir is generally well tolerated, with headache (2%) and insomnia (3%) being the most common adverse effects reported in clinical trials. Dolutegravir decreases tubular secretion of creatinine, leading to an increase in serum creatinine concentration, without having an effect on glomerular filtration. This serum creatinine increase is often seen within the first 4 weeks of therapy. Dolutegravir has several unique advantages over the available INSTIs, including the tolerability profile and virologic potency in both treatment-naïve and experienced patients (including patients failing elvitegravir- or raltegravir-based regimens) and its low potential for drug interactions. Although it is the newest agent on the market with the least clinical experience, dolutegravir shows promise to be the preferred INSTI for some patients.

Elvitegravir

Elvitegravir is only available within the fixed-dose combination INSTI + NRTI one-pill, once-a-day formulation Stribild. Stribild contains elvitegravir 150 mg, cobicistat 150 mg, emtricitabine 200 mg, and tenofovir 300 mg. Elvitegravir is a substrate of CYP3A4 and requires pharmacokinetic enhancement to increase its systemic exposure. Cobicistat is a new CYP3A4 inhibitor without antiretroviral activity. The absorption of elvitegravir is increased with food. It is highly protein bound (99%) and is metabolized not only by CYP3A but also undergoes glucuronidation via UGT1A1/3.[53]

The drug-interaction profile of this coformulated product elvitegravir/cobicistat/tenofovir/emtricitabine is an important consideration when given with other medications primarily because of the various enzymes and drug transporters that mediate the metabolism of components of this formulation elvitegravir/cobicistat/tenofovir/emtricitabine. Elvitegravir is a substrate of CYP3A4 and UGT1A1/3. Cobicistat, being a potent inhibitor of CYP3A4, a moderate inhibitor of CYP2D6, and an inhibitor of

Table 7
Characteristics of INSTIs

	Dolutegravir (Tivicay)	Elvitegravir	Raltegravir (Isentress)
Abbreviation	DTG	EVG	RAL
US FDA approval year	2013	2012	2007
US FDA indications for HIV-infected adults	ART-naïve and experienced patients	ART-naïve patients	ART-naïve and experienced patients
US FDA indications for HIV-infected children	12 y of age and older	Not recommended for children	4 wk and older
Generic formulation	No	No	No
Usual dose (adult)	50 mg PO once daily or 50 mg PO twice daily for the following situations: • For INSTI-naïve patients given with potent UGT1A1/CYP3A4 inducers[a] or • For INSTI-experienced patients with certain INSTI mutations (see product label) or with clinically suspected INSTI resistance	EVG only available in a coformulated single-tablet regimen with cobicistat/emtricitabine/tenofovir: STRIBILD One tablet once daily Not recommended for patients with CrCl <70 mL/min	400 mg PO twice daily
Adjust dose in renal dysfunction	No	Yes	No
Formulations	Oral tablet: 50 mg	Single tablet: elvitegravir 150 mg/cobicistat 150 mg/emtricitabine 200 mg/tenofovir 300 mg	Oral tablet: 400 mg Chewable tablets: 25 mg, 100 mg
Daily pill burden	1 pill, once-daily administration	1 pill, once-daily administration (full regimen)	2 pills, twice-daily administration

Significant and/or common adverse effects	Insomnia Headache	Nausea Diarrhea Renal impairment (caused by cobicistat and tenofovir)	Rash Nausea Insomnia CPK elevations
Major drug interactions[b]	Mediated mainly by UGT1A1 and to a lesser extent CYP3A: dosage adjustments required when given concomitantly with UGT1A1/CYP3A4 inducers[a] Inhibits tubular secretion of creatinine via inhibition of OCT2: use with dofetilide contraindicated; use metformin with caution Chelation: administration should be separated (2 h) when giving DTG with polyvalent cations containing Mg, Al, Fe, Ca	Mediated mainly by CYP3A and UGT1A1/3 Potent CYP3A4 inhibition (by cobicistat): cautionary use with drugs that are major CYP3A4 substrates Chelation: administration should be separated (2 h) when giving EVG with polyvalent cations containing Mg, Al, Fe, Ca	Mediated mainly by UGT1A1: cautionary use with drugs that induce UGT1A1, including rifamycins Chelation: administration should be avoided when giving RAL with polyvalent cations containing Mg, Al, Fe. Antacids containing calcium carbonate may be given without dosage adjustment
Primary resistance mutations[61]	E138A/K, G140S, Q148	T66A/I, E92G/Q, S147G, Q148R, N155H	Y143C/H/R, Q148H/K/R, N155H
Special considerations		Should be discontinued in patients with a CrCl <50 mL/min while on therapy	

Abbreviations: Al, aluminum; ART, antiretroviral therapy; Ca, calcium; CPK, creatine kinase; CrCl, creatinine clearance; Fe, iron; Mg, magnesium.

[a] Efavirenz, fosamprenavir/ritonavir, tipranavir/ritonavir, or rifampin.

[b] Please refer to http://aidsinfo.nih.gov/guidelines/html/1/adult-and-adolescent-arv-guidelines/32/drug-interactions for a comprehensive list of drug-drug interactions.

multiple drug transporters, including P-gp, BCRP, OATP1B1 and OATP1B3, increases the overall potential for drug interactions.

Toxicities associated with elvitegravir/cobicistat/tenofovir/emtricitabine include those observed with tenofovir therapy, including decreased bone mineral density and renal tubular damage, as well as diarrhea, nausea, and headache. Cobicistat may falsely increase serum creatinine and decrease creatinine clearance by inhibiting the tubular secretion of creatinine. This increase largely occurs early in treatment and does not affect glomerular function. Stribild should only be initiated in patients with an estimated creatinine clearance of 70 mL/min or higher and be promptly discontinued in those whose creatinine clearance decreases less than 50 mL/min while on therapy. The coformulated product of elvitegravir/cobicistat/tenofovir/emtricitabine is currently recommended as a preferred option in treatment-naïve patients.[51] It is available as a one-pill, once-a-day regimen, which is attractive from a medication adherence stand-point. It is relatively well tolerated; however, its potential effects on renal function when given with other renally eliminated medications and the high likelihood for significant drug interactions are some limitations.

Raltegravir

Raltegravir is the first INSTI to be introduced to the market.[54] It was initially studied and approved for use in treatment-experienced patients at a dosage of 400 mg twice daily.[56] It was later studied and approved for use in treatment-naïve patients at the same dosage.[57] The lower potential for drug interactions is attributed to raltegravir being principally metabolized via glucuronidation mediated by UGT1A1 and not via the CYP enzyme system. Its concentrations may increase/decrease if given concomitantly with potent inhibitors or inducers of UGT1A1, such as rifampin. It is excreted into both feces (51%) and urine (32%) as unchanged drug.

Raltegravir is well tolerated, with the most common side effects reported being headache, nausea, and fatigue. There have been case reports of creatinine kinase elevations, rhabdomyolysis, and myopathy in postmarketing surveillance.[50,58] The exact mechanism as to how this occurs is unknown. It is also unclear what predisposes patients to a higher risk of developing these toxicities including factors such as age, sex, duration of raltegravir therapy, or background regimen. Raltegravir should be used with caution in patients who are at an increased risk of rhabdomyolysis or myopathy.

Raltegravir is an attractive option in both treatment-naïve and experienced patients because of its potency and low potential for side effects and drug interactions. With the advent of newer once-daily integrase inhibitors, raltegravir, which requires twice-daily dosing, may be less preferred in patients who prefer a once-daily regimen. Raltegravir remains as a preferred INSTI because of the longer clinical trial and postmarketing experience compared with that of newer-generation INSTIs.[51]

CCR5 ANTAGONIST

Maraviroc is the only CCR5 antagonist approved for use in treatment-naïve or treatment-experienced patients with CCR5-using virus. It selectively binds to the human CCR5 receptor on the cell membrane, thus, blocking the interaction of the HIV gp120 and the CCR5 receptor for CCR5-tropic HIV. However, it does not block the viral entry of CXCR4-tropic HIV or HIV that uses both CCR5 and CXCR4 for cell entry. Before the prescription of maraviroc, viral tropism testing must be performed to confirm that the patient's virus only uses the CCR5 coreceptor.[8,59] As coreceptor usage may change over time of the HIV infection, it should be performed as close to the initiation of maraviroc as possible. Tropism testing should also be done in patients who fail to achieve viral suppression while receiving a maraviroc-based regimen, to assess whether there is a switch from CCR5-using to CXCR4 or dual-mix virus. Maraviroc is a substrate of CYP3A4 but does not cause enzyme induction or inhibition. The usual dosage is 300 mg orally twice daily, but the dosage has to be modified if it is used with a CYP3A4 inhibitor or inducer. Hepatotoxicity (sometimes as a manifestation of a hypersensitivity reaction), upper respiratory tract infections, and fever have

Table 8
Characteristics of CCR5 antagonist and fusion inhibitor

	CCR5 Antagonist	Fusion Inhibitor
Drug name	Maraviroc (Selzentry)	Enfuvirtide (Fuzeon)
Abbreviation	MVC	T-20
US FDA approval year	2007	2003
US FDA indications for HIV-1 infected adults	ART-naïve and ART-experienced patients, with only CCR5-tropic HIV	ART-experienced patients with HIV replication despite ongoing antiretroviral therapy
Approval for HIV-1 infected children	Not approved for children	6 y and older
Generic formulation	No	No
Usual dose (adult)	Usual dosage: 300 mg PO twice daily With potent CYP3A4 inhibitor: 150 mg PO twice daily With potent CYP3A4 inducer: 600 mg PO twice daily	90 mg subcutaneously injection twice daily
Adjust dose in renal insufficiency	Yes	Yes
Formulations (as individual drugs)	Oral tablet: 150 mg, 300 mg	Lyophilized powder for injection: 108 mg per vial
Significant and/or common adverse effects	Hepatoxicity with hypersensitivity reactions, may be in conjunction with severe systemic symptoms, such as fever, rash, eosinophilia Postural hypotension: reported in patients with renal insufficiency	Local injection site reactions (pain, induration, erythema, nodule formation) Hypersensitivity reaction Increased rate of pneumonia in clinical trials
CYP3A4 interaction	CYP3A4 substrate, dosage adjustment needed in patients receiving potent CYP3A4 inhibitor or inducer	None
Special considerations	Viral tropism testing should be done before initiation of maraviroc; can only be performed if HIV RNA is >1000 copies per milliliter Maraviroc should not be used if patients with CXCR4 using HIV-1 or with dual/mixed receptor usage Tropism DNA assay may be useful in patients with HIV RNA <1000 copies per milliliter	

Abbreviation: ART, antiretroviral therapy.

been reported in the clinical trials. Orthostatic hypotension has been reported, especially in patients with renal impairment. Because of the need for obtaining an expensive tropism testing before initiation, the drug interaction potential, and twice-daily dosing, maraviroc is not commonly used in clinical practice (**Table 8**).

FUSION INHIBITOR

The fusion inhibitor enfuvirtide interferes with this fusion process by binding to the first heptad-repeat (HR1) in the viral envelope glycoprotein gp41, thus, preventing conformational changes necessary for the fusion of the viral and cellular membrane.[60] Because of its unique mechanism of action, there is no cross resistance with other antiretroviral drugs; thus, most patients who have not received enfuvirtide have found virologic benefit when enfuvirtide is added as part of a salvage regimen in patients with multiple drug class resistance. Enfuvirtide is only available in an injectable formulation and needs to be given as a subcutaneous injection twice daily. Almost all patients experience some degree of injection-site reaction, manifested as pain, erythema, induration, nodules, ecchymoses. Because of the profound loss of subcutaneous fat in some HIV-infected patients, some have found it difficult to locate and rotate the injection sites. Hypersensitivity reactions have also been reported. An increase in incidence of pneumonia was observed in clinical trials in subjects who received enfuvirtide, although the mechanism of this association is not known. Because of the need of a twice-daily injection, enfuvirtide is generally reserved for patients with multiple drug resistance whereby at least 2 or 3 orally active agents cannot be used (see **Table 8**).

SUMMARY

The advances in antiretroviral drug development have dramatically changed the face of HIV infection worldwide from a deadly disease to a manageable chronic condition. Currently available antiretroviral drugs have greater potency, tolerability, and less pill burden than earlier agents. Understanding the potency of the drugs and drug regimens, toxicity profile, drug interaction potential, and resistance potential will help clinicians select a regimen most suitable for a specific patient.

REFERENCES

1. Fischl MA, Richman DD, Grieco MH, et al. The efficacy of azidothymidine (AZT) in the treatment of patients with AIDS and AIDS-related complex. A double-blind, placebo-controlled trial. N Engl J Med 1987;317:185–91.
2. Lederman MM, Connick E, Landay A, et al. Immunologic responses associated with 12 weeks of combination antiretroviral therapy consisting of zidovudine, lamivudine, and ritonavir: results of AIDS clinical trials group protocol 315. J Infect Dis 1998;178:70–9.
3. Cattelan AM, Calabro ML, Gasperini P, et al. Acquired immunodeficiency syndrome-related Kaposi's sarcoma regression after highly active antiretroviral therapy: biologic correlates of clinical outcome. J Natl Cancer Inst Monogr 2001;28:44–9.
4. De Luca A, Giancola ML, Ammassari A, et al. The effect of potent antiretroviral therapy and JC virus load in cerebrospinal fluid on clinical outcome of patients with AIDS-associated progressive multifocal leukoencephalopathy. The Journal of infectious diseases 2000;182:1077–83.

5. Palella FJ Jr, Delaney KM, Moorman AC, et al. Declining morbidity and mortality among patients with advanced human immunodeficiency virus infection. HIV Outpatient Study Investigators. N Engl J Med 1998;338:853–60.

6. Davey RT Jr, Bhat N, Yoder C, et al. HIV-1 and T cell dynamics after interruption of highly active antiretroviral therapy (HAART) in patients with a history of sustained viral suppression. Proc Natl Acad Sci U S A 1999;96:15109–14.

7. HIV replication cycle. 2012. Available at: http://www.niaid.nih.gov/topics/HIV AIDS/Understanding/Biology/pages/hivreplicationcycle.aspx. Accessed March 10, 2014.

8. Panel on Antiretroviral Guidelines for Adults and Adolescents. Guidelines for the use of antiretroviral agents in HIV-1-infected adults and adolescents. Department of Health and Human Services. 2013. Available at: http://aidsinfo.nih.gov/contentfiles/lvguidelines/AdultandAdolescentGL.pdf. Accessed March 10, 2014.

9. Nolan D, Mallal S. Complications associated with NRTI therapy: update on clinical features and possible pathogenic mechanisms. Antivir Ther 2004;9:849–63.

10. Moyle G. Mechanisms of HIV and nucleoside reverse transcriptase inhibitor injury to mitochondria. Antivir Ther 2005;10(Suppl 2):M47–52.

11. Food and Drug Administration. Ziagen (product label). 2013. Available at: http://www.accessdata.fda.gov/drugsatfda_docs/label/2013/020977s026,020978s030lbl.pdf. Accessed March 10, 2014.

12. Gulick RM, Ribaudo HJ, Shikuma CM, et al. Triple-nucleoside regimens versus efavirenz-containing regimens for the initial treatment of HIV-1 infection. N Engl J Med 2004;350:1850–61.

13. Hetherington S, McGuirk S, Powell G, et al. Hypersensitivity reactions during therapy with the nucleoside reverse transcriptase inhibitor abacavir. Clin Ther 2001;23:1603–14.

14. Frissen PH, de Vries J, Weigel HM, et al. Severe anaphylactic shock after rechallenge with abacavir without preceding hypersensitivity. AIDS 2001;15:289.

15. Walensky RP, Goldberg JH, Daily JP. Anaphylaxis after rechallenge with abacavir. AIDS 1999;13:999–1000.

16. Mallal S, Phillips E, Carosi G, et al. HLA-B*5701 screening for hypersensitivity to abacavir. N Engl J Med 2008;358:568–79.

17. Saag M, Balu R, Phillips E, et al. High sensitivity of human leukocyte antigen-b*5701 as a marker for immunologically confirmed abacavir hypersensitivity in white and black patients. Clin Infect Dis 2008;46:1111–8.

18. Sabin CA, Worm SW, Weber R, et al. Use of nucleoside reverse transcriptase inhibitors and risk of myocardial infarction in HIV-infected patients enrolled in the D:A:D study: a multi-cohort collaboration. Lancet 2008;371:1417–26.

19. Ding X, Andraca-Carrera E, Cooper C, et al. No association of abacavir use with myocardial infarction: findings of an FDA meta-analysis. J Acquir Immune Defic Syndr 2012;61:441–7.

20. Ofotokun I, Smithson SE, Lu C, et al. Liver enzymes elevation and immune reconstitution among treatment-naive HIV-infected patients instituting antiretroviral therapy. Am J Med Sci 2007;334:334–41.

21. Bellini C, Keiser O, Chave JP, et al. Liver enzyme elevation after lamivudine withdrawal in HIV-hepatitis B virus co-infected patients: the Swiss HIV cohort study. HIV Med 2009;10:12–8.

22. Food and Drug Administration. Truvada (product label). 2013. Available at: http://www.accessdata.fda.gov/drugsatfda_docs/label/2013/021752s043lbl.pdf. Accessed March 10, 2014.

23. Hall AM, Hendry BM, Nitsch D, et al. Tenofovir-associated kidney toxicity in HIV-infected patients: a review of the evidence. Am J Kidney Dis 2011;57: 773–80.

24. Morlat P, Vivot A, Vandenhende MA, et al. Role of traditional risk factors and antiretroviral drugs in the incidence of chronic kidney disease, ANRS CO3 Aquitaine cohort, France, 2004-2012. PLos One 2013;8:e66223.

25. Kalayjian RC, Lau B, Mechekano RN, et al. Risk factors for chronic kidney disease in a large cohort of HIV-1 infected individuals initiating antiretroviral therapy in routine care. AIDS 2012;26:1907–15.

26. Huang JS, Hughes MD, Riddler SA, et al. Bone mineral density effects of randomized regimen and nucleoside reverse transcriptase inhibitor selection from ACTG A5142. HIV Clin Trials 2013;14:224–34.

27. Havens PL, Kiser JJ, Stephensen CB, et al. Association of higher plasma vitamin d binding protein and lower free calcitriol levels with tenofovir disoproxil fumarate use and plasma and intracellular tenofovir pharmacokinetics: cause of a functional vitamin D deficiency? Antimicrob Agents Chemother 2013;57: 5619–28.

28. Perrot S, Aslangul E, Szwebel T, et al. Bone pain due to fractures revealing osteomalacia related to tenofovir-induced proximal renal tubular dysfunction in a human immunodeficiency virus-infected patient. J Clin Rheumatol 2009;15: 72–4.

29. Haverkort ME, van der Spek BW, Lips P, et al. Tenofovir-induced Fanconi syndrome and osteomalacia in two HIV-infected patients: role of intracellular tenofovir diphosphate levels and review of the literature. Scand J Infect Dis 2011;43: 821–6.

30. Connor EM, Sperling RS, Gelber R, et al. Reduction of maternal-infant transmission of human immunodeficiency virus type 1 with zidovudine treatment. Pediatric AIDS clinical trials group protocol 076 study group. N Engl J Med 1994;331: 1173–80.

31. Food and Drug Administration. Sustiva (product label). 2013. Available at: http://www.accessdata.fda.gov/drugsatfda_docs/label/2013/020972s043021360s031 lbl.pdf. Accessed March 10, 2014.

32. Mollan K, Smurzynski M, Na L, et al. Hazard of suicidality in patients randomly assigned to efavirenz for initial treatment of HIV-1: a cross study analysis conducted by the AIDS Clinical Trials Group (ACTG). Abs #670. ID week 2013. San Francisco (CA): 2013. PMID: 24979445.

33. Panel on Treatment of HIV-Infected Pregnant Women and Prevention of Perinatal Transmission. Recommendations for use of antiretroviral drugs in pregnant HIV-1-infected women for maternal health and interventions to reduce perinatal HIV transmission in the United States. 2012. Available at: http://aidsinfo.nih.gov/contentfiles/lvguidelines/PerinatalGL.pdf. Accessed March 10, 2014.

34. World Health Organization. Consolidated guidelines on the use of antiretroviral drugs for treating and preventing HIV infection. Recommendations for a public health approach. 2013. Available at: http://www.who.int/entity/hiv/pub/guidelines/arv2013/download/en/index.html. Accessed March 10, 2014.

35. Food and Drug Administration. Intelence (product label). 2013. Available at: http://www.accessdata.fda.gov/drugsatfda_docs/label/2013/022187s011s012s 014lbl.pdf. Accessed March 10, 2014.

36. Asahchop EL, Wainberg MA, Oliveira M, et al. Distinct resistance patterns to etravirine and rilpivirine in viruses containing nonnucleoside reverse transcriptase inhibitor mutations at baseline. AIDS 2013;27:879–87.

37. Food and Drug Administration. Viramune (product label). 2014. Available at: http://www.accessdata.fda.gov/drugsatfda_docs/label/2014/020636s044,0209 33s035lbl.pdf. Accessed March 10, 2014.

38. Food and Drug Administration. Edurant (product label). 2013. Available at: http://www.accessdata.fda.gov/drugsatfda_docs/label/2013/202022s005lbl.pdf. Accessed March 10, 2014.

39. Nelson MR, Elion RA, Cohen CJ, et al. Rilpivirine versus efavirenz in HIV-1-infected subjects receiving emtricitabine/tenofovir DF: pooled 96-week data from ECHO and THRIVE Studies. HIV Clin Trials 2013;14:81–91.

40. Food and Drug Administration. Reyataz (product label). 2013. Available at: http://www.accessdata.fda.gov/drugsatfda_docs/label/2013/021567s032s033 lbl.pdf. Accessed March 10, 2014.

41. Nishijima T, Shimbo T, Komatsu H, et al. Cumulative exposure to ritonavir-boosted atazanavir is associated with cholelithiasis in patients with HIV-1 infection. J Antimicrob Chemother 2014;69(5):1385–9.

42. Rockwood N, Mandalia S, Bower M, et al. Ritonavir-boosted atazanavir exposure is associated with an increased rate of renal stones compared with efavirenz, ritonavir-boosted lopinavir and ritonavir-boosted darunavir. AIDS 2011;25: 1671–3.

43. Food and Drug Administration. Prezista (product label). 2013. Available at: http://www.accessdata.fda.gov/drugsatfda_docs/label/2013/021976s033_2028 95s010lbl.pdf. Accessed March 10, 2014.

44. Orkin C, DeJesus E, Khanlou H, et al. Final 192-week efficacy and safety of once-daily darunavir/ritonavir compared with lopinavir/ritonavir in HIV-1-infected treatment-naive patients in the ARTEMIS trial. HIV Med 2013;14: 49–59.

45. Food and Drug Administration. Kaletra (product label). 2013. Available at: http://www.accessdata.fda.gov/drugsatfda_docs/label/2013/021226s038lbl.pdf. Accessed March 10, 2014.

46. Food and Drug Administration. Invirase (product label). 2012. Available at: http://www.accessdata.fda.gov/drugsatfda_docs/label/2012/020628s034-0217 85s011lbl.pdf. Accessed March 10, 2014

47. Zhang X, Jordan P, Cristea L, et al. Thorough QT/QTc study of ritonavir-boosted saquinavir following multiple-dose administration of therapeutic and supratherapeutic doses in healthy participants. J Clin Pharmacol 2012;52:520–9.

48. Food and Drug Administration. Aptivus (product label). 2012. Available at: http://www.accessdata.fda.gov/drugsatfda_docs/label/2012/021814s013,0222 92s006lbl.pdf. Accessed March 10, 2014.

49. Chan-Tack KM, Struble KA, Birnkrant DB. Intracranial hemorrhage and liver-associated deaths associated with tipranavir/ritonavir: review of cases from the FDA's Adverse Event Reporting System. AIDS Patient Care STDs 2008;22: 843–50.

50. Hicks C, Gulick RM. Raltegravir: the first HIV type 1 integrase inhibitor. Clin Infect Dis 2009;48:931–9.

51. HHS Panel on Antiretroviral Guidelines for Adults and Adolescents. Recommendation on integrase inhibitor use in antiretroviral treatment-naive HIV-infected individuals. 2013. Available at: http://aidsinfo.nih.gov/contentfiles/upload/Adult ARV_INSTIRecommendations.pdf. Accessed March 10, 2014.

52. Food and Drug Administration. Tivicay (product label). 2013. Available at: http://www.accessdata.fda.gov/drugsatfda_docs/label/2013/204790lbl.pdf. Accessed March 10, 2014.

53. Food and Drug Administration. Stribild (product label). 2013. Available at: http://www.accessdata.fda.gov/drugsatfda_docs/label/2013/203100s009lbl.pdf. Accessed March 10, 2014.

54. Food and Drug Administration. Isentress (product label). 2013. Available at: http://www.accessdata.fda.gov/drugsatfda_docs/label/2013/205786s000,022145s031,203045s009lbl.pdf. Accessed March 10, 2014.

55. Castagna A, Maggiolo F, Penco G, et al. Dolutegravir in antiretroviral-experienced patients with raltegravir- and/or elvitegravir-resistant HIV-1: 24-week results of the phase III VIKING-3 Study. J Infect Dis 2014. [Epub ahead of print].

56. Steigbigel RT, Cooper DA, Kumar PN, et al. Raltegravir with optimized background therapy for resistant HIV-1 infection. N Engl J Med 2008;359:339–54.

57. Lennox JL, Dejesus E, Berger DS, et al. Raltegravir versus efavirenz regimens in treatment-naive HIV-1-infected patients: 96-week efficacy, durability, subgroup, safety, and metabolic analyses. J Acquir Immune Defic Syndr 2010;55:39–48.

58. Lee FJ, Amin J, Bloch M, et al. Skeletal muscle toxicity associated with raltegravir-based combination antiretroviral therapy in HIV-infected adults. J Acquir Immune Defic Syndr 2013;62:525–33.

59. Food and Drug Administration. Selzentry (product label). 2013. Available at: http://www.accessdata.fda.gov/drugsatfda_docs/label/2013/022128s011lbl.pdf. Accessed March 10, 2014.

60. Food and Drug Administration. Fuzeon (product label). 2013. Available at: http://www.accessdata.fda.gov/drugsatfda_docs/label/2013/021481s027lbl.pdf. Accessed March 10, 2014.

61. Johnson VA, Calvez V, Gunthard HF, et al. Update of the drug resistance mutations in HIV-1: March 2013. Top Antivir Med 2013;21:6–14.

Antiretroviral Therapy
When to Start

Christopher J. Sellers, MD, David A. Wohl, MD*

KEYWORDS

- Human immunodeficiency virus • Antiretroviral • Initiation • CD4 • Start • Timing
- Therapy

KEY POINTS

- Despite incomplete and in some cases conflicting cohort data regarding the mortality benefit to ART at CD4+ cell counts higher than 500/mm^3, there is evidence to reasonably suggest the existence of harm with untreated HIV, even at high CD4+ cell counts.
- In the absence of evidence of significant harm due to early ART initiation, there are clear reasons to recommend initiation of ART at any CD4 count.

INTRODUCTION

The development of effective antiretroviral therapy (ART) in response to the emerging epidemic of human immunodeficiency virus (HIV) ranks as one of the most remarkable achievements of modern medicine. However, it was not long after the first of these medications became available that the issue of when is the optimal time in the disease course to use these agents was raised: a question that continues to be asked today. The answer, framed in terms of a balance between the potential benefits of therapy and its risks and costs, has evolved along with HIV therapy and our understanding of its benefits and disadvantages.

At lower CD4+ cell counts, there is irrefutable evidence that the benefits of ART outweigh the harms. For individuals with less advanced infection, the balance between the hazards of unchecked viral replication and the possibility of long-term drug toxicities, development of drug resistance, and expense of treatment of many years seemed to favor delaying HIV therapy. As the potency, tolerability, and

Disclosures: C.J. Sellers has no disclosures. D.A. Wohl has served on advisory boards for Gilead and Janssen and payments to the University of North Carolina have been made by Merck, ViiV, and Gilead to fund research he has led.
Support: Dr C.J. Sellers supported by NIH/NIAID Training in Infectious Disease Epidemiology Grant (National Institutes of Health 5T32AI070114-08).
Division of Infectious Diseases, School of Medicine, University of North Carolina, 130 Mason Farm Road, CB# 7030, Chapel Hill, NC 27599-7030, USA
* Corresponding author.
E-mail address: david_wohl@med.unc.edu

convenience of ART regimens have improved and the deleterious effects of even moderate CD4+ cell depletion have been shown, the calculus of ART initiation has shifted, and the rationale for deferring therapy until a specific CD4+ count threshold has become vulnerable to challenge. However, the evidence supporting the initiation of ART at high CD4+ counts is less robust than that available for those with lower counts, and within this data vacuum, controversy has emerged.

In this article, current expert panels' recommendations on when to start ART are reviewed, and the strengths and weaknesses are discussed of the rationale to treat earlier rather than later in the course of HIV infection.

HIV TREATMENT GUIDELINES

Current recommendations by both major US HIV treatment guideline panels, the Department of Health and Human Services (DHHS) and the International Antiviral Society-USA (IAS-USA), call for the initiation of ART in practically all patients with HIV infection willing and able to take these medications. This position abandons any deferral of treatment until a set CD4+ cell count threshold (a substantial departure from earlier recommendations to hold ART until immunosuppression became evident). The history of the evolution of the guidelines from advocating a cautious application of ART to a near universal approach to HIV therapy is also a history of the evolution of HIV therapeutics and our use of these medications (**Fig. 1**).

The first edition of the DHHS guidelines, published in 1998, recommended ART initiation for asymptomatic individuals with CD4+ counts up to 500 cells/mm^3, underscoring the urgency at the time of what was a dire public health emergency.[1] However, the only therapeutic option available at that time, zidovudine, has low potency and high-level toxicity. With data from the CONCORDE study, a large trial of high-dose zidovudine monotherapy in those with earlier versus more advanced HIV disease, showing no survival or disease progression benefit of this nucleoside,[2] the guidelines downshifted to a more stringent CD4+ count threshold for ART initiation

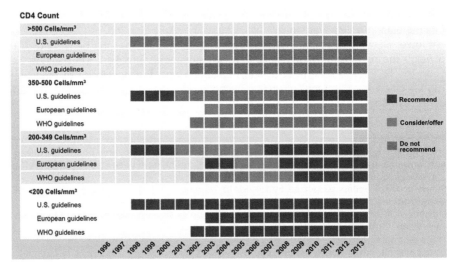

Fig. 1. Evolution of CD4+ count criteria for starting ART in asymptomatic persons with HIV infection, according to different guidelines. (*From* De Cock KM, El-Sadr WM. When to start ART in Africa–an urgent research priority. N Engl J Med 2013;368:887; with permission.)

of less than 200 cells/mm^3.[2,3] For years, a count of 200/mm^3 stood as a tipping point at which the benefits of therapy started to outweigh its liabilities. As ART became more effective, durable, and tolerable, this line in the sand began to move. In 2007, the CD4+ cell count criterion at which ART initiation was recommended began a steady increase in both the DHHS[4] and the IAS-USA guidelines, increasing to 350 cells/mm^3 after observational cohorts reported an association between deferral of ART until counts less than 200 cells/mm^3 and a heightened risk of opportunistic conditions and death.[5–7] Subsequent guideline revisions have seen the initiation of ART grow more inclusive, extending to those with counts of 500 cells/mm^3 or less in 2009[8] and in 2012 to include all CD4+ counts (a recommendation based on many different lines of evidence, as discussed later).[9]

The latest DHHS guidelines in explaining the use of ART for all patients infected with patients regardless of CD4+ count make clear that the strength of the recommendation increases with decreasing CD4+ cell counts (**Table 1**).[10] In addition, these guidelines introduce the use of ART in individuals infected with HIV to prevent transmission after the announcement of findings from a large randomized clinical trial reporting the efficacy of ART as prevention.[11] The guidelines advise that "Patients starting ART should be willing and able to commit to treatment and understand the benefits and risks of therapy and the importance of adherence."

As detailed later, several conditions are also specified in the DHHS and IAS-USA guidelines as favoring more rapid or urgent initiation of ART (**Box 1**).[10] AIDS-defining conditions have long been recognized as an indication for prompt ART initiation, and joining them are comorbidities, such as coinfection with hepatitis B and hepatitis C and HIV-associated nephropathy (HIVAN), as well as pregnancy, high viral load, and acute HIV infection.

The current US guidelines differ significantly from those from outside the United States, including those issued by the World Health Organization (WHO), and the British

Table 1	
2014 DHHS guidelines on initiation of ART in treatment-naive patients	
Indication	**Recommendation Rating[a]**
Pretreatment CD4+ count (cells/mm^3)	
<350	AI
350–500	AII
>500	BIII
To prevent:	
Perinatal transmission	AI
Heterosexual transmission	AI
Other transmission risk group	AIII

ART is recommended for all HIV-infected individuals to reduce the risk of disease progression.

[a] Rating scheme

Strength of recommendation: A, strong recommendation for the statement; B, moderate recommendation for the statement; C, optional recommendation for the statement I: one or more randomized trials with clinical outcomes.

Evidence of recommendation: I, one or more randomized trials with clinical outcomes or validated laboratory end points; II, one or more well-designed, nonrandomized trials or observational cohort studies with long-term clinical outcomes; III, expert opinion.

From Panel on Antiretroviral Guidelines for Adults and Adolescents. Guidelines for the use of antiretroviral agents in HIV-1-infected adults and adolescents. Department of Health and Human Services. Available at: http://aidsinfo.nih.gov/contentfiles/lvguidelines/AdultandAdolescentGL.pdf. Accessed July 1, 2014.

Box 1
2014 DHHS guidelines: conditions favoring more rapid ART initiation

Pregnancy (AI[a])

AIDS-defining conditions (AI)

Acute opportunistic infections[b]

Lower CD4+ counts (eg, <200 cells/mm^3) (AI)

HIVAN (AII)

Acute/early infection (BII)

HIV/hepatitis B virus coinfection (AII)

HIV/hepatitis C virus coinfection (BII)

Rapidly declining CD4+ counts (eg, 100 cells/mm^3 decrease per year) (AIII)

Higher viral loads (eg, >100,000 copies/mL) (BII)

[a] Rating scheme
Strength of recommendation: A, strong recommendation for the statement; B, moderate recommendation for the statement; C, optional recommendation for the statement I: one or more randomized trials with clinical outcomes.
Evidence of recommendation: I, one or more randomized trials with clinical outcomes or validated laboratory end points; II, one or more well-designed, nonrandomized trials or observational cohort studies with long-term clinical outcomes; III, expert opinion.

[b] Recommendation rating varies by specific pathogen and OI disease site. See article elsewhere in this issue for details.
From Panel on Antiretroviral Guidelines for Adults and Adolescents. Guidelines for the use of antiretroviral agents in HIV-1-infected adults and adolescents. Department of Health and Human Services. Available at: http://aidsinfo.nih.gov/contentfiles/lvguidelines/AdultandAdolescentGL. pdf. Accessed July 1, 2014.

---

and European guidelines on the timing of ART (see **Fig. 1**). The 2013 British HIV Association guidelines recommend ART initiation at a CD4+ cell count of 350 cells/mm^3 or lower in asymptomatic individuals without relevant comorbidities but suggest offering ART to patients at higher CD4+ cell counts who wish to reduce their risk of transmission to others.[12] Likewise, the European AIDS Clinical Society guidelines also published in 2013 recommend ART initiation at CD4+ counts less than 350 cells/mm^3 and for those with a CD4+ count greater than 350 cells/mm^3, ART can be considered, particularly to reduce infectiousness.[13] The most recent WHO guidelines recommend ART initiation at CD4+ count of 500 cells/mm^3 or lower, prioritizing those with CD4+ counts of 350 cells/mm^3 or lower.[14] In contrast, 2013 French guidelines recommend ART initiation regardless of CD4+ count.[15] The differences between these guidelines are a reflection of several considerations, including interpretation of the data regarding the benefits of ART earlier in the HIV disease course as well as regional availability and affordability of ART.

EVIDENCE INFORMING THE QUESTION OF WHEN TO START ART

The gradual creep in the CD4+ cell count threshold for ART initiation reflects an increasing body of data indicating that even modest degrees of immunosuppression and ongoing viral replication carry significant risks to health. However, the strength of any association between adverse outcomes and CD4+ cell count wanes when it comes to the benefits of ART in those with normal or near normal counts. Large randomized trials of ART initiation at such high CD4+ cell counts (ie, >500 cells/mm^3) have not been conducted. A multinational trial comparing immediate ART versus deferral of treatment until declines in CD4+ cell count to less than 350 cells/mm^3 is ongoing but may face some limitations in fully addressing the essential question of when to start ART if those referred to the study, by virtue of entry viral load or other characteristics, are at low risk for disease progression.[16] Therefore, support for the use of ART earlier in the HIV disease course relies on data from alternative sources, including observational cohort studies, other types of ART trials, and pathogenesis studies.

Observational Data

Several large HIV cohorts have reported a benefit of modern ART initiated at CD4+ counts between 350 cells/mm^3 and 500 cells/mm^3 in terms of decreased progression to AIDS[17–19] and lower rates of death.[20] For example, analyses from both MACS (Multicenter AIDS Cohort Study) and WHIS (Women's Interagency HIV Study) reported that individuals initiating ART at CD4+ cell counts higher than 350 cells/mm^3 have a nearly identical hazard of non-AIDS death as HIV-uninfected individuals (hazard ratio [HR] of 1.01), whereas HIV-positive individuals initiating at CD4+ cell counts 201 to 350 cells/mm^3 and lower than 200 cells/mm^3 have HRs of 1.66 and 2.15, respectively, compared with HIV-positive early initiators of ART.[21]

Investigations of the potential mortality and HIV disease progression benefits of ART initiation at CD4+ counts higher than 500 cells/mm^3 have been addressed in large cohort studies, producing mixed results and provoking much discussion (**Table 2**). Analyses of data from 2 cohorts, the European ART-CC (ART Cohort Collaboration) and HIV-CAUSAL (HIV Cohorts Analyzed Using Structural Approaches to Longitudinal) data,[18,19] did not show a significant difference in all-cause mortality using an ART

Table 2
Results of major prospective cohort studies on the timing of ART initiation[a]

Outcome and CD4+ Threshold	NA-ACCORD[20]	HIV-CAUSAL[19]	ART-CC[18]
All-cause mortality			
CD4+ 450 or 500	Yes[b] RR 1.94 (1.37, 2.79)	No HR 1.03 (0.92–1.14)[b]	No HR 0.93 (0.60, 1.44)
CD4+ 350	Yes RR 1.69 (1.26, 2.26)	No HR 1.01 (0.84, 1.22)	No HR 1.13 (0.80, 1.60)
CD4+ 200		Yes HR 1.20 (0.97, 1.48)	Yes HR 1.34 (1.05, 1.71)
AIDS-defining illness or death			
CD4+ 450		Yes 1.14 (1.07, 1.22)	No HR 0.99 (0.76, 1.29)
CD4+ 350		Yes HR 1.38 (1.23, 1.56)	Yes HR 1.28 (1.04, 1.57)
CD4+ 200		Yes HR 1.90 (1.67, 2.15)	Yes HR 2.21 (1.91, 2.56)

Abbreviation: RR, relative risk.
[a] The CASCADE study examined the hazards associated with ART delay vs initiation, stratified by CD4+ count using a different statistical methodology and reference standard. Results showed benefit to immediate initiation at CD4+ count <500/mm^3 but not >500/mm^3.[22]
[b] CD4+ threshold of 500/mm^3 used in NA-ACCORD, 450/mm^3 used in HIV-CAUSAL and ART-CC.

initiation threshold of 450 cells/mm³, although both found benefits when death and progression to AIDS were used as a combined end point. In stark contrast, NA-ACCORD (North American AIDS Cohort Collaboration on Research and Design)[20] reported significantly lower adjusted mortality in those who initiate ART higher than a count of 500/mm³. The CASCADE (Concerted Action on Sero-Conversion to AIDS and Death in Europe) cohort[22] showed slower disease progression when initiating ART at CD4+ thresholds of 500 and lower, but did not report benefit to starting at counts of 500 to 799/mm³. Differences in populations, study design, and analysis techniques can be implicated to account for these discrepant results.

Other observational studies have explored the relationship between CD4+ cell count and well-being. An analysis of more than 200,000 individuals enrolled in the COHERE (Collaboration of Observational HIV Epidemiological Research Europe) study[23] examined the incidence of the 18 most common AIDS-defining illnesses across the CD4+ cell count spectrum, ranging from 200/mm³ to greater than 1000/mm³. As expected, the incidence rates of AIDS-defining illnesses were highest in those with lower CD4+ cell counts of 200 to 349/mm³, with the rate of new AIDS-defining illnesses decreasing as the CD4+ cell count examined increased. However, even at the higher CD4+ cell counts, when in smaller studies, such associations often become tenuous, those with a current CD4+ cell count of 750 to 999 cells/mm³ had a significantly higher rate of new AIDS-defining conditions compared with those with counts of 500 to 749 cells/mm³ (adjusted incidence rate ratio, 1.20 [95% confidence interval [CI], 1.10–1.32], $P<.0001$). The incidence of these conditions among those with current CD4+ counts of greater than 1000 cells/mm³ was not significantly different from those with counts of 750 to 999 cells/mm³. The relationship between CD4+ cell count and disease development was stronger for malignant than nonmalignant conditions. The investigators' conclusion that persons with HIV infection are not fully immune reconstituted until the CD4+ count increases to greater than 750 cells/mm³, although expressly not intended to address the question of when to start ART, does suggest that avoidance of even modest levels of immunosuppression can be expected to be beneficial in terms of protection from AIDS-defining conditions, including certain cancers.

Studies of cardiovascular, neurocognitive, and bone health in persons living with HIV also show a link between end-organ damage and reduction of the CD4+ cell count pool. Most have been consistent in identifying nadir (lowest) CD4+ cell count as a marker of increased risk for disease. In a large cohort of patients enrolled in the Kaiser Permanente managed care system in California,[24] lower CD4+ count nadir was associated with a significantly increased incidence of myocardial infarction (MI); those with counts that never decreased lower than 500 cells/mm³ had rates of MI that were similar to patients without HIV infection. Investigators from the CNICS (Centers for AIDS Research Network of Integrated Clinical Systems) study,[25] a US multiclinic cohort, presented similar findings of a relationship between CD4+ cell count and cardiovascular disease, especially when the presence of viremia was considered. Those with a recent CD4+ cell count of greater than 500/mm³ had an increased risk of MI when virus was not controlled compared with those with similar counts and undetectable viremia after adjustment for age, sex, tobacco, injection drug use, diabetes, male sex as HIV risk factor, statin use, treated hypertension, renal function, and ART.

Data from the CHARTER (CNS HIV Anti-Retroviral Therapy Effects Research) cohort, a longitudinal study of the neurocognition HIV-infected persons, found an association between nadir CD4+ cell count and cognitive impairment.[26] A greater prevalence of impairment was observed among those with nadir counts lower than 500 cells/mm³ compared with those with lower nadir counts; there were too few participants with counts higher than 500/mm^3 to examine trends among those with higher CD4+ cell count. Likewise, studies of bone density also point to deleterious effects of CD4+ cell count depletion on skeletal health, including fracture risk.[27,28]

Observations of an association between abnormal CD4+ cell counts and adverse outcomes are concerning given findings of an attenuated immunologic response to HIV therapy in those initiating ART at lower CD4+ cell counts (**Fig. 2**). Slower and truncated gains in CD4+ cells over time were evident in a recently presented study of more than 1300 participants in HOPS (HIV Outpatient Study) in the United States.[29] In this analysis, the likelihood of achieving a CD4+ cell count higher than 750/mm^3 (the level higher than which the COHERE study suggests is protective against AIDS-defining illnesses) by 4 years after initiation of ART increased with each higher stratum of CD4+ cell count at the start of therapy, ranging from 4.3% for those with nadir CD4+ counts lower than 50/mm^3 to 83.6% for those with counts higher than 500/mm^3. However, only 65.8% of those with counts 350 to 499 achieved immune reconstitution, as indicated by a CD4+ cell count of 750/mm^3 or greater.

Observational studies have their inherent limitations. Unmeasured confounding, channeling bias, limited numbers of outcomes of interest in those at higher CD4+ cell counts, and other issues can challenge confidence in the conclusions reached. Although the association between undesired outcomes and lower CD4+ cell counts has been strong and is convincing, these limitations and the mixed findings from the larger cohort studies regarding the benefits of ART at high CD4+ cell counts fuel the ongoing debate of when to start ART.

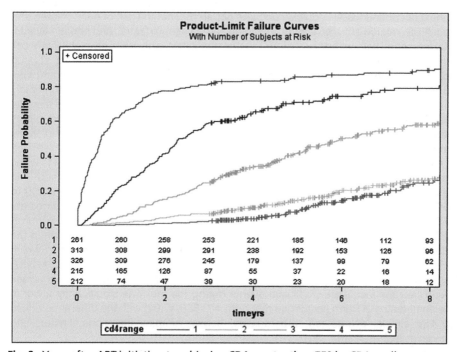

Fig. 2. Years after ART initiation to achieving CD4 greater than 750 by CD4+ cell count stratum at ART initiation: HOPS Cohort 1996-2012 (N = 1327). (*From* Palella F, Armon C, Chmiel J, et al. Higher CD4 at ART initiation predicts greater long term likelihood of CD4 normalization. Presented at the 21th Conference on Retroviruses and Opportunistic Infections. Poster 560. Boston, March 3–6, 2014; with permission.)

Clinical Trials

Given the shortcomings of observational data, well-designed randomized clinical trials are looked at to guide standards of care. Although the results of a trial directly comparing the initiation of ART at counts that are nearer to normal versus more profoundly depleted does not exist, examination of trials of when to start at lower counts have been used to support a strategy of early HIV therapy. The CIPRA (Comprehensive International Program of Research on AIDS) study HT 01[30] was a randomized controlled trial of immediate ART versus deferral of ART until the CD4+ count decreased lower than 200 cells/mm^3 in patients in Haiti with baseline CD4+ counts between 200 cells/mm^3 and 350 cells/mm^3. This trial found higher rates of death (23 vs 6 deaths; HR = 4.0; 95% CI: 1.6–9.8) and tuberculosis (HR = 2.0, 95% CI: 1.2–3.6) in those who deferred ART compared with those randomized to immediate ART initiation. Although far from addressing the timing of ART for those with higher CD4+ cell counts, the trial reported a striking benefit of HIV therapy that many believe extends to higher counts.

The SMART (Strategies for Management of Antiretroviral Therapy) trial[5,31] was not designed to address the timing of the initiation of ART but has been important in understanding the potential hazards of uncontrolled HIV infection. This study randomized 5472 patients with baseline CD4+ counts higher than 350 cells/mm^3 (median CD4+ cell count at baseline was 597 cells/mm^3) to continuous ART or to a strategy of CD4+ cell count guided ART interruption, wherein treatment was stopped, restarted when counts decreased lower than 250 cells/mm^3, and then withdrawn again when counts rebounded more than 350 cells/mm^3. The trial was halted early after a survival benefit of continuous ART quickly became apparent. That the risk of AIDS-related and non-AIDS–related adverse events, including cardiovascular, renal, and hepatic events, was increased with withdrawal of ART in this population with relatively high CD4+ cell counts has been interpreted to suggest a benefit of starting HIV treatment at such counts. A subgroup analysis of the 249 participants (median CD4+ cell count was 437 cells/mm^3) who were ART-naive at entry and randomized to start ART immediately of defer ART until counts reached 250 cells/mm^3 looked at this question more directly. Although uncommon, the rate of serious AIDS-related and non-AIDS–related events was higher among the arm randomized to defer ART initiation than among those who started ART immediately (7 vs 2 events, HR: 4.6; 95% CI: 1.0–22.2).

Additional indirect support for earlier initiation of HIV therapy came in 2011, when data from the HPTN (HIV Prevention Trials Network) 052 study were released.[11] In this trial, more than 1700 individuals infected with HIV with CD4+ counts of 350 to 550 cells/mm^3 with partners uninfected with HIV were randomized to immediate ART versus ART initiation when CD4+ cell count decreased to less than 250/mm^3. ART profoundly reduced transmission of HIV, with only 1 linked transmission in the 886 couples randomized to immediate ART compared with 27 in the arm in which ART was delayed, an HR in the early-therapy group of 0.04 (95% CI, 0.01–0.27; $P<.001$), which showed a 96% reduction in transmission risk. Additional analyses found that the incidence of clinical events during the trial was significantly lower in the immediate ART arm (incidence rate ratio = 0.8, $P = .02$) with the difference driven by HIV clinical events (eg, tuberculosis, herpes simplex infections, zoster, and candidiasis).[32]

Studies of Pathogenesis and End-Organ Disease

An increasing body of work explores the very early and persistent effects of HIV infection on activation of the immune system, levels of inflammation, and integrity of the gastrointestinal mucosa. Ongoing viremia has been shown in the CNICS cohort to be a risk factor for mortality independent of CD4+ cell count.[33] Similarly, in the COHERE analysis, controlled viremia (HIV RNA <400 copies/mL) was associated with a reduced risk of development of AIDS-defining illness.[23]

Other studies have described increased levels of markers of inflammation and coagulation in patients with uncontrolled HIV infection. In the SMART trial, baseline levels of interleukin 6 and D-dimer were significantly associated with subsequent mortality.[34] This heightened inflammatory state begins soon after infection with HIV and persists if viral replication continues unchecked. ART has been reported to significantly reduce markers of immune activation, inflammation, and coagulation as well as those for endothelial dysfunction and microbial translocation.[35,36] However, studies comparing ART treated patients with control individuals uninfected with HIV[37] suggest that this improvement may be incomplete and that a residual level of excess inflammation persists. The extent of such residual inflammation during ART may be a function of the nadir CD4+ cell count.[38–40] Therefore, an argument for early initiation of ART holds that ongoing inflammation, fed by immune activation and microbial translocation, starts early, is harmful, and is addressed by ART, potentially reducing the risk of subsequent disease.

Treatment as Prevention

Recently, the public health benefits of ART have entered into the discussion of when to start ART. The dramatic effect of ART on reducing HIV transmission found in the HPTN 052 study established ART as prevention.[11] Subsequent studies including the results from the PARTNER study, a Western European study of HIV discordant couples that found no linked transmission events when the infected partner's HIV was controlled despite unprotected sex, has further fueled broader use of ART to reduce the spread of the virus.[41]

Modeling of the effects of early ART in serodiscordant couples (including individual benefit and prevention benefits) in South Africa and India has suggested cost saving and cost-effectiveness, respectively, over a 5-year period, and cost-effectiveness over a lifetime.[42] As with any communicable disease, there is a responsibility for a treating clinician to take into account transmission risks in treating HIV infection, a consideration reflected in recent US and European ART treatment guidelines. Although few are advocating universal ART strictly for its public health benefits, the impact of ART on transmission, coupled with the proven and potential personal health benefits of HIV therapy, has strengthened arguments for broader and earlier use of treatment to suppress viral replication.

ART Toxicity

HIV remains incurable, and once begun, HIV therapy can be anticipated to be lifelong. There are concerns regarding the long-term effects of ART. In the antiretroviral agents in widespread use, several toxicities have been recognized. These are discussed elsewhere in this issue in the article by Alice Pau. Major concerns center on the effects of ART on major organ systems, including the circulatory, renal, and skeletal systems. The D:A:D (Data Collection on Adverse Events of Anti-HIV Drugs) study, other observational studies, and 1 randomized controlled trial[17,43–45] have reported an association between abacavir-containing ART regimens and increased risk of MI, although other cohort analyses,[46] secondary analyses of randomized trials, and meta-analyses have not found such an association.[47–49] Although the relative risk of cardiovascular disease associated with common ART is concerning, it should be recognized that the absolute risk of MI and stroke remains low in the D:A:D and other cohorts. A recent report from the Kaiser Permanente group found that in recent years, the incidence rates of both MI and stroke in patients infected and uninfected with HIV had converged, whereas previously, patients infected with HIV had higher rates of both. These investigators attributed the reduced incidence of cardiovascular disease in patients infected with HIV to better lipid management, lifestyle interventions, and, importantly, to earlier use of ART.[50,51]

Tenofovir is an integral component of the most commonly used ART regimens. This nucleotide analogue can produce renal tubular damage, and rarely proximal tubulopathy with features of Fanconi syndrome, including increasing serum creatinine levels, glycosuria, hypophosphatemia, and acute tubular necrosis. It is estimated that less than 2% of treated patients can be expected to develop tubulopathy from tenofovir.[52] The protease inhibitor (PI) atazanavir has also been linked in the D:A:D and EuroSIDA cohorts to renal issues, including chronic kidney disease.[53] This drug can crystallize in the urine, causing nephrolithiasis. Recent reports[54,55] have also documented atazanavir stones as a cause of cholelithiasis.

Decreases in bone mineral density (BMD) are well described after initiation of ART, perhaps a consequence of an immune reconstitution phenomenon. In recent clinical trials, declines in BMD have been observed to be greater for both tenofovir and atazanavir than other antiretrovirals. There are limited data suggesting an association between pathologic fractures and ART-mediated reductions in BMD.[52,56–58]

Additional potential adverse events accompany these and other antiretroviral agents and are detailed in each package insert. However, recent clinical trials of modern ART have found relatively low levels of treatment discontinuations as a result of toxicity or treatment intolerance.[59–61] Although the support provided to patients within the context of a research study may be more robust than that provided in clinical settings, the overall tolerability of these agents is reassuring and indicates the dramatic improvement in these therapies from the days of the CONCORDE trial.

Antiretroviral Resistance

Development of antiretroviral resistance is a well-recognized limitation of HIV treatment. Expanding the number of people receiving ART could result in an at least proportionate increase in the development of drug resistance. There are limited data on whether rates of developing resistance differ depending on CD4+ cell count or HIV disease stage at initiation, although 1 study[62] has suggested initiation at CD4+ count higher than 350 cells/mm^3 was associated with a lower frequency of resistance mutations. Higher rates of acute illness in those with advanced HIV could plausibly increase likelihood of treatment interruption and poor absorption of ART and might result in an increased need for non-HIV medications, with potential for drug-drug interaction.

In addition, advances in ART have enhanced not only potency, tolerability, and convenience but also durability. Drug resistance to PIs boosted with ritonavir or cobicistat is rarely detected. The integrase inhibitor dolutegravir also appears in clinical trials to have a high barrier to drug resistance.[61] Therefore, although the risk of drug resistance will never be completely eliminated, it has been reduced, and newer-generation agents provide the ability to control even drug-resistant strains of HIV.

CONDITIONS STRONGLY FAVORING ART INITIATION

Outside the debate over whether or not to start ART at high CD4+ cell counts are a variety of conditions in which the benefit of prompt and, in some cases, urgent initiation of ART, regardless of CD4+ count, is clear.

Pregnancy

The management of HIV in pregnancy is a major topic in its own right, for which the current US guidelines are a useful starting point.[63] ART is indicated in pregnancy because of dramatic and repeatedly proven benefits in reducing perinatal transmission of HIV.[64] Current US guidelines recommend initiation during pregnancy and state that deciding whether to start during the first trimester should involve weighing risk of potential fetal toxicities of first-trimester ART exposure against benefits, with maternal CD4+ cell count, HIV RNA level, and other maternal conditions.[63] Lack of early viral control is noted to be a risk factor for perinatal transmission.[65]

Acute Opportunistic Infections

Initiation of ART in the setting of opportunistic infections (OIs) is covered more fully elsewhere in this issue in the article by Rajesh Gandhi. Presence of an acute opportunistic condition is generally an indication for ART initiation, but the urgency, optimal timing of initiation, and mechanism of benefit varies by infection. Concern for severe immune reconstitution inflammatory syndrome (IRIS) exists with certain opportunistic conditions, including tuberculosis and cryptococcosis. For tuberculosis, several clinical trials have shown mortality and other health benefits to prompt ART initiation.[66–68] In tuberculous meningitis, there is some evidence to suggest higher rates of adverse events with immediate ART compared with ART delayed 2 months,[69] although the high rate of adverse events in both groups in this international trial has prompted concerns about generalizability. IRIS can also occur with other manifestations of tuberculosis. Current DHHS guidelines recommend close monitoring and caution when initiating ART in patients with tuberculous meningitis, and, for tuberculosis in general, recommend initiating ART within 2 weeks when CD4+ count is lower than 50/mm^3 and within 8 to 12 weeks with counts higher than 50/mm^3. For severe cryptococcosis, concern also exists that immediate ART may lead to worse outcomes via IRIS, and these guidelines state that "it may be prudent to delay initiation of ART until induction (the first two weeks) or the total induction/consolidation phase (10 weeks) has been completed."[70]

For most other opportunistic conditions, there is a consensus on the benefits of early ART. For infections such as progressive multifocal leukoencephalopathy (PML) and cryptosporidiosis, for which no effective targeted therapy exists, ART is a means to potentially improve outcomes by improving immune function, although IRIS is common among those with PML who receive ART, and monitoring for this outcome is recommended.[10] Even for infections with effective treatment, there is often a benefit to ART. The ACTG 5164 study randomized patients to early ART (defined as starting within 14 days of acute OI treatment) versus deferred ART given after acute treatment of the infection was completed. There were lower rates of death and progression to AIDS in the early ART arm compared with the deferred ART arm. In that study, tuberculosis was excluded, pneumocystis was responsible for most infections, and there were few cases of cryptococcal meningitis.[71]

Other Comorbid Conditions

ART initiation is indicated after the diagnosis of AIDS-defining malignancies (ADMs). For HIV-associated lymphomas, higher cumulative HIV viremia in the 6 months after lymphoma diagnosis was associated with increased mortality.[72] Additional observational data suggested that a lower CD4+ cell count was predictive of death from ADMs.[6]

Coinfection with hepatitis B and C viruses are also indications for prompt initiation of ART, as discussed in the article elsewhere in this issue. HIV-associated neurocognitive disorders and HIVAN are also indications for ART initiation and are discussed at greater length in the article elsewhere in this issue.

Acute HIV Infection

Acute or primary HIV infection is another indication for rapid ART initiation, for a variety of reasons. There is considerable evidence of immunologic benefits of ART initiated in acute HIV infection, including improved CD4+ reconstitution,[73,74] faster decline of HIV reservoir compared with later ART initiation,[73,75,76] and greater preservation of T-cell[77,78] and B-cell function.[79] Decreased HIV sequence diversity has also been seen with ART initiation in primary infection.[80,81]

Randomized controlled trials have evaluated whether limited duration courses of ART initiated early in the disease course were of benefit. The ACTG Setpoint Study, the Primo-SHM trial, and the SPARTAC trial found benefits of early HIV therapy, including transient decreasing of viral set point and delay in initiation of long-term ART. However, CD4+ count decline occurred after cessation of ART in all of these trials.[82–84] Thus, early treatment does not obviate lifelong ART.

The disproportionate contribution of the recently infected to HIV transmission also suggests that treatment in this population could have a significant impact on the prevention of HIV transmission.[85] Therefore, initiation of ART during primary infection seems to provide benefits both to individual and to public health.

CHALLENGES AND CONSIDERATIONS

A major and often underacknowledged fact is that most HIV-positive individuals present with CD4+ cell counts lower than $500/mm^3$.[86] Furthermore, rates of loss to follow-up (on and off ART) as well as attrition from routine HIV care are high, with recent national estimates showing only 24% and 33% of all persons in the United States infected with HIV receive effective ART.[87,88]

Adherence to ART is a struggle for many patients. Although ART has become simpler and more forgiving of lapses in adherence, mental health and substance abuse disorders, in particular, remain impediments to long-term control of HIV infection and reduced infectiousness. Better tools to assess for risk of nonadherence and improved interventions to enhance adherence and retention in care are critical to decreasing the risks of developing ART resistance and to reducing the potential harms of erratic and interrupted HIV care. Expanded mental health and substance abuse treatment will be essential to the success of a substantial proportion of those living with HIV.

An increasing challenge to the use of ART is affordability. Changes to the health care landscape in the United States have had ramifications for many individuals infected with HIV with and without insurance. As the Affordable Care Act is implemented, access to health insurance, including via expansion of Medicaid in some states, has provided much needed services to the underinsured and uninsured. However, for others, insurance companies have responded by increasing ART copays and deductibles: a devastating burden for patients struggling with limited resources.

SUMMARY

There are many circumstances, including low CD4+ cell count, development of an acute opportunistic condition, and presence of an AIDS-defining condition, in which the benefits of prompt ART initiation are unambiguous. In contrast, whether to recommend routine ART initiation at CD4+ cell counts that are closer to normal remains a subject of some debate. Despite conflicting cohort data regarding the mortality benefit to ART at CD4+ cell counts higher than $500/mm^3$, there is evidence to reasonably suggest the existence of harm with untreated HIV, even at high CD4+ cell counts. In contrast, no data, cohort or otherwise, exist that show harm from earlier initiation of ART. The robust clinical data of the benefits of ART at low CD4+ cell counts and a clear biological plausibility for benefits that extend to high-count individuals compels many to advocate for ART for all. The reduction in infectiousness with effective ART adds further support to the earlier is better enthusiasts.

Critics of this approach can justifiably point to the notable limitations of the available data. However, perhaps the greater drag on the use of ART at higher CD4+ cell counts is operational. Despite ambitious HIV screening programs, most infected individuals are still diagnosed long after their CD4+ cell counts have declined to 50% or more from normal. Among those who are diagnosed, the massive logistical challenges of diagnosing, retaining in care, and supporting medication adherence remains a major and daunting undertaking, especially in the United States, where access to health care is uneven and often unaffordable. Until those who are infected with HIV can be identified and their continued engagement in care is supported, the debate of when to start ART will be moot for most affected by its outcome.

REFERENCES

1. Centers for Disease Control and Prevention. Report of the NIH panel to define principles of therapy of HIV infection and guidelines for the use of antiretroviral agents in HIV-infected adults and adolescents. 1998. Available at: http://Aidsinfo.nih.gov/ContentFiles/AdultandAdolescentGL04241998014.pdf. Accessed February 16, 2014.
2. Aboulker J, Swart A. Preliminary analysis of the CONCORDE trial. Lancet 1993; 341(8849):889–90.
3. Panel on Antiretroviral Guidelines for Adults and Adolescents. Guidelines for the use of antiretroviral agents in HIV-infected adults and adolescents. Department of Health and Human Services. 2001. Available at: http://Aidsinfo.nih.gov/ContentFiles/AdultandAdolescentGL02052001009.pdf. Accessed February 16, 2014.
4. Panel on antiretroviral guidelines for adults and adolescents. Guidelines for the use of antiretroviral agents in HIV-1-infected adults and adolescents. Department of Health and Human services. 2007. Available at: http://Aidsinfo.nih.gov/contentfiles/AdultandAdolescentGL000721.pdf. Accessed February 16, 2014.
5. Strategies for Management of Antiretroviral Therapy (SMART) Study Group. Major clinical outcomes in antiretroviral therapy (ART)-naive participants and in those not receiving ART at baseline in the SMART study. J Infect Dis 2008; 197:1133–44.
6. Data Collection on Adverse Events of Anti-HIV Drugs (D:A:D) Study Group, d'Arminio Monforte A, Abrams D, Pradier C, et al. HIV-induced immunodeficiency and risk of fatal AIDS-defining and non-AIDS defining malignancies. AIDS 2007;22(16):2143.
7. May M, Sterne JA, Sabin C, et al. Prognosis of HIV-1-infected patients up to 5 years after initiation of HAART: collaborative analysis of prospective studies. AIDS 2007;21(9):1185–97.
8. Panel on antiretroviral guidelines for adults and adolescents. Guidelines for the use of antiretroviral agents in HIV-1-infected adults and adolescents. Department of Health and Human Services. 2009. Available at: http://Aidsinfo.nih.gov/contentfiles/AdultandAdolescentGL001561.pdf. Accessed February 16, 2014.

9. Panel on Antiretroviral Guidelines for Adults and Adolescents. Guidelines for the use of antiretroviral agents in HIV-1-infected adults and adolescents. Department of Health and Human Services. 2012. Available at: http://Aidsinfo.nih.gov/contentfiles/AdultandAdolescentGL003093.pdf. Accessed February 16, 2014.

10. Panel on Antiretroviral Guidelines for Adults and Adolescents. Guidelines for the use of antiretroviral agents in HIV-1-infected adults and adolescents. Department of Health and Human Services. Available at: http://aidsinfo.nih.gov/contentfiles/lvguidelines/AdultandAdolescentGL.pdf. Accessed July 1, 2014.

11. Cohen MS, Chen YQ, McCauley M, et al. Prevention of HIV-1 infection with early antiretroviral therapy. N Engl J Med 2011;365(6):493–505.

12. Williams I, Churchill D, Anderson J, et al. British HIV association guidelines for the treatment of HIV-1-positive adults with antiretroviral therapy 2012. HIV Med 2012;13(S2):1–6.

13. EACS European AIDS Clinical Society Guidelines. 2013. Available at: http://www.eacsociety.org/guidelines.aspx. Accessed February 16, 2014.

14. World Health Organization. Consolidated guidelines on general HIV care and the use of antiretroviral drugs for treating and preventing HIV infection: recommendations for a public health approach. 2013.

15. Ministère des Affaires Sociales et de la Santé, Conseil National du SIDA, Agence Nationale de Recherches sur le SIDA et les Hépatites Virales. Prise en charge médicale des personnes vivant avec le VIH. Recommandations du groupe d'experts. Rapport. 2013. Available at: http://www.sante.gouv.fr/IMG/pdf/Rapport_Morlat_2013_Mise_en_ligne.pdf. Accessed February 16, 2014.

16. Available at: http://insight.ccbr.umn.edu/start/. Accessed March 29, 2014.

17. Opravil M, Ledergerber B, Furrer H, et al. Clinical efficacy of early initiation of HAART in patients with asymptomatic HIV infection and CD4 cell count >350 × 106/L. AIDS 2002;16(10):1371–81.

18. When To Start Consortium, Sterne JA, May M, Costagliola D, et al. Timing of initiation of antiretroviral therapy in AIDS-free HIV-1-infected patients: a collaborative analysis of 18 HIV cohort studies. Lancet 2009;373(9672):1352–63.

19. HIV-CAUSAL Collaboration, Cain LE, Logan R, Robins JM, et al. When to initiate combined antiretroviral therapy to reduce mortality and AIDS-defining illness in HIV-infected persons in developed countries: an observational study. Ann Intern Med 2011;154(8):509–15.

20. Kitahata MM, Gange SJ, Abraham AG, et al. Effect of early versus deferred antiretroviral therapy for HIV on survival. N Engl J Med 2009;360(18):1815–26.

21. Wada N, Jacobson LP, Cohen M, et al. Cause-specific life expectancies after 35 years of age for human immunodeficiency syndrome-infected and human immunodeficiency syndrome-negative individuals followed simultaneously in long-term cohort studies, 1984-2008. Am J Epidemiol 2013;177(2):116–25.

22. Writing Committee for the CASCADE Collaboration. Timing of HAART initiation and clinical outcomes in human immunodeficiency virus type 1 seroconverters. Arch Intern Med 2011;171(17):1560–9.

23. Mocroft A, Furrer HJ, Miro JM, et al. The incidence of AIDS-defining illnesses at a current CD4 count >/= 200 cells/muL in the post-combination antiretroviral therapy era. Clin Infect Dis 2013;57(7):1038–47.

24. Silverberg MJ, Leyden WA, Xu L, et al. Immunodeficiency and risk of myocardial infarction among HIV-positive individuals with access to care. J Acquir Immune Defic Syndr 2014;65(2):160–6.

25. Drozd D, Nance R, Delaney J, et al. Lower CD4 count and higher viral load are associated with increased risk of myocardial infarction. Presented at the

21th Conference on Retroviruses and Opportunistic Infections. Poster 739. Boston, March 3–6, 2014.

26. Ellis RJ, Badiee J, Vaida F, et al. CD4 nadir is a predictor of HIV neurocognitive impairment in the era of combination antiretroviral therapy. AIDS 2011;25(14): 1747–51.

27. Mary-Krause M, Viard J, Ename-Mkoumazok B, et al. Prevalence of low bone mineral density in men and women infected with human immunodeficiency virus 1 and a proposal for screening strategy. J Clin Densitom 2012;15(4):422–33.

28. Young B, Dao CN, Buchacz K, et al, HIV Outpatient Study (HOPS) Investigators. Increased rates of bone fracture among HIV-infected persons in the HIV outpatient study (HOPS) compared with the US general population, 2000-2006. Clin Infect Dis 2011;52(8):1061–8.

29. Palella F, Armon C, Chmiel J, et al. Higher CD4 at ART initiation predicts greater long term likelihood of CD4 normalization. Presented at the 21th Conference on Retroviruses and Opportunistic Infections. Poster 560. Boston, March 3–6, 2014.

30. Severe P, Jean Juste MA, Ambroise A, et al. Early versus standard antiretroviral therapy for HIV-infected adults in Haiti. N Engl J Med 2010;363(3):257–65.

31. El-Sadr W, Lundgren JD, Neaton J, et al. CD4 count-guided interruption of antiretroviral treatment. N Engl J Med 2006;355(22):2283–96.

32. Grinsztejn B, Hosseinipour MC, Ribaudo HJ, et al. Effects of early versus delayed initiation of antiretroviral treatment on clinical outcomes of HIV-1 infection: results from the phase 3 HPTN 052 randomised controlled trial. Lancet Infect Dis 2014;14(4):281–90.

33. Mugavero M, Westfall A, Gill M, et al. Cumulative viral load predicts all-cause and AIDS-related mortality after initiation of ART. Presented at the 21th Conference on Retroviruses and Opportunistic Infections. Poster 565. Boston, March 3–6, 2014.

34. Kuller LH, Tracy R, Belloso W, et al. Inflammatory and coagulation biomarkers and mortality in patients with HIV infection. PLoS Med 2008;5(10):e203.

35. Torriani FJ, Komarow L, Parker RA, et al. Endothelial function in human immunodeficiency virus-infected antiretroviral-naive subjects before and after starting potent antiretroviral Therapy. The ACTG (AIDS Clinical Trials Group) study 5152s. J Am Coll Cardiol 2008;52(7):569–76.

36. McComsey GA, Smith KY, Patel P, et al. Similar reductions in markers of inflammation and endothelial activation after initiation of abacavir/lamivudine (ABC/3TC) or tenofovir/emtricitabine (TDF/FTC) in the HEAT study. RNA 2009;4:1.

37. Neuhaus J, Jacobs DR Jr, Baker JV, et al. Markers of inflammation, coagulation, and renal function are elevated in adults with HIV infection. J Infect Dis 2010; 201(12):1788–95.

38. Robbins GK, Spritzler JG, Chan ES, et al. Incomplete reconstitution of T cell subsets on combination antiretroviral therapy in the AIDS clinical trials group protocol 384. Clin Infect Dis 2009;48(3):350–61.

39. Lange CG, Lederman MM, Madero JS, et al. Impact of suppression of viral replication by highly active antiretroviral therapy on immune function and phenotype in chronic HIV-1 infection. J Acquir Immune Defic Syndr 2002;30(1):33–40.

40. Hunt PW, Martin JN, Sinclair E, et al. T cell activation is associated with lower CD4+ T cell gains in human immunodeficiency virus-infected patients with sustained viral suppression during antiretroviral therapy. J Infect Dis 2003;187(10): 1534–43.

41. Rodger A, Bruun T, Cambiano V, et al. HIV transmission risk through condomless sex if HIV+ partner on suppressive ART: PARTNER study. Presented at the

21th Conference on Retroviruses and Opportunistic Infections. Abstract: 153LB. Boston, March 3–6, 2014.

42. Walensky RP, Ross EL, Kumarasamy N, et al. Cost-effectiveness of HIV treatment as prevention in serodiscordant couples. N Engl J Med 2013;369(18): 1715–25.

43. Worm SW, Sabin C, Weber R, et al. Risk of myocardial infarction in patients with HIV infection exposed to specific individual antiretroviral drugs from the 3 major drug classes: the data collection on adverse events of anti-HIV drugs (D:A:D) study. J Infect Dis 2010;201(3):318–30.

44. Strategies for Management of Anti-Retroviral Therapy/INSIGHT, DAD Study Groups. Use of nucleoside reverse transcriptase inhibitors and risk of myocardial infarction in HIV-infected patients. AIDS 2008;22(14):F17–24.

45. D:A:D Study Group, Sabin CA, Worm SW, et al. Use of nucleoside reverse transcriptase inhibitors and risk of myocardial infarction in HIV-infected patients enrolled in the D:A:D study: a multi-cohort collaboration. Lancet 2008; 371(9622):1417–26.

46. Bedimo RJ, Westfall AO, Drechsler H, et al. Abacavir use and risk of acute myocardial infarction and cerebrovascular events in the highly active antiretroviral therapy era. Clin Infect Dis 2011;53(1):84–91.

47. Brothers CH, Hernandez JE, Cutrell AG, et al. Risk of myocardial infarction and abacavir therapy: no increased risk across 52 GlaxoSmithKline-sponsored clinical trials in adult subjects. J Acquir Immune Defic Syndr 2009;51(1):20–8.

48. Ribaudo HJ, Benson CA, Zheng Y, et al. No risk of myocardial infarction associated with initial antiretroviral treatment containing abacavir: short and long-term results from ACTG A5001/ALLRT. Clin Infect Dis 2011;52(7):929–40.

49. Cruciani M, Zanichelli V, Serpelloni G, et al. Abacavir use and cardiovascular disease events: a meta-analysis of published and unpublished data. AIDS 2011;25(16):1993–2004.

50. Klein D, Leyden W, Chao C, et al. No difference in incidence of myocardial infarction for HIV+ and HIV- individuals in recent years. Presented at the 21th Conference on Retroviruses and Opportunistic Infections. Poster 737. Boston, March 3–6, 2014.

51. Marcus J, Leyden W, Chao C, et al. HIV infection and immunodeficiency as risk factors for ischemic stroke. Presented at the 21th Conference on Retroviruses and Opportunistic Infections. Poster 741. Boston, March 3–6, 2014.

52. Wyatt CM. The kidney in HIV infection: beyond HIV-associated nephropathy. Top Antivir Med 2012;20(3):106–10.

53. Mocroft A, Kirk O, Reiss P, et al. Estimated glomerular filtration rate, chronic kidney disease and antiretroviral drug use in HIV-positive patients. AIDS 2010; 24(11):1667–78.

54. Nishijima T, Shimbo T, Komatsu H, et al. Cumulative exposure to ritonavir-boosted atazanavir is associated with cholelithiasis in patients with HIV-1 infection. J Antimicrob Chemother 2013;69(5):1385–9.

55. Rakotondravelo S, Poinsignon Y, Borsa-Lebas F, et al. Complicated atazanavir-associated cholelithiasis: a report of 14 cases. Clin Infect Dis 2012;55(9): 1270–2.

56. McComsey GA, Kitch D, Daar ES, et al. Bone mineral density and fractures in antiretroviral-naive persons randomized to receive abacavir-lamivudine or tenofovir disoproxil fumarate-emtricitabine along with efavirenz or atazanavir-ritonavir: AIDS Clinical Trials Group A5224s, a substudy of ACTG A5202. J Infect Dis 2011;203(12):1791–801.

57. Stellbrink HJ, Orkin C, Arribas JR, et al. Comparison of changes in bone density and turnover with abacavir-lamivudine versus tenofovir-emtricitabine in HIV-infected adults: 48-week results from the ASSERT study. Clin Infect Dis 2010; 51(8):963–72.

58. Brown T, Moser C, Currier J, et al. Bone density changes after antiretroviral initiation with protease inhibitors or raltegravir. Presented at the 21th Conference on Retroviruses and Opportunistic Infections. Poster 779LB. Boston, March 3–6, 2014.

59. Landovitz R, Ribaudo H, Ofotokun I, et al. Efficacy and tolerability of atazanavir, raltegravir, or darunavir with FTC/tenofovir: ACTG 5257. Presented at the 21th Conference on Retroviruses and Opportunistic Infections. Oral abstract 85. Boston, March 3–6, 2014.

60. Sax PE, DeJesus E, Mills A, et al. Co-formulated elvitegravir, cobicistat, emtricitabine, and tenofovir versus co-formulated efavirenz, emtricitabine, and tenofovir for initial treatment of HIV-1 infection: a randomised, double-blind, phase 3 trial, analysis of results after 48 weeks. Lancet 2012;379(9835):2439–48.

61. Walmsley SL, Antela A, Clumeck N, et al. Dolutegravir plus abacavir–lamivudine for the treatment of HIV-1 infection. N Engl J Med 2013;369(19):1807–18.

62. Uy J, Armon C, Buchacz K, et al, HOPS Investigators. Initiation of HAART at higher CD4 cell counts is associated with a lower frequency of antiretroviral drug resistance mutations at virologic failure. J Acquir Immune Defic Syndr 2009;51(4):450–3.

63. Panel on Treatment of HIV-Infected Pregnant Women and Prevention of Perinatal Transmission. Recommendations for use of antiretroviral drugs in pregnant HIV-1- infected women for maternal health and interventions to reduce perinatal HIV transmission in the United States. 2012. Available at: http://Aidsinfo.nih.gov/contentfiles/lvguidelines/PerinatalGL.pdf. Accessed February 17, 2014.

64. Townsend CL, Cortina-Borja M, Peckham CS, et al. Low rates of mother-to-child transmission of HIV following effective pregnancy interventions in the United Kingdom and Ireland, 2000-2006. AIDS 2008;22(8):973–81.

65. Warszawski J, Tubiana R, Le Chenadec J, et al. Mother-to-child HIV transmission despite antiretroviral therapy in the ANRS French perinatal cohort. AIDS 2008;22(2):289–99.

66. Abdool Karim SS, Naidoo K, Grobler A, et al. Integration of antiretroviral therapy with tuberculosis treatment. N Engl J Med 2011;365(16):1492–501.

67. Blanc F, Sok T, Laureillard D, et al. Earlier versus later start of antiretroviral therapy in HIV-infected adults with tuberculosis. N Engl J Med 2011;365(16):1471–81.

68. Havlir DV, Kendall MA, Ive P, et al. Timing of antiretroviral therapy for HIV-1 infection and tuberculosis. N Engl J Med 2011;365(16):1482–91.

69. Torok ME, Yen NT, Chau TT, et al. Timing of initiation of antiretroviral therapy in human immunodeficiency virus (HIV)–associated tuberculous meningitis. Clin Infect Dis 2011;52(11):1374–83.

70. Panel on Opportunistic Infections in HIV-Infected Adults and Adolescents. Guidelines for the prevention and treatment of opportunistic infections in HIV-infected adults and adolescents: Recommendations from the Centers for Disease Control and Prevention, the National Institutes of Health, and the HIV Medicine Association of the Infectious Diseases Society of America. 2013. Available at: http://Aidsinfo.nih.gov/contentfiles/lvguidelines/adult_oi.pdf. Accessed March 27, 2014.

71. Zolopa AR, Andersen J, Komarow L, et al. Early antiretroviral therapy reduces AIDS progression/death in individuals with acute opportunistic infections: a multicenter randomized strategy trial. PLoS One 2009;4(5):e5575.

72. Gopal S, Patel MR, Yanik EL, et al. Association of early HIV viremia with mortality after HIV-associated lymphoma. AIDS 2013;27(15):2365–73.
73. Ananworanich J, Schuetz A, Vandergeeten C, et al. Impact of multi-targeted antiretroviral treatment on gut T cell depletion and HIV reservoir seeding during acute HIV infection. PLoS One 2012;7(3):e33948.
74. Le T, Wright EJ, Smith DM, et al. Enhanced CD4 T-cell recovery with earlier HIV-1 antiretroviral therapy. N Engl J Med 2013;368(3):218–30.
75. Chun TW, Justement JS, Moir S, et al. Decay of the HIV reservoir in patients receiving antiretroviral therapy for extended periods: implications for eradication of virus. J Infect Dis 2007;195(12):1762–4.
76. Strain MC, Little SJ, Daar ES, et al. Effect of treatment, during primary infection, on establishment and clearance of cellular reservoirs of HIV-1. J Infect Dis 2005; 191(9):1410–8.
77. Rosenberg ES, Altfeld M, Poon SH, et al. Immune control of HIV-1 after early treatment of acute infection. Nature 2000;407(6803):523–6.
78. Oxenius A, Price DA, Easterbrook PJ, et al. Early highly active antiretroviral therapy for acute HIV-1 infection preserves immune function of CD8+ and CD4+ T lymphocytes. Proc Natl Acad Sci U S A 2000;97(7):3382–7.
79. Titanji K, Chiodi F, Bellocco R, et al. Primary HIV-1 infection sets the stage for important B lymphocyte dysfunctions. AIDS 2005;19(17):1947–55.
80. Gall A, Kaye S, Hué S, et al. Restriction of V3 region sequence divergence in the HIV-1 envelope gene during antiretroviral treatment in a cohort of recent sero-converters. Retrovirology 2013;10(1):8.1–8.15.
81. Evering TH, Mehandru S, Racz P, et al. Absence of HIV-1 evolution in the gut-associated lymphoid tissue from patients on combination antiviral therapy initiated during primary infection. PLoS Pathog 2012;8(2):e1002506.
82. Walker BD, Hirsch MS. Antiretroviral therapy in early HIV infection. N Engl J Med 2013;368(3):279–81.
83. Grijsen ML, Steingrover R, Wit FW, et al. No treatment versus 24 or 60 weeks of antiretroviral treatment during primary HIV infection: the randomized primo-SHM trial. PLoS Med 2012;9(3):e1001196.
84. Hogan CM, Degruttola V, Sun X, et al. The setpoint study (ACTG A5217): effect of immediate versus deferred antiretroviral therapy on virologic set point in recently HIV-1-infected individuals. J Infect Dis 2012;205(1):87–96.
85. Powers KA, Ghani AC, Miller WC, et al. The role of acute and early HIV infection in the spread of HIV and implications for transmission prevention strategies in Lilongwe, Malawi: a modelling study. Lancet 2011;378(9787):256–68.
86. Lesko CR, Cole SR, Zinski A, et al. A systematic review and meta-regression of temporal trends in adult CD4(+) cell count at presentation to HIV care, 1992-2011. Clin Infect Dis 2013;57(7):1027–37.
87. Gardner EM, McLees MP, Steiner JF, et al. The spectrum of engagement in HIV care and its relevance to test-and-treat strategies for prevention of HIV infection. Clin Infect Dis 2011;52(6):793–800.
88. Hall HI, Gray KM, Tang T, et al. Retention in care of adults and adolescents living with HIV in 13 US areas. J Acquir Immune Defic Syndr 2012;60(1):77–82.

Beginning Antiretroviral Therapy for Patients with HIV

Jennifer A. Johnson, MD*, Paul E. Sax, MD

KEYWORDS

- HIV • Antiretroviral therapy (ART) • Treatment-naïve
- Nucleoside/nucleotide reverse transcriptase inhibitor (NRTI)
- Nonnucleoside reverse transcriptase inhibitor (NNRTI) • Protease inhibitor (PI)
- Integrase strand transfer inhibitor (INSTI)

KEY POINTS

- There are many effective options for initial antiretroviral therapy (ART) available, with significantly less toxicity than older regimens.
- Of the many choices, most patients will prefer 1 of the 3 currently available single-tablet, once-daily regimens. A fourth single-tablet, once-daily regimen is anticipated soon.
- Because maintenance of virologic suppression is critical to achieve the benefits of ART, it is important to select a regimen enables the patient to continue on lifelong treatment with minimal toxicities and minimal barriers to adherence.

INTRODUCTION

Antiretroviral (ARV) therapy (ART) has come a long way since the early, nonsuppressive regimens and the challenging 10- to 20-pill regimens of the late 1990s. Persons with HIV can now expect to start an ARV regimen of no more than 3 pills per day, usually all taken once daily. Many patients will prefer 1 of the 3 single-daily tablet regimens. With this single-daily tablet, if taken faithfully with appropriate monitoring, HIV-infected patients can expect survival approaching that of the general population, especially if treatment is started before severe immunosuppression.[1,2] Effective ART also reduces the incidence of HIV- and non–HIV-related complications, including opportunistic infections, malignancies, nephropathy, neurologic complications, cardiovascular disease, and liver disease among persons coinfected with hepatitis B (HBV) and/or C.[3–16] Beyond these many benefits to the HIV-infected individual,

Division of Infectious Diseases, Brigham and Women's Hospital, Harvard Medical School, 75 Francis Street, PBBA4, Boston, MA 02115, USA
* Corresponding author.
E-mail address: jjohnson30@partners.org

Infect Dis Clin N Am 28 (2014) 421–438
http://dx.doi.org/10.1016/j.idc.2014.06.003   id.theclinics.com

effective ART nearly eliminates the risk of HIV transmission, playing an important role in HIV prevention.[17–20] These benefits are realized by the collaborative efforts of the patient and medical team to select, initiate, and then maintain treatment on the optimal ART regimen for that individual, thus achieving and maintaining virologic suppression. Because maintenance of virologic suppression is critical to achieve the benefits of ART, it is important to select a regimen that enables the patient to continue on long-term treatment with minimal toxicities and minimal barriers to adherence. Factors to consider in determining when to start ART are addressed elsewhere. Here we review the options for initial ART, including data from clinical trials to support these choices, and the factors to consider in selection of a regimen to best fit each patient.

PHARMACOLOGIC STRATEGIES

Selection of initial therapy depends on individual patient characteristics. Providers should assess the following factors for each patient before discussing options for initial ART, to select the best fit:

- Pretreatment plasma HIV RNA (viral load) and CD4 cell count
- Baseline drug resistance as determined by HIV genotypic drug-resistance testing, preferably at the time of HIV diagnosis
- Preexisting conditions, such as cardiovascular disease, liver disease, renal disease, and psychiatric illness
- Coinfections, such as HBV, hepatitis C, and tuberculosis
- Concurrent medications that may have interactions with certain agents, such as proton pump inhibitors, warfarin, methadone, and inhaled corticosteroids
- Any symptomatic complaints at baseline that might augment known adverse effects of treatment, such as diarrhea, heartburn, and depression
- Current pregnancy or desire/potential for pregnancy in the future
- Patient past experience with chronic medications and estimated capacity for medication adherence
- Patient lifestyle and work schedule, as it relates to medication dosing frequency, food and fluid requirements with medication dosing, and overall pill burden
- Factors specific to certain drugs:
  - Results of HLA-B*5701 testing, when considering treatment with abacavir (ABC)
  - Results of coreceptor tropism assay, when considering treatment with maraviroc
  - Pretreatment HIV RNA and CD4 cell count when considering treatment with rilpivirine (RPV) or ABC.

These factors, if assessed thoroughly during discussion of initiation of ART, can then be considered along with the characteristics of each regimen (eg, adverse effects, dosing frequency, food restrictions, barrier to resistance) to find the best patient–regimen match. This promotes sustained medication adherence and virologic suppression, with all of the associated clinical benefits.

This article focuses primarily on the Guidelines for the Use of Antiretroviral Agents in HIV-1–Infected Adults and Adolescents as issued by the US Department of Health and Human Services, with additional information from the ARV treatment guidelines by the International Antiviral Society-USA. The recommended and alternative initial ART regimens, as recommended by the US Department of Health and Human Services and International Antiviral Society-USA, all include 2 drugs from the nucleoside/nucleotide reverse transcriptase inhibitor (NRTI) class, along with a third drug from either the nonnucleoside reverse transcriptase inhibitor (NNRTI), protease inhibitor (PI), or integrase strand transfer inhibitor (INSTI) class (**Table 1**).[21,22]

RECOMMENDED INITIAL REGIMENS: TENOFOVIR VERSUS ABC
Tenofovir

Most of the recommended initial regimens and, as of early 2014, all of the single tablet once-daily ART options include the NRTIs tenofovir disoproxil fumarate (TDF) and emtricitabine (FTC; see **Table 1**).[21] When combined with efavirenz (EFV) or ritonavir (RTV)-boosted atazanavir (ATV/r), TDF/FTC has been shown to be more effective than ABC/lamivudine (3TC) for patients with pretreatment plasma HIV RNA of 100,000 copies/mL or greater.[23] By contrast, when combined with RTV-boosted lopinavir (LPV/r), there was no difference in virologic efficacy between TDF/FTC and ABC/3TC.[24] Furthermore, a subsequent study of a regimen of dolutegravir (DTG) plus ABC/3TC compared with EFV/TDF/FTC did not show a difference in virologic efficacy, even for patients with high pretreatment plasma HIV RNA levels.[25]

TDF is potentially nephrotoxic, especially for those with preexisting kidney disease.[26,27] The TDF dose must be adjusted for those with significant renal dysfunction,

Table 1	
Recommended and alternative initial antiretroviral therapy (ART) regimens, as per US Department of Health and Human Services guidelines	
Recommended initial ART regimens	Efavirenz/tenofovir disoproxil fumarate/emtricitabine (EFV/TDF/FTC)
	Ritonavir-boosted darunavir + tenofovir disoproxil fumarate/emtricitabine (DRV/r + TDF/FTC)
	Ritonavir-boosted atazanavir + tenofovir disoproxil fumarate/emtricitabine (ATV/r + TDF/FTC)
	Dolutegravir + tenofovir disoproxil fumarate/emtricitabine (DTG + TDF/FTC)
	Dolutegravir + abacavir/lamivudine (DTG + ABC/3TC)[a]
	Raltegravir + tenofovir disoproxil fumarate/emtricitabine (RAL + TDF/FTC)
Recommended initial ART regimens for patients with pretreatment plasma HIV RNA <100,000 copies/mL	Elvitegravir/cobicistat/tenofovir disoproxil fumarate/emtricitabine (EVG/COBI/TDF/FTC)[b]
	Rilpivirine/tenofovir disoproxil fumarate/emtricitabine (RPV/TDF/FTC)[c]
	Efavirenz + abacavir/lamivudine (EFV + ABC/3TC)[a]
	Ritonavir-boosted atazanavir + abacavir/lamivudine (ATV/r + ABC/3TC)[a]
Alternative initial ART regimens	Ritonavir-boosted darunavir + abacavir/lamivudine (DRV/r + ABC/3TC)[a]
	Ritonavir-boosted lopinavir + tenofovir disoproxil fumarate/emtricitabine (LPV/r + TDF/FTC)
	Ritonavir-boosted lopinavir + abacavir/lamivudine (LPV/r + ABC/3TC)[a]
	Raltegravir + abacavir/lamivudine (RAL + ABC/3TC)[a]

[a] Abacavir-containing regimens should only be chosen for patients who are HLA-B*5701 negative.
[b] EVG/COBI/TDF/FTC should only be used for patients with estimated creatinine clearance ≥70 mL/min.
[c] RPV/TDF/FTC should only be used for patients with CD4 count >200 cells/mm[3].

From The Panel on Antiretroviral Guidelines for Adults and Adolescents. Guidelines for the use of antiretroviral agents in HIV-1-infected adults and adolescents. Department of Health and Human Services. Available at: http://aidsinfo.nih.gov/contentfiles/lvguidelines/AdultandAdolescentGL.pdf. Accessed August 2, 2014.

and kidney function must be monitored for all patients on TDF. Regimens containing TDF may not be appropriate for patients with significant kidney disease at baseline.

TDF leads to loss of bone mineral density more than ABC/3TC, and several studies demonstrate an increase in markers of bone metabolism for those receiving the drug.[28,29] Although this is rarely a contraindication to TDF use in young and otherwise healthy patients, individuals with preexisting low bone mineral density may be more optimally treated with non–TDF-containing regimens.

The availability of single-tablet, once-daily options and the long track record of efficacy and tolerability in clinical practice often leads to the choice of TDF-containing regimens over ABC-containing options. Patients with HBV coinfection will also be preferentially treated with TDF/FTC rather than ABC/3TC, because both TDF and FTC effectively treat HBV, whereas ABC is not active against HBV.[30]

ABC

ABC can cause a hypersensitivity reaction manifesting most commonly as fever and rash, sometimes with accompanying end-organ symptoms such as diarrhea or shortness of breath. Rechallenge after ABC hypersensitivity can lead to rapid cardiovascular collapse. Fortunately, this syndrome can be prevented by screening for HLA B*5701. This test should be done for all patients before ABC treatment, and ABC treatment should not be initiated for any patients who screen positive for this allele.[31] Concerns have been raised about a potential association of ABC with an increased risk of myocardial infarction based on some (but not all) observational studies.[32–34] However a metaanalysis by the US Food and Drug Administration (FDA) found no association between ABC use and myocardial infarction.[35] Nonetheless, our practice is to avoid use of ABC in patients at high cardiovascular risk if there are suitable alternatives. ABC is available as a coformulated combination tablet with 3TC, but at the time of this writing, none of the currently available single-tablet, once-daily regimens contain ABC. A single-tablet regimen (STR) of ABC, 3TC, and DTG is in development, with approval expected in 2014.

RECOMMENDED INITIAL ART REGIMENS: SINGLE-TABLET, ONCE-DAILY REGIMENS

Of the 10 regimens that are currently listed as "recommended" options for initial ART (including those recommended only for patients with pretreatment plasma HIV RNA <100,000 copies/mL), 3 are coformulated into single-tablet, once-daily regimens (**Table 2**). Many patients express a preference for STRs for multiple reasons, including simplicity of dosing, refills, sometimes a lower prescription copayment, and easier pill management during travel. These improvements in the patient experience of medication management may translate into higher rates of medication adherence, and thus better outcomes.[36] In observational studies, STRs have been associated with lower pharmacy and total health care costs, as well as fewer hospitalizations.[37,38] At the time of this writing, all of the available STRs include TDF/FTC. These TDF-containing, STRs are not appropriate for most patients with significant renal disease, given the potential for TDF-related nephrotoxicity and the need for dose adjustment with TDF in renal dysfunction.

EFV/TDF/FTC

The combination of EFV with TDF/FTC (Atripla, Gilead, Foster City, CA, USA) has the longest track record of all of the recommended options for initial ART, and for many years was the standard against which other strategies were compared. Several randomized trials have documented the efficacy and tolerability of this regimen.[39–43]

Table 2
Choosing a single-tablet, once-daily regimen for initial antiretroviral therapy (ART)

Regimen	Distinguishing Characteristics Among Single-Tablet Art Regimens
EFV/TDF/FTC	Consider alternatives in women who are planning to become pregnant or not using effective contraception. Neuropsychiatric side effects including depression and sleep disturbances; consider alternatives in patients with preexisting depression or neurologic disease. Monitor for rash and dyslipidemia. Lower barrier to resistance than boosted PI-based regimens; reinforce the importance of adherence. Check for drug–drug interactions owing to induction of cytochrome p450 pathway (eg, methadone).
EVG/COBI/TDF/FTC	No known teratogenicity, but minimal data during pregnancy; consider alternatives for pregnant women. Well tolerated; neuropsychiatric side effects and rash not as common as with EFV/TDF/FTC. Many drug–drug interactions owing to COBI's inhibition of cytochrome p450 pathway (more than with EFV/TDF/FTC); screen concurrent medications for possible interactions before initiating. Lower barrier to resistance than boosted PI-based regimens.
RPV/TDF/FTC	Only for patients with pretreatment plasma HIV RNA 100,000 copies/mL and CD4 count >200 cells/mm^3. No known teratogenicity, but minimal data during pregnancy; consider alternatives for pregnant women. Well tolerated; dyslipidemia and significant neuropsychiatric side effects not as common as with EFV/TDF/FTC. Must be taken with a meal ($\geq$400 kcal with 13 g of fat). Do not use for patients taking proton pump inhibitors, and use only with caution and explicit dose-staggering guidelines for patients on other acid blockers, owing to need for stomach acid for absorption. Lower barrier to resistance than boosted PI-based regimens.
DTG/ABC/3TC[a]	Only for patients who are HLA B*5701 negative. No data during pregnancy, but no known teratogenicity; consider only if other options are not available. Higher barrier to resistance than raltegravir and EFV-based regimens. DTG inhibition of tubular secretion of creatinine may cause increased serum creatinine. ABC may be associated with increased cardiovascular events.

For all of the single-tablet regimens, TDF is associated with nephrotoxicity, may not be appropriate for patients with significant renal dysfunction, and must be dose reduced if administered to those with renal dysfunction, which is not feasible with fixed-dose combination tablets.

Abbreviations: ABC, abacavir; COBI, cobicistat; DTG, dolutegravir; EFV, efavirenz; EVG, elvitegravir; FTC, emtricitabine; PI, protease inhibitor; RPV, rilpivirine; TDF, tenofovir disoproxil fumarate; 3TC, lamivudine.

[a] DTG/ABC/3TC is not currently available coformulated, but is expected soon.

EFV has been shown to be teratogenic in nonhuman primates, but recent data suggest that even first-trimester exposure to EFV does not necessarily increase birth defects above the background rate of the general population.[44,45] Despite these reassuring data, current US guidelines recommend considering alternatives to EFV in women who are planning to become pregnant or not using effective contraception, although women who are already stable on EFV-based treatment when presenting for prenatal care may continue their current ART.[46] Notably, treatment guidelines from the World

Health Organization recommend use of EFV-based initial therapy for all patients, including women of childbearing potential and during pregnancy.[47]

Although generally well tolerated, EFV is associated with neuropsychiatric side effects, including depression and sleep disturbances. These usually resolve over the first couple of months of treatment, but persist and may be problematic for patients with preexisting depression or other psychiatric disease. One recent study found an excess of suicidality among those randomized to EFV-based regimens in clinical trials.[48] EFV also confers a higher incidence of rash, from mild transient maculopapular eruptions to less commonly severe skin reactions, including Stevens-Johnson syndrome. EFV can increase lipids more than then other recommended regimens, although no adverse cardiovascular outcomes with EFV treatment have been reported. There are fewer drug–drug interactions with EFV than with boosted PI-containing or cobicistat (COBI)-containing regimens, but there are a few important interactions owing to the induction of the cytochrome p450 pathway. For example, patients on methadone maintenance who begin EFV may require a change in methadone dose, and those receiving certain statins may need a higher dose.

Although EFV-based treatment generally yields high rates of virologic suppression, there is also a relatively high incidence of resistance mutations at the time of virologic failure for those experiencing virologic rebound; this phenomenon is often referred to as a "low barrier to resistance." The most common resistance mutation to emerge is K103N, which leads to cross-resistance with nevirapine but retained susceptibility to etravirine. The lower barrier to resistance with EFV compared with RTV-boosted, PI-containing regimens leads many clinicians to avoid EFV-based treatments as first line in patients who have an high likelihood of intermittent therapy or nonadherence.

EVG/COBI/TDF/FTC

A single-tablet, once-daily regimen combining elvitegravir (EVG) with COBI and TDF/FTC (Stribild, Gilead) was approved by the FDA in August 2012. EVG is an INSTI that requires pharmacologic boosting to be given once daily. Like RTV, COBI boosts EVG levels by inhibition the cytochrome p450 pathway; unlike RTV, COBI has no independent anti-HIV activity. Coformulated EVG/COBI/TDF/FTC has been shown to be as effective and well tolerated as other recommended initial ART regimens (EFV/TDF/FTC and ATV/r + TDF/FTC) in clinical trials.[49,50] This regimen is not thought to be teratogenic, although there are limited data on safety in pregnancy to date. It is currently recommended for use in pregnancy only if the potential benefit justifies the potential uncertain risk to the fetus.[46,51] A clinical trial of this regimen exclusively in women is now fully enrolled. This study will yield additional data both on women receiving this regimen (few had enrolled in the original clinical trials) and on any pregnancies occurring during the study.[52]

In the pivotal phase III clinical trial, fewer patients discontinued EVG/COBI/TDF/FTC owing to neuropsychiatric side effects or rash than EFV/TDF/FTC.[49] However, there were numerically more renal events in the EVG/COBI/TDF/FTC group, including some patients who developed TDF-related tubular toxicity. In addition, COBI decreases tubular secretion of creatinine, leading to an average 0.15-mg/dL increase in serum creatinine; clinicians should be concerned about possible TDF nephrotoxicity if there is a rise of 0.4 mg/dL or more. Because of these renal issues, EVG/COBI/TDF/FTC should only be used in patients with an estimated creatinine clearance of 70 mL/min or more.[53] As with RTV, there are many drug–drug interactions with COBI, so screening concurrent medications for possible interactions is important before initiation of this regimen. Cationic supplements (calcium, magnesium, aluminum, and iron) can bind INSTIs and decrease efficacy, so dosing of such supplements and INSTI-containing ART should be separated by a few hours.

RPV/TDF/FTC

The STR of RPV with TDF/FTC (Complera, Gilead) is well tolerated and effective for most patients. However, in studies comparing RPV with EFV (with either TDF/FTC or ABC/3TC), there was an increased rate of virologic failure in the RPV group among patients with pretreatment plasma HIV RNA greater than 100,000 copies/mL or pretreatment CD4 count less than 200 cells/mm³.[54–56] A second open-label study compared the STRs of RPV/TDF/FTC with EFV/TDF/FTC and, although there were fewer discontinuations owing to adverse events in the RPV arm, again there were more virologic failures in the RPV arm.[57] As a result, RPV/TDF/FTC should not be used for patients with pretreatment plasma HIV RNA 100,000 copies/mL or more or pretreatment CD4 counts of less than 200 cells/mm³. On a positive note, RPV is better tolerated than EFV, with fewer rash and adverse lipid effects, and fewer drug discontinuations owing to neuropsychiatric side effects than EFV/TDF/FTC. There is no evidence of teratogenicity with RPV/TDF/FTC, but because there are few data on use of this regimen in pregnant women, it is currently recommended for use during pregnancy only when alternatives are not available.[46,51]

Adequate absorption of RPV depends on coadministration with a meal, defined as approximately 400 kcal with 13 g of fat, and on the presence of stomach acid.[58] Patients taking proton pump inhibitors cannot take RPV/TDF/FTC, and other acid blockers such as H2 blockers can only be used concurrently with staggered dosing. These dosing requirements can make adherence more difficult for some patients. As with TDF/FTC/EFV, the regimen of TDF/FTC/RPV has a relatively low barrier to resistance, with new mutations common with virologic failure. Importantly, RPV may select for the E138K mutation, which confers resistance to all available NNRTIs, including etravirine.[57]

DTG/ABC/3TC

A coformulated STR with DTG, ABC, and 3TC (no trade name yet) is anticipated soon. The features of this regimen are discussed in the next section in the context of reviewing data on DTG.

RECOMMENDED INITIAL ART REGIMENS: MULTIPLE-TABLET REGIMENS

All of the recommended initial regimens have been shown to have potent virologic efficacy in clinical trials, so other factors will be considered in choosing the best option for each patient. There are 7 recommended options for initial ART that are multiple-tablet regimens; fortunately, all are 3 or fewer pills per day and all but the raltegravir (RAL)-based regimen are taken once daily (see **Table 1**). The characteristics of each drug to consider in constructing a regimen for the recommended and alternative ART regimens are presented in **Table 3**.

Boosted PI-Based Regimens

The primary advantage of the boosted PI-based regimens is that virologic failure is rarely associated with the development of resistance. This high genetic barrier to resistance is particularly notable with regard to PI resistance, but regimens with boosted PIs seem to reduce the risk of NRTI resistance at failure as well. In contrast with many other ARVs, including EFV, RPV, RAL and EVG, multiple mutations are required to generate significant resistance to the boosted PIs. This characteristic makes the boosted-PI

Table 3
Distinguishing characteristics of individual antiretroviral components of the multiple-tablet recommended and alternative initial antiretroviral therapy (ART) regimens

Antiretroviral Agent	Distinguishing Characteristics
TDF/FTC	• Highly efficacious in all clinical trials. • Provides effective treatment for HBV for patients coinfected with HBV and HIV. • Once daily dosing, well tolerated. • Alternative option during pregnancy. • Potential for nephrotoxicity with TDF, requires ongoing monitoring of renal function and screening for proteinuria. • Cannot use for some patients with significant renal dysfunction. • Regimens with TDF reduce bone mineral density more than those without the drug.
ABC/3TC	• Once daily dosing, well tolerated. • Alternative option during pregnancy. • Requires HLA B*5701 testing before initiation to prevent potentially fatal hypersensitivity reaction. • When combined with EFV or ATV/r, inferior virologic efficacy for patients with pretreatment plasma HIV RNA $\geq$100,000 copies/mL. • Concerns about increased risk of myocardial infarction, although data are conflicting.
DRV/r	• Alternative regimen option during pregnancy. • High barrier to resistance. • Many drug–drug interactions owing to inhibition of cytochrome p450 pathway (more than with EFV/TDF/FTC); screen concurrent medications for possible interactions before initiating. • Well tolerated; may rarely cause rash. • Can be given with acid-reducing agents; unlike ATV/r, is not associated with hyperbilirubinemia or nephrolithiasis. • Potential GI side effects (eg, diarrhea, nausea) in some patients, but generally well tolerated. • Dosing schedule with TDF/FTC or ABC/3TC: 3 separate pills, all taken together once daily.
ATV/r	• For pregnant women, ATV/r is a preferred option. • High barrier to resistance. • Many drug–drug interactions owing to inhibition of cytochrome p450 pathway; screen concurrent medications for possible interactions before initiating. • Absorption depends on gastric acidity, follow dosing guidelines carefully when coadministering with acid-reducing medications, or consider other ART options if acid-reducing medications must be continued. • Causes nontoxic reversible indirect hyperbilirubinemia; may be cosmetically unappealing. • Has been associated with nephrolithiasis, cholelithiasis, and nephrotoxicity. • Potential GI side effects (eg, diarrhea, nausea) in some patients. • Dosing schedule with TDF/FTC or ABC/3TC: 3 separate pills, all taken together once daily.

(continued on next page)

Table 3 (continued)	
Antiretroviral Agent	**Distinguishing Characteristics**
RAL	• Minimal data during pregnancy but no known teratogenicity; consider if no other preferred or alternative options. • Well tolerated; minimal GI side effects compared with boosted-PI options and minimal neuropsychiatric side effects compared with EFV-containing options. • Rare incidence of myopathy and rhabdomyolysis. • Fewer drug–drug interactions than the boosted-PI regimens, EFV-based regimens and EVG/COBI/TDF/FTC. • Lower barrier to resistance than with boosted PI-based regimens. • Twice daily dosing may be a barrier to adherence for some patients. • Dosing schedule: TDF/FTC or ABC/3TC taken as 1 pill daily, and RAL is 1 pill taken twice daily.
DTG	• No data during pregnancy, but no known teratogenicity; consider only if other options are not available. • Well-tolerated, minimal side effects reported in multiple studies. • DTG inhibition of tubular secretion of creatinine may cause increased serum creatinine. • Effective with either TDF/FTC or ABC/3TC even for patients with pretreatment plasma HIV RNA >100,000 copies/mL. • No selection of drug resistance to DTG on virologic failure in clinical trials of treatment-naïve patients. • Dosing schedule with either TDF/FTC or ABC/3TC: 2 separate pills taken together once daily. • Once-daily coformulation of DTG/ABC/3TC[a] is anticipated soon.
EFV	• Consider alternatives in women who are planning to become pregnant or not using effective contraception. • Neuropsychiatric side effects including depression and sleep disturbances; consider alternatives in patients with preexisting depression or neurologic disease. • Monitor for rash and dyslipidemia. • Lower barrier to resistance than boosted PI-based regimens. • Check for drug–drug interactions owing to induction of cytochrome p450 pathway (eg, methadone). • Dosing schedule with ABC/3TC: 2 separate pills taken together once daily.
LPV/r	• MANY drug–drug interactions owing to inhibition of cytochrome p450 pathway. • LPV/r is a preferred option during pregnancy. • Higher rate of toxicities, primarily GI toxicities (diarrhea), which may be treatment limiting. • Daily dose of ritonavir is 200 mg, twice the dose of recommended PI options. • Dosing schedule with TDF/FTC or ABC/3TC: 5 pills per day; the 4 LPV/r tablets may be taken once daily (except for pregnant women), or as 2 pills twice daily.

Abbreviations: ABC, abacavir; COBI, cobicistat; DTG, dolutegravir; EFV, efavirenz; EVG, elvitegravir; FTC, emtricitabine; GI, gastrointestinal; HBV, hepatitis B virus. PI, protease inhibitor; RPV, rilpivirine; TDF, tenofovir disoproxil fumarate; 3TC, lamivudine.
[a] DTG/ABC/3TC is not currently available coformulated, but is expected to be available soon.

regimens attractive for patients who may be at high risk of medication nonadherence, although this is balanced against the increased pill burden compared with the single-tablet, once-daily regimens. The low rate of transmitted drug resistance to PIs makes boosted PI-based regimens the preferred options when treating acute HIV infection before the availability of results of genotypic HIV resistance testing.[21]

All of the PI-based recommended initial ART options include the use of RTV boosting to increase drug levels and enable once-daily dosing. RTV is a potent inhibitor of the cytochrome p450 pathway, so drug–drug interactions are common and screening concurrent medications for interactions is important before initiation of a boosted-PI regimen. RTV is also associated with gastrointestinal side effects, including diarrhea, which is usually mild but for some individuals may be particularly troublesome. RTV is available in both a capsule formulation, which must be maintained at 78°F or lower, and a heat-stable tablet formulation, which is generally easier for travel and is preferred in warmer climates.

Among the boosted PI-based options, ATV/r has been compared with EFV and found to be equally efficacious and well-tolerated, with a lower incidence of neuropsychiatric side effects, rash, and dyslipidemia within the ATV/r group.[41] ATV/r was also shown to be efficacious and well tolerated compared with LPV/r when each was taken with TDF/FTC.[59] Although generally well tolerated, the most important and frequent toxicity of ATV is indirect hyperbilirubinemia. Although not associated with liver dysfunction and rapidly reversible on cessation of the drug, this may result in visible scleral icterus or jaundice, which some patients may find cosmetically unappealing. In ACTG 5257, ATV-related hyperbilirubinemia led to a significantly greater number of treatment discontinuations than those treated with darunavir or RAL.[60] Atazanavir has also been associated with nephrolithiasis, cholelithiasis, and nephrotoxicity. Similar to RPV, atazanavir absorption depends on gastric acidity, so the efficacy of this regimen may be reduced in patients taking acid-reducing medications. There are dosing guidelines to facilitate use of this regimen in patients taking acid-reducing medications, but the staggered dosing schedule may create a barrier to consistent medication adherence for some patients. In a randomized comparison of ATV/r with TDF/FTC or ABC/3TC, there was an increased rate of virologic failure among those receiving ATV/r + ABC/3TC if the pretreatment HIV RNA level was 100,000 copies/mL or greater.[23]

Ritonavir-boosted darunavir (DRV/r) shares with ATV/r the resistance benefit cited. In addition, DRV/r is not associated with hyperbilirubinemia, nephrolithiasis, or cholelithiasis, and it can be given effectively with acid-reducing medications. Based on these toxicity benefits and the results of ACTG 5257, DRV/r is our preferred boosted PI for initial treatment. Treatment-related rash is reported infrequently with DRV/r; severe rash with fever and systemic drug reaction is rare. The efficacy and tolerability of DRV/r with TDF/FTC has been documented compared with LPV/r with TDF/FTC, but DRV/r has not been studied extensively in combination with ABC/3TC.[61] As a result, the combination of DRV/r with ABC/3TC is listed as an alternative initial regimen.

INSTI Options

Raltegravir was the first FDA-approved INSTI, and the first to be added to the US Department of Health and Human Services guidelines for initial ART. When studied in comparison with EFV plus TDF/FTC, RAL with TDF/FTC was found to be noninferior and well tolerated, with fewer neuropsychiatric side effects and a lower incidence of rash and dyslipidemia.[40,62] In combination with TDF/FTC, RAL was also compared with ATV/r and DRV/r in ACTG 5257; at 96 weeks, RAL was superior to both comparator arms using a combined virologic and tolerability endpoint.[60]

Myopathy and rhabdomyolysis have been reported with RAL, so patients at risk for these conditions may require additional monitoring, but these events are rare. In addition to the low rate of side effects, RAL has few drug–drug interactions, making it a better option than boosted-PI, COBI-containing, or even EFV-containing regimens for patients with complex concurrent medication regimens. However, RAL must be administered twice daily to maintain efficacy, which may be a significant barrier to adherence for some patients.[63] As with EFV-based and EVG/COBI-based regimens, virologic failure with RAL is more commonly associated with new drug resistance mutations than with boosted-PI regimens. Cationic supplements (calcium, magnesium, aluminum, and iron) can bind INSTIs and decrease efficacy, so dosing of such supplements with RAL, EVG, or DTG, should be separated by a few hours.

Dolutegravir is the newest INSTI, with FDA approval in August 2013. DTG is also the only INSTI that is dosed once daily without requiring pharmacokinetic boosting, which is helpful for the ease of dosing and for limiting drug–drug interactions. Three randomized clinical trials have been conducted with DTG comparing it with other recommended regimens:

- SPRING-2: DTG was noninferior to RAL; both were given with either TDF/FTC or ABC/3TC.[64]
- SINGLE: DTG plus ABC/3TC was superior to coformulated TDF/FTC/EFV, with the result largely driven by more drug discontinuations in the TDF/FTC/EFV arm.[25]
- FLAMINGO: When given with TDF/FTC or ABC/3TC, DTG was superior to DRV/r; results again were largely the result of more discontinuations in the DRV/r arm.[65]

A notable observation thus far in the DTG studies is that there were no treatment-associated, integrase inhibitor mutations observed in DTG-treated patients in these studies after regimen failure, suggesting that DTG has a greater barrier to resistance than NNRTIs and other INSTIs. In addition, ABC/3TC plus DTG maintains virologic efficacy in patients with pretreatment plasma HIV RNA greater than 100,000 copies/mL. As a result, both DTG + TDF/FTC and DTG + ABC/3TC are currently listed as recommended options for initial ART; the ABC/3TC + DTG option will become more attractive with the upcoming approval of a STR containing these drugs.

Overall, DTG is well tolerated. Insomnia has been reported with DTG, but has not led to treatment discontinuation in clinical trials. In addition, hypersensitivity to DTG has rarely been reported. As with COBI, it decreases tubular secretion of creatinine, causing a mild increase in serum creatinine; however, there have been no discontinuations owing to DTG-related renal adverse events reported to date. It shares with RAL a relative paucity of drug–drug interactions: The dose of the drug should be doubled to 50 mg twice daily when given with strong cytochrome3A4 inducers such as rifampin or EFV.

NNRTI with ABC Option

The final remaining recommended option for initial ART is EFV + ABC/3TC. As described, EFV-based treatment has been extensively studied. For patients who cannot take TDF, EFV + ABC/3TC may be an appropriate option. EFV is not available coformulated with ABC/3TC, but the components may be taken together once daily. The combination of EFV + ABC/3TC has been shown to be efficacious and well tolerated for most patients. However, an increased rate of virologic failure, compared with EFV/TDF/FTC, has been documented for patients with pretreatment plasma HIV RNA 100,000 copies/mL or greater, so EFV + ABC/3TC should not be used in this group.[23] A second study also demonstrated a higher rate of virologic failure when EFV + ABC/3TC was compared with EFV + TDF/FTC.[66]

ALTERNATIVE INITIAL REGIMENS

If the recommended initial ART regimens are not appropriate for a particular patient owing to drug toxicities, interactions, or preexisting conditions, then there are additional options. Given the large number of recommended regimens now available, these "alternative" regimens should be selected relatively infrequently. Now that many less toxic, effective options are available, several ARVs that were previously commonly used are no longer recommended as part of an initial ART regimen (**Table 4**). The alternative regimens for initial ART are listed in **Table 1**, and the distinguishing characteristics of the components of these regimens are presented in **Table 3**. Some of the alternative regimens are classified as such owing to their being fewer clinical trial data on the particular regimen. For example, there are limited comparative prospective clinical trial data on the regimens of ABC/3TC plus DRV/r, RAL, or RPV.[67] LPV/r has been studied extensively. However, the high pill burden (4 pills per day) and higher rates of adverse events (possibly secondary to a greater daily dose of RTV) with LPV/r make it a less attractive option.[61,68–70]

NRTI-SPARING OR NRTI-LIMITING OPTIONS

If a patient cannot take TDF or ABC, it may be necessary to consider other initial ART options. Unfortunately, most studies of NRTI-sparing regimens have yielded disappointing results with either inferior virologic efficacy, high rates of toxicity, or both. The hopes for a successful regimen with RAL with DRV/r were dampened when this regimen was shown to yield a high rate of virologic failure, especially for those with pretreatment plasma HIV RNA greater than 100,000 copies/mL.[71,72] Another recent study found that the combination of RAL with DRV/r was noninferior to TDF/FTC

Table 4
Antiretrovirals not recommended for initial antiretroviral therapy (ART)

Drug Class	Antiretroviral Drugs	Reasons Not Recommended for Initial ART
NRTIs	ddI, d4T, ZDV and the combination pill ZDV/3TC[a]	All agents: Lipoatrophy, lactic acidosis, hepatic steatosis ddI and d4T: Neuropathy, pancreatitis, noncirrhotic portal hypertension ZDV: Bone marrow suppression
NNRTIs	NVP	NVP: Severe rashes and potentially fatal hepatic events, especially in women with CD4 >250, men CD4 >400
	ETR	ETR: Not well studied in initial ART; used for treatment-experienced patients
PIs	FPV, IDV, NFV, SQV, and TPV	Higher pill burden, increased toxicities and/or lower virologic efficacy than other available agents Fosamprenavir may select for darunavir resistance
CCR5 antagonist	MVC	No benefit over other options and requires CCR5 tropism assay before initiation

Abbreviations: d4T, stavudine; ddI, didanosine; ETR, etravirine; FPV, fosamprenavir; IDV, indinavir; MVC, maraviroc; NFV, nelfinavir; NNRTI, nonnucleoside reverse transcriptase inhibitor; NRTI, nucleoside/nucleotide reverse transcriptase inhibitor; NVP, nevirapine; PI, protease inhibitor; SQV, saquinavir; TPV, tipranavir; ZDV, zidovudine; 3TC, lamivudine.
[a] ZDV and the combination pill ZDV/3TC are still used for initial ART for pregnant women.

with DRV/r, with minimal toxicities, but there was a trend toward decreased virologic efficacy as well as more new resistance mutations in the NRTI-sparing arm when the regimen failed.[73] One study demonstrated that the 2-drug regimen of LPV/r plus 3TC was as effective and better tolerated than LPV/r plus 2 NRTI.[74] However, practical application of this study's results is limited given the use of twice daily LPV/r. It is hoped that better NRTI-sparing or NRTI-limiting options will be available in the future.

SUMMARY AND FUTURE DIRECTIONS

There are now numerous safe and effective options for initial therapy. Clinicians and patients have the luxury of choosing between 10 recommended regimens, all of which have shown durable virologic suppression and favorable safety profiles. The optimal initial choice for therapy should take into consideration individual patient characteristics, which will improve long-term outcomes. Many patients will prefer 1 of the 3 single-tablet once daily regimens, which have been shown to improve adherence and may decrease health care costs; we recommend these options for most patients. As noted, coformulated DTG/ABC/3TC will be available soon.

Because of the success of existing strategies for initial therapy, investigational treatments must offer substantial benefits—safety/tolerability, efficacy, or cost—before being adopted as part of recommended regimens. Although 1 modeling analysis found that using separate generic versions of coformulated TDF/FTC/EFV would be a cost-effective strategy,[75] thus far the impact of generic ARVs on HIV prescribing practices in the United States is relatively modest—that could change as further agents go off patent. A prodrug of TDF, tenofovir alafenamide, achieves higher intracellular concentrations of TDF diphosphate (the active component) with lower plasma exposures. This strategy allows lower milligram dosing with comparable antiviral potency, as well as lower renal and bone toxicity.[76] It is currently in Phase III clinical trials. An investigational NNRTI, doravirine, can be given once daily and may have the antiviral potency of EFV and a more favorable tolerability profile.[77] Phase III studies are about to begin. Finally, long-acting antivirals, such as 744 and reformulated RPV, offer the possibility of once-monthly dosing, by injection; proof-of-concept studies have been conducted with this combination.[78] Such a strategy could conceivably be adopted by community workers for patients who struggle to adhere to daily treatment and doctor's visits.

REFERENCES

1. Van Sighem A, Gras LA, Reiss P, et al. Life expectancy of recently diagnosed asymptomatic HIV-infected patients approaches that of uninfected individuals. AIDS 2010;24(10):1527–35.
2. Rodger AJ, Lodwick R, Schechter M, et al. Mortality in well controlled HIV in the continuous antiretroviral therapy arms of the SMART and ESPRIT trials compared with the general population. AIDS 2013;27(6):973–9.
3. Vittinghoff E, Scheer S, O'Malley P, et al. Combination antiretroviral therapy and recent declines in AIDS incidence and mortality. J Infect Dis 1999;179(3): 717–20.
4. Palella FJ Jr, Delaney KM, Moorman AC, et al. Declining morbidity and mortality among patients with advanced human immunodeficiency virus infection. HIV Outpatient Study Investigators. N Engl J Med 1998;338(13):853–60.
5. Reekie J, Gatell JM, Yust I, et al. Fatal and nonfatal AIDS and non-AIDS events in HIV-1-positive individuals with high CD4 cell counts according to viral load strata. AIDS 2011;25(18):2259–68.

6. Kalayjian RC, Franceschini N, Gupta SK, et al. Suppression of HIV-1 replication by antiretroviral therapy improves renal function in persons with low CD4 counts and chronic kidney disease. AIDS 2008;22(4):481–7.

7. Estrella M, Fine DM, Gallant JE, et al. HIV type 1 RNA level as a clinical indicator of renal pathology in HIV-infected patients. Clin Infect Dis 2006;43(3): 377–80.

8. Zoufaly A, Stellbrink HJ, Heiden MA, et al. Cumulative HIV viremia during highly active antiretroviral therapy is a strong predictor of AIDS-related lymphoma. J Infect Dis 2009;200(1):79–87.

9. Silverberg MJ, Neuhaus J, Bower M, et al. Risk of cancers during interrupted antiretroviral therapy in the SMART study. AIDS 2007;21(14):1957–63.

10. Neuhaus J, Jacobs DR Jr, Baker JV, et al. Markers of inflammation, coagulation, and renal function are elevated in adults with HIV infection. J Infect Dis 2010; 201(12):1788–95.

11. Bhaskaran K, Mussini C, Antinori A, et al. Changes in the incidence and predictors of human immunodeficiency virus-associated dementia in the era of highly active antiretroviral therapy. Ann Neurol 2008;63(2):213–21.

12. Peters MG, Andersen J, Lynch P, et al. Randomized controlled study of tenofovir and adefovir in chronic hepatitis B virus and HIV infection: ACTG A5127. Hepatology 2006;44(5):1110–6.

13. Strategies for Management of Antiretroviral Therapy (SMART) Study Group, El-Sadr WM, Lundgren J, et al. CD4+ count-guided interruption of antiretroviral treatment. N Engl J Med 2006;355(22):2283–96.

14. Islam FM, Wu J, Jansson J, et al. Relative risk of cardiovascular disease among people living with HIV: a systematic review and meta-analysis. HIV Med 2012; 13(8):453–68.

15. Kuller LH, Tracy R, Belloso W, et al. Inflammatory and coagulation biomarkers and mortality in patients with HIV infection. PLoS Med 2008;5(10):e203.

16. Sandler NG, Wand H, Roque A, et al. Plasma levels of soluble CD14 independently predict mortality in HIV infection. J Infect Dis 2011;203(6):780–90.

17. Mofenson LM, Lambert JS, Stiehm ER, et al. Risk factors for perinatal transmission of human immunodeficiency virus type 1 in women treated with zidovudine. Pediatric AIDS Clinical Trials Group Study 185 Team. N Engl J Med 1999;341(6): 385–93.

18. Wood E, Kerr T, Marshall BD, et al. Longitudinal community plasma HIV-1 RNA concentrations and incidence of HIV-1 among injecting drug users: prospective cohort study. BMJ 2009;338:b1649.

19. Cohen MS, Chen YQ, McCauley M, et al. Prevention of HIV-1 infection with early antiretroviral therapy. N Engl J Med 2011;365(6):493–505.

20. Granich RM, Gilks CF, Dye C, et al. Universal voluntary HIV testing with immediate antiretroviral therapy as a strategy for elimination of HIV transmission: a mathematical model. Lancet 2009;373(9657):48–57.

21. Panel on Antiretroviral Guidelines for Adults and Adolescents. Guidelines for the use of antiretroviral agents in HIV-1-infected adults and adolescents. Department of Health and Human Services. Available at: http://aidsinfo.nih.gov/ContentFiles/AdultandAdolescentGL.pdf. Accessed August 2, 2014.

22. Thompson MA, Aberg JA, Hoy JF, et al. Antiretroviral treatment of adult HIV infection: 2012 recommendations of the International Antiviral Society-USA panel. JAMA 2012;308(4):387–402.

23. Sax PE, Tierney C, Collier AC, et al. Abacavir-lamivudine versus tenofovir-emtricitabine for initial HIV-1 therapy. N Engl J Med 2009;361(23):2230–40.

24. Smith KY, Patel P, Fine D, et al. Randomized double-blind, placebo-matched, multi-center trial of abacavir/lamivudine or tenofovir/emtricitabine with lopinavir/ritonavir for initial HIV treatment. AIDS 2009;23(12):1547–56.

25. Walmsley SL, Antela A, Clumeck N, et al. Dolutegravir plus abacavir-lamivudine for the treatment of HIV-1 infection. N Engl J Med 2013;369(19):1807–18.

26. Mocroft A, Kirk O, Reiss P, et al. Estimated glomerular filtration rate, chronic kidney disease and antiretroviral drug use in HIV-positive patients. AIDS 2010; 24(11):1667–78.

27. Zimmermann AE, Pizzoferrato T, Bedford J, et al. Tenofovir-associated acute and chronic kidney disease: a case of multiple drug interactions. Clin Infect Dis 2006; 42(2):283–90.

28. McComsey GA, Kitch D, Daar ES, et al. Bone mineral density and fractures in antiretroviral-naive persons randomized to receive abacavir-lamivudine or tenofovir disoproxil fumarate-emtricitabine along with efavirenz or atazanavir-ritonavir: AIDS Clinical Trials Group A5224s, a substudy of ACTG A5202. J Infect Dis 2011;203(12):1791–801.

29. Haskelberg H, Hoy JF, Amin J, et al. Changes in bone turnover and bone loss in HIV-infected patients changing treatment to tenofovir-emtricitabine or abacavir-lamivudine. PLoS One 2012;7:e38377.

30. Kosi L, Reiberger T, Payer BA, et al. Five-year on-treatment efficacy of lamivudine-, tenofovir- and tenofovir + emtricitabine-based HAART in HBV-HIV-coinfected patients. J Viral Hepat 2012;19(11):801–10.

31. Mallal S, Phillips E, Carosi G, et al. HLA-B*5701 screening for hypersensitivity to abacavir. N Engl J Med 2008;358(6):568–79.

32. D:A:D Study Group, Sabin CA, Worm SW, et al. Use of nucleoside reverse transcriptase inhibitors and risk of myocardial infarction in HIV-infected patients enrolled in the D:A:D study: a multi-cohort collaboration. Lancet 2008; 371(9622):1417–26.

33. Obel N, Farkas DK, Kronborg G, et al. Abacavir and risk of myocardial infarction in HIV-infected patients on highly active antiretroviral therapy: a population-based nationwide cohort study. HIV Med 2010;11(2):130–6.

34. Choi AI, Vittinghoff E, Deeks SG, et al. Cardiovascular risks associated with abacavir and tenofovir exposure in HIV-infected persons. AIDS 2011;25(10): 1289–98.

35. Ding X, Andraca-Carrera E, Cooper C, et al. No association of abacavir use with myocardial infarction: findings of an FDA meta-analysis. J Acquir Immune Defic Syndr 2012;61(4):441–7.

36. Aldir I, Horta A, Serrado M. Single-tablet regimens in HIV: does it really make a difference? Curr Med Res Opin 2014;30(1):89–97.

37. Cohen CJ, Meyers JL, Davis KL. Association between daily antiretroviral pill burden and treatment adherence, hospitalisation risk, and other healthcare utilisation and costs in a US Medicaid population with HIV. BMJ Open 2013;3(8): e003028.

38. Sax PE, Meyers JL, Mugavero M, et al. Adherence to antiretroviral treatment and correlation with risk of hospitalization among commercially insured HIV patients in the United States. PLoS One 2012;7(2):e31591.

39. Gallant JE, DeJesus E, Arribas JR, et al. Tenofovir DF, emtricitabine, and efavirenz vs. zidovudine, lamivudine, and efavirenz for HIV. N Engl J Med 2006;354(3): 251–60.

40. Lennox JL, DeJesus E, Lazzarin A, et al. Safety and efficacy of raltegravir-based versus efavirenz-based combination therapy in treatment-naïve patients with

HIV-1 infection: a multicenter, double-blind randomized controlled trial. Lancet 2009;374(9692):796–806.

41. Daar ES, Tierney C, Fischl MA, et al. Atazanavir plus ritonavir or efavirenz as part of a 3-drug regimen for initial treatment of HIV-1. Ann Intern Med 2011;154(7): 445–56.

42. Cohen CJ, Molina JM, Cahn P, et al. Efficacy and safety of rilpivirine (TMC278) versus efavirenz at 48 weeks in treatment-naïve HIV-1 infected patients: pooled results from the phase 3 double-blind randomized ECHO and THRIVE Trials. J Acquir Immune Defic Syndr 2012;60(1):33–42.

43. Sax PE, DeJesus E, Mills A, et al. Co-formulated elvitegravir, cobicistat, emtricitabine, and tenofovir versus co-formulated efavirenz, emtricitabine, and tenofovir for initial treatment of HIV-1 infection: a randomized, double-blind, phase 3 trial, analysis of results after 48 weeks. Lancet 2012;379(9835):2439–48.

44. Ford N, Mofenson L, Kranzer K, et al. Safety of efavirenz in first-trimester of pregnancy: a systematic review and meta-analysis of outcomes from observational cohorts. AIDS 2010;24(1):1461–70.

45. Ford N, Calmy A, Mofenson L. Safety of efavirenz in the first trimester of pregnancy: an updated systematic review and meta-analysis. AIDS 2011;25(18):2301–4.

46. Panel on Treatment of HIV-Infected Pregnant Women and Prevention of Perinatal Transmission. Recommendations for use of antiretroviral drugs in pregnant hiv-1-infected women for maternal health and interventions to reduce perinatal HIV transmission in the United States. Available at: http://aidsinfo.nih.gov/contentfiles/lvguidelines/PerinatalGL.pdf. Accessed August 2, 2014.

47. World Health Organization. Consolidated guidelines on the use of antiretroviral drugs for treating and preventing HIV infection. 2013. Available at: http://www.who.int/hiv/pub/guidelines/arv2013/en/. Accessed August 2, 2014.

48. Mollan K, Smurzynski M, Eron JJ, et al. Association between efavirenz as initial therapy for HIV-1 infection and increased risk for suicidal ideation or attempted or completed suicide: An Analysis of Trial Data. Annals of Internal Medicine 2014;161:1–10.

49. Wohl DA, Cohen C, Gallant JE, et al. A randomized, double-blind comparison of single-tablet regimen elvitegravir/cobicistat/emtricitabine/tenofovir DF versus single-tablet regimen efavirenz/emtricitabine/tenofovir DF for initial treatment of HIV-1 infection: analysis of week 144 results. J Acquir Immune Defic Syndr 2014;65(3):e118–20.

50. Clumeck N, Molina JM, Henry K, et al. A randomized, double-blind comparison of single-tablet regimen elvitegravir/cobicistat/emtricitabine/tenofovir DF vs ritonavir-boosted atazanavir plus emtricitabine/tenofovir/DF for initial treatment of HIV-1 infection: analysis of week 144 results. J Acquir Immune Defic Syndr 2014;65(3):e121–4.

51. Antiretroviral Pregnancy Registry Steering Committee. Antiretroviral Pregnancy Registry international interim report for 1 January 1989 through 31 July 2013. Wilmington (NC): Registry Coordinating Center; 2013. Available at: www.APRegistry.com. Accessed August 2, 2014.

52. Gilead Sciences. Phase 3B study to evaluate the safety and efficacy of elvitegravir/cobicistat/emtricitabine/tenofovir disoproxil fumarate versus ritonavir-boosted atazanavir plus emtricitabine/tenofovir disoproxil fumarate in HIV-1 infected, antiretroviral treatment-naïve women (WAVES). In ClinicalTrials.gov [Internet]. Bethesda (MD): National Library of Medicine (US); 2000. NLM Identifier NCT01705574. Available at: http://clinicaltrials.gov/ct2/show/NCT01705574?term=nct01705574&rank=1. Accessed March 8, 2014.

53. Gilead Sciences. STRIBILD Package Insert (Prescribing Information). Reference ID: 3179895. Available at: http://www.accessdata.fda.gov/drugsatfda_docs/label/2012/203100s000lbl.pdf. Accessed August 2, 2014.

54. Cohen C, Wohl D, Arribas JR, et al. Week 48 results from a randomized clinical trial of rilpivirine/emtricitabine/tenofovir disoproxil fumarate vs. efavirenz/emtricitabine/tenofovir disoproxil fumarate in treatment-naïve HIV-1-infected adults. AIDS 2014; 28:989–97.

55. Cohen CJ, Andrade-Villanueva J, Clotet B, et al. Rilpivirine versus efavirenz with two background nucleoside or nucleotide reverse transcriptase inhibitors in treatment-naïve adults infected with HIV-1 (THRIVE): a phase 3, randomized, non-inferiority trial. Lancet 2011;378(9787):229–37.

56. Molina JM, Cahn P, Grinsztejn B, et al. Rilpivirine versus efavirenz with tenofovir and emtricitabine in treatment-naïve adults infected with HIV-1 (ECHO): a phase 3 randomised double-blind active-controlled trial. Lancet 2011;378(9787): 238–46.

57. Cohen C, Wohl D, Arribas JR, et al. Week 48 results from a randomized clinical trial of rilpivirine/emtricitabine/tenofovir disoproxil fumarate vs. efavirenz/emtricitabine/tenofovir disoproxil fumarate in treatment-naive HIV-1-infected adults. AIDS 2014;28(7):989–97.

58. Gilead Sciences. COMPLERA Package Insert (Prescribing Information). Available at: http://www.gilead.com/~/media/Files/pdfs/medicines/hiv/complera/complera_pi.PDF. Accessed December, 2013.

59. Molina JM, Andrade-Villanueva J, Echevarria J, et al. Once-daily atazanavir/ritonavir compared with twice-daily lopinavir/ritonavir, each in combination with tenofovir and emtricitabine, for management of antiretroviral-naïve HIV-1-infected patients: 96-week efficacy and safety results of the CASTLE study. J Acquir Immune Defic Syndr 2010;53(3):323–32.

60. Landovitz RL, Ribaudo HJ, Ofotokun I, et al. Efficacy and tolerability of atazanavir, raltegravir or darunavir with FTC/tenofovir: ACTG 5257. CROI 2014. Conference on Retroviruses and Opportunistic Infections [abstract: 85]. Boston, March 3–6, 2014.

61. Mills AM, Nelson M, Jayaweera D, et al. Once-daily darunavir/ritonavir vs. lopinavir/ritonavir in treatment-naïve, HIV-1-infected patients: 96-week analysis. AIDS 2009;23(13):1679–88.

62. Rockstroh JK, DeJesus E, Lennox JL, et al. Durable efficacy and safety of raltegravir versus efavirenz when combined with tenofovir/emtricitabine in treatment-naïve HIV-1-infected patients: final 5-year results from STARTMRK. J Acquir Immune Defic Syndr 2013;63(1):77–85.

63. Eron JJ Jr, Rockstroh JK, Reynes J, et al. Raltegravir once daily or twice daily in previously untreated patients with HIV-1: a randomized, active-controlled phase 3 non-inferiority trial. Lancet Infect Dis 2011;11(12):907–15.

64. Raffi F, Jaeger H, Quiros-Roldan E, et al. Once-daily dolutegravir versus twice-daily raltegravir in antiretroviral-naïve adults with HIV-1 infection (SPRING-2 study): 96 week results from a randomized, double blind, non-inferiority trial. Lancet Infect Dis 2013;13(11):927–35.

65. Clotet B, Feinberg J, van Lunzen J, et al. Once-daily dolutegravir versus darunavir plus ritonavir in antiretroviral-naive adults with HIV-1 infection (FLAMINGO): 48 week results from the randomised open-label phase 3b study. Lancet 2014;383(9936):2222–31.

66. Moyle GJ, Stellbrink HJ, Compston J, et al. 96-week results of abacavir/lamivudine versus tenofovir/emtricitabine, plus efavirenz, in antiretroviral-naïve, HIV-1 infected adults: ASSERT study. Antivir Ther 2013;18(7):905–13.

67. De los Santos I, Gomez-Berrocal A, Valencia E, et al. Efficacy and tolerability of darunavir/ritonavir in combination with abacavir/lamivudine: an option in selected HIV-infected patients. HIV Clin Trials 2013;14(5):254–9.

68. Orkin C, DeJesus E, Khanlou H, et al. Final 192-week efficacy and safety of once-daily darunavir/ritonavir compared with lopinavir/ritonavir in HIV-1-infected treatment-naïve patients in the ARTEMIS trial. HIV Med 2013;14(1):49–59.

69. Worm SW, Sabin C, Weber R, et al. Risk of myocardial infarction in patients with HIV infection exposed to specific individual antiretroviral drugs from the 3 major drug classes: the data collection on adverse events of anti-HIV drugs (D:A:D) study. J Infect Dis 2010;201(3):318–30.

70. Lang S, Mary-Krause M, Cotte L, et al. Impact of individual antiretroviral drugs on the risk of myocardial infarction in human immunodeficiency virus-infected patients: a case-control study nested within the French Hospital Database on HIV ANRS cohort CO4. Arch Intern Med 2010;170(14):1228–38.

71. Taiwo B, Zheng L, Gallien S, et al. Efficacy of a nucleoside-sparing regimen of darunavir/ritonavir plus raltegravir in treatment-naïve HIV-1 infected patients (ACTG A5262). AIDS 2011;25(17):2113–22.

72. Bedimo R, Drechsler H, Cutrell J, et al. RADAR study: week 48 safety and efficacy of raltegravir combined with boosted darunavir compared to tenofovir/emtricitabine combined with boosted darunavir in antiretroviral-naïve patients: impact on bone health. 7th IAS Conference on HIV Pathogenesis, Treatment and Prevention [abstract: WEPE512]. Kuala Lumpur, June 20–July 3, 2013.

73. Raffi F, Babiker AG, Richert L, et al. First-line RAL + DRV/r is non-inferior to TDF/FTC + DRV/r: the NEAT001/ANRS 143 randomised trial. 21st Conference on Retroviruses and Opportunistic Infections (CROI 2014) [abstract: 84LB]. Boston, March 3–6, 2014.

74. Cahn P, Andrade-Villanueva J, Arribas JR, et al. Dual therapy with lopinavir and ritonavir plus lamivudine versus triple therapy with lopinavir and ritonavir plus two nucleoside reverse transcriptase inhibitors in antiretroviral-therapy-naive adults with HIV-1 infection: 48 week results of the randomised, open label, non-inferiority GARDEL trial. Lancet Infect Dis 2014;14(7):572–80.

75. Walensky RP, Sax PE, Nakamura YM, et al. Economic savings versus health losses: the cost-effectiveness of generic antiretroviral therapy in the United States. Ann Intern Med 2013;158(2):84–92.

76. Sax PE, Zolopa A, Brar I, et al. Tenofovir alafenamide vs. Tenofovir disoproxil fumarate in single tablet regimens for initial HIV-1 therapy: a randomized phase 2 study. J Acquir Immune Defic Syndr May 27, 2014. [Epub ahead of print].

77. Morales-Ramirez JO, Gatell JM, Hagins DP, et al. Safety and antiviral activity of MK-1439, a novel NNRTI, in treatment-naïve HIV+ patients. 21st Conference on Retroviruses and Opportunistic Infections (CROI 2014) [abstract: 92LB]. Boston, March 3–6, 2014.

78. Margolis DA, Brinson CC, Eron JJ, et al. 744 and rilpivirine as two drug oral maintenance therapy: LAI116482 (LATTE) week 48 results. 20th Conference on Retroviruses and Opportunistic Infections (CROI 2014) [abstract: 91LB]. Boston, March 3–6, 2014.

Antiretroviral Therapy

Treatment-experienced Individuals

Katya R. Calvo, MD[a], Eric S. Daar, MD[b],*

KEYWORDS

- Treatment experienced • HIV resistance • Treatment simplification
- Antiretroviral failure

KEY POINTS

- Modifying antiretroviral therapy (ART) requires knowledge of efficacy and tolerability of prior regimens, resistance test results, and careful assessment of ART adherence.
- Individuals experiencing suboptimal virologic response on ART should be assessed for modifiable factors that relate to the individual (eg, adherence) and the drugs (eg, absorption, drug-drug and drug-food interactions) before treatment modification.
- Once suboptimal virologic response is confirmed, a delay in modifying therapy is associated with worse virologic and clinical outcomes.
- There are strategic differences in modifying therapy in individuals failing first-line failure versus those who are highly treatment experienced.
- ART simplification in virologically suppressed individuals should take into consideration potential or known archived drug-resistant virus.

INTRODUCTION

Managing antiretroviral therapy (ART)–experienced individuals requires a systematic approach in order to optimize outcomes. Consideration must be given to the different reasons for switching or modifying therapy in a given person. These reasons range from the management of suboptimal virologic response, poor tolerability, to enhance convenience, or to minimize interactions with other medications or food. This article categorizes individuals as those planning to modify therapy for suboptimal virologic response or while maintaining virologic suppression.

[a] Division of HIV Medicine, Department of Internal Medicine, Harbor-UCLA Medical Center, David Geffen School of Medicine at UCLA, 1124 West Carson Street, CDCRC 203, Torrance, CA 90502, USA; [b] Division of HIV Medicine, Department of Internal Medicine, Harbor-UCLA Medical Center, David Geffen School of Medicine at UCLA, 1124 West Carson Street, CDCRC 205, Torrance, CA 90502, USA
* Corresponding author.
E-mail address: edaar@labiomed.org

Infect Dis Clin N Am 28 (2014) 439–456
http://dx.doi.org/10.1016/j.idc.2014.06.005
0891-5520/14/$ – see front matter © 2014 Elsevier Inc. All rights reserved.

id.theclinics.com

The goal of therapy for ART-experienced individuals remains the same as for those who are starting therapy for the first time: to suppress plasma human immunodeficiency virus (HIV) RNA to undetectable levels. There are numerous highly effective and well-tolerated options for those initiating therapy for the first time.[1,2] This therapeutic goal becomes more challenging in ART-experienced persons with histories of drug intolerance or resistance. This article provides guidance for clinicians managing ART-experienced individuals.

ART-EXPERIENCED INDIVIDUALS WITH SUBOPTIMAL VIROLOGIC RESPONSE

Although there are no standardized definitions for virologic response, there is a consensus that plasma HIV RNA should ideally be suppressed to below the limits of detection of the available assays. Nevertheless, responses vary and each situation needs to be defined in order to address specific management strategies. Although such definitions may change with time, conceptualizing what is meant by each is important and they have been proposed in the current treatment guidelines and are summarized in **Table 1**.[1]

For the purposes of this article, suboptimal virologic response is defined as incomplete virologic response or rebound. The causes of suboptimal virologic response can be separated into factors related to the individual and those related to the antiretroviral regimen.[6–8]

Table 1
Definitions of virologic response

Term	Definition	Comment
Virologic suppression	Plasma HIV RNA below the lower limits of detection of the available assay	—
Virologic failure	Inability to achieve or maintain suppression of plasma HIV RNA levels to <200 copies/mL	With newer assays, level of detection is much less than 200 copies/mL. Although the goal is to maintain an undetectable viral load, some patients do not achieve this goal but maintain levels less than 200 copies/mL. Although these persons may be at risk for virologic failure,[3,4] the risk seems to be low and the optimal management in this situation is not defined[1,5]
Incomplete virologic response	Two consecutive plasma HIV RNA levels >200 copies/mL after 24 wk of ART	The time to this goal may vary depending on baseline plasma HIV RNA and type of ART initiated
Virologic rebound	Confirmed plasma HIV RNA >200 copies/mL after virologic suppression is achieved	—
Virologic blip	Isolated detectable plasma HIV RNA level after virologic suppression, followed by return to virologic suppression	This does not seem to be an increased risk for virologic failure

Causes of Suboptimal Virologic Response

The causes of suboptimal virologic response may vary from person to person and require different management approaches, some of which are summarized in **Table 2** and later in this article.

- Starting with higher plasma HIV RNA, with which it may take longer than 24 weeks to achieve full virologic suppression[9]
- Having inadequate drug levels resulting from poor adherence, or drug-drug or drug-food interactions
- Using a regimen with inadequate potency either because of intrinsic properties of the drugs or the presence of drug-resistant virus acquired at the time of infection and/or selected for during the course of therapy

Defining which of these factors may be contributing to suboptimal virologic response is a critical first step in the management of these individuals. If the suboptimal response is a result of taking the medication incorrectly then further instruction and adherence counseling may suffice. It is critical to identify reasons for poor adherence so that they can be managed. Common barriers to adherence include substance abuse, psychiatric illnesses, or unstable living situations, which need to be addressed as soon as possible or there is a risk of jeopardizing success with future regimens. If poor adherence is related to medication intolerance, then substitution of another drug usually is sufficient.

Suspected Drug Resistance

If suboptimal virologic response persists after careful review and management of the modifiable causes outlined earlier, drug resistance testing should be obtained while patients are taking their current regimens or within 4 weeks after regimen discontinuation.[1] Resistance tests are most reliable when plasma viral load is greater than 1000 copies/mL; however, testing can sometimes be performed successfully in patients with plasma HIV RNA less than 1000 copies/mL,[10] although for technical and logistical reasons this is not always possible.

Genotypic drug resistance testing is preferred for patients failing first-line or second-line regimens. Genotypic testing yields pertinent results regarding protease inhibitor (PI), non-nucleoside reverse transcriptase inhibitor (NNRTI), and nucleoside reverse transcriptase inhibitor (NRTI) resistance. The same is true for integrase strand transfer inhibitor (InSTI) resistance, although often this needs to be ordered separately. The role of phenotypic drug resistance testing is limited to patients with complex drug resistance patterns, especially to the PIs. In select situations additional testing may be ordered to assess resistance to the fusion inhibitor enfuvirtide or for viral tropism in

Table 2
Common reasons for suboptimal virologic response

Drug Related	Patient/Virus Related
Intolerance	High baseline plasma HIV RNA
Pharmacologic (eg, drug-drug or drug-food interactions)	Low baseline CD4 cell count
	Transmitted or acquired drug resistance mutations
Complex dosing schedule	Comorbidities (eg, substance abuse, psychiatric illnesses, neurocognitive deficits)
Suboptimal potency	Poor adherence
	Missed appointments
	Poor access to medications

patients considering the use of, or experiencing virologic failure on, a CCR5 antagonist. Useful resources to assist clinicians in interpreting the results of drug resistance testing are available from the International Antiviral Society–USA (iasusa.org) and Stanford University Drug Resistance Database (hivdb.stanford.edu).

Management of Suboptimal Virologic Response

Confirmed persistent plasma HIV RNA, especially when greater than 200 copies/mL, often results in the emergence of drug-resistant virus. A delay in treatment modification can be associated with increasing accumulation of resistance conferring mutations to drugs in the current regimen that often are cross-resistant to drugs not in the current regimen.[11] As a result, viral suppression is more likely to occur when a therapeutic switch occurs in patients with low plasma HIV RNA and/or high CD4 T-cell counts.[12] Once a decision is made to modify ART, guidelines traditionally recommend that patients with suboptimal virologic response be changed to a regimen that includes at least 2, and preferable 3, fully active drugs.[1,13,14] The less potent the regimen (ie, <3 fully active drugs), the higher the rate of subsequent virologic failure.[3] The optimal new regimen is defined by careful review of the given individual's treatment history, prior drug resistance testing, and, when appropriate, tropism results.

Strategies for the management of suboptimal virologic response in patients with plasma HIV persistently greater than 200 copies/mL after at least 24 weeks of therapy can be stratified by the following clinical scenarios:

1. First-line regimen
2. Failed multiple regimens with drug-resistant virus
3. Resistance testing cannot be performed, such as when plasma HIV RNA is less than 500 to 1000 copies/mL
4. Testing shows no significant resistance
5. The individual has a history of suboptimal virologic response but has been off all therapy for months

Clinical scenario: suboptimal virologic response on first-line therapy

Based on currently preferred treatment options most of these individuals are on 2 NRTIs, one of which is a cytosine analogue (ie, lamivudine or emtricitabine) with an NNRTI, pharmacologically boosted PI, or an InSTI. Management of suboptimal virologic response in each of these cases is addressed later and summarized in **Table 3**.

NRTIs plus NNRTI Resistance testing typically shows either no detectable drug resistance, which can occur on any regimen and is discussed later, or resistance limited to the NNRTI, or the NNRTI plus the cytosine analogue.[15,16]

Following first-line NNRTI-based regimen failure, 2 to 3 NRTIs plus ritonavir-boosted lopinavir typically results in high levels of virologic suppression.[17–19] Two studies compared this strategy with ritonavir-boosted lopinavir monotherapy, showing inferior outcomes in therapy not including NRTIs.[17,19] The excellent response to NRTIs plus the ritonavir-boosted PI occurred despite the frequent presence of extensive NRTI resistance, consistent with findings in an observational cohort study.[20] Ritonavir-boosted lopinavir plus twice-daily raltegravir yielded similar levels of viral suppression to the NRTIs combined with the ritonavir-boosted PI.[18,19] Thus, an optimal management strategy for these individuals is to use a pharmacologically boosted PI with NRTIs[1,21] or to use raltegravir with a pharmacologically boosted PI, although it is not known whether similar results would be achieved with alternative PIs or InSTIs. In choosing between these options consideration must be given to dosing frequency,

Table 3
Management of suboptimal virologic response on first-line antiretroviral therapy

NRTI Plus NNRTI with Suboptimal Virologic Response	
No resistance	Adherence counseling Switch to any alternative first-line preferred option
NNRTI with or without NRTI resistance	2–3 NRTIs plus pharmacologically boosted PI InSTI plus pharmacologically boosted PI
NRTI Plus Pharmacologically Boosted PI with Suboptimal Virologic Response	
No resistance	Adherence counseling Switch to any alternative first-line preferred option

NRTI resistance	Adherence counseling
	Switch to alternative NRTIs and/or
	  pharmacologically boosted PI to enhance
	  convenience and/or tolerability

NRTI plus InSTI with Suboptimal Virologic Response	
No resistance	Adherence counseling Switch to any alternative first-line preferred option
Resistance	2–3 NRTIs plus a pharmacologically boosted PI Susceptible InSTI plus a pharmacologically boosted PI

overall tolerability, the reasons for failure of the prior regimen, the consequences of failure (such as InSTI resistance), and the cost of therapy.

Second-generation NNRTIs, such as etravirine and rilpivirine, remain active against some strains that are resistant to efavirenz and nevirapine, in particular strains with the K103N mutation. Nevertheless, a switch to an alternative NNRTI must be made with caution because the presence of underlying NRTI resistance can result in inferior virologic response.[22] Although several recent InSTI-based first-line studies included subjects with transmitted NNRTI resistance, consideration of switching patients failing an NNRTI-based regimen to NRTIs plus an InSTI should be done with caution because concomitant NRTI resistance can limit efficacy.[23,24]

NRTIs plus pharmacologically boosted PIs In this setting, clinically relevant PI resistance is extremely rare and NRTI resistance occurs at a variable rate.[15,25,26] Plasma HIV RNA levels persistently greater than 200 copies/mL in this setting are most likely a result of poor adherence, or drug-drug or drug-food interactions. Clinical experience and a recent systematic review of multiple randomized controlled trials of ritonavir-boosted PI first-line failure suggest that, in this setting, reinforcing adherence and maintaining the current regimen is as likely to result in virologic suppression as a modification in therapy.[27]

NRTIs plus InSTI Patients experiencing virologic failure on NRTIs plus either raltegravir or elvitegravir frequently have either no detectable drug resistance or resistance to the cytosine analogue with or without to the InSTI.[23,28–30] In contrast, patients failing NRTIs plus dolutegravir as a first-line regimen have not been shown to develop InSTI resistance.[31–33] Although there are very few data defining how patients failing NRTIs plus InSTI-based first-line therapy should be managed, it is reasonable to extrapolate from the data in first-line NNRTI failures in which a regimen of NRTIs plus a ritonavir-boosted PI is highly effective. A ritonavir-boosted PI plus a susceptible InSTI is also a reasonable option.

Clinical scenario: suboptimal virologic response after having failed multiple regimens with drug-resistant virus

Designing a new regimen for patients who have experienced virologic failure on multiple drug classes is a complex situation that frequently requires expert consultation. The guiding principle is that at least 2, and preferably 3, fully active agents representing at least 2 different classes be included in any new regimen. A detailed ART history along with review of prior and current genotypic and phenotypic drug resistance studies, along with the possible use of tropism testing, should be collected. Once this information is gathered the clinician can determine which drugs are likely to be fully or partially active for inclusion in the next regimen.

For patients with single-class–resistant virus, or resistance limited to NRTIs with either NNRTIs or InSTIs, treatment strategies may mirror those outlined earlier for first-line therapy failure. The focus here is on the management of patients with more complicated multiclass resistance. The discussion of treatment strategies is separated based on whether options do or do not exist to achieve full virologic suppression.

Treatment strategies when a fully suppressive regimen is likely to be achievable Most regimens used in highly treatment-experienced individuals include a combination of NRTIs, a pharmacologically boosted PI, and some combination of other drugs such as an InSTI, enfuvirtide, and/or a CCR5 antagonist. The activity of these drugs is determined by genotypic and/or phenotypic drug resistance testing and a tropism assay. Patients who have never been exposed to enfuvirtide or an InSTI are likely to have viruses fully susceptible to these agents.

The TRIO study showed the outcome associated with using multiple active drugs in highly treatment-experienced individuals. InSTI-naive and darunavir-naive individuals received ritonavir-boosted darunavir with raltegravir and the second-generation NNRTI, etravirine, along with other drugs at the discretion of the investigator, with resultant high levels of viral suppression.[34] Data from this study along with those from other treatment-experienced trials using novel drugs have reinforced the importance of attempting to incorporate at least 2, and preferably 3, fully active agents into a new regimen, including individual studies in which new drugs such as raltegravir, maraviroc, enfuvirtide, elvitegravir, and dolutegravir were included as part of a new regimen in treatment-experienced individuals.[28,35–42]

The same applies when using second-generation drugs in existing classes that often, but not always, lack cross-resistance with first-generation drugs in the class. These drugs include the PIs tipranavir[43] and darunavir[13,44] as well as the NNRTI etravirine[14] and the InSTI dolutegravir.[45,46] These studies further showed how susceptibility can be predicted for these second-generation agents.

The second-generation NNRTI etravirine maintains activity against select NNRTI-resistant viruses,[47] with clinical trials showing that, when used in combination with darunavir plus ritonavir and an optimized background regimen, there was better virologic responses than the same regimens without etravirine.[14,48,49] It was further shown that 17 reverse transcriptase mutations were associated with reduced response to etravirine[50] with a weighted scoring system developed to assist in evaluating when etravirine is likely to be active (**Table 4**).

Second-generation PIs have also been shown to have antiviral activity against select PI-resistant viruses, including ritonavir-boosted tipranavir for which activity can be predicted based on genotypic pattern.[43,51] Similar data exist for ritonavir-boosted darunavir.[13,52,53] Early data from darunavir studies showed that optimal response to twice-daily darunavir boosted by ritonavir (600 mg and 100 mg, respectively) was seen when fewer than 3 of a list of mutations were present (ie, V11I, V32I,

Table 4
Predicting susceptibility to etravirine

Weight for Individual Etravirine Mutations			
1	1.5	2.5	3
V90I	V106I	L100I	Y181I/V
A98	E138A	K101P′	—
K101E/H	V179F	Y181C	—
V179D/T	G190S	M230L	—
G190A	—	—	—

Weighted score is calculated by adding numbers based on presence of specific mutations. Patients with a score that is less than or equal to 2.0 are likely to be fully susceptible, those from 2.5 to 3.5 are partially susceptible, and those great than 3.5 derive little if any antiviral activity from this drug.

L33F, I47V, I50V, I54L/M, T74P, L76V, I84V, L89V).[54] In addition, the drug maintains good activity when given as darunavir plus ritonavir once daily (800 mg and 100 mg, respectively) if none of these mutations are present.[55] Optimizing PI use in patients with extensive drug resistance may be further facilitated by the use of phenotypic drug resistance testing.[56,57]

The second-generation InSTI dolutegravir has been shown to have activity in patients with resistance to first-generation drugs in this class,[45,46] although in this setting it must be dosed at 50 mg twice daily rather than 50 mg once daily as used in InSTI-naive individuals. Data from these studies have further shown that dolutegravir activity is attenuated in patients with the Q148H/R mutations combined with 2 or more secondary mutations at L74I/M, E138A/D/K/T, G140A/S, Y143H/R, E157Q, G163E/K/Q/R/S, or G193E/R.[45]

Treatment strategies when a fully suppressive regimen is unlikely to be achievable The goal in this setting is to preserve immunologic function, prevent clinical progression, and minimize the development of further drug-resistant virus that will limit future treatment options. If full suppression is unlikely to be achieved with currently available medications, it is important to consider alternative strategies in order to avoid adding 1 new drug to a failing regimen. One such strategy is to continue the current regimen until new therapies become available. Continued immunologic and clinical benefits may still be seen even if the HIV RNA level is maintained at less than 10,000 to 20,000 copies/mL.[58,59] Treatment discontinuation is not recommended because it is associated with increased clinical progression.[60] In patients with a high likelihood for clinical progression who have limited treatment options, consultation with an ART expert is strongly advised.

Clinical scenario: drug resistance testing cannot be performed
This situation most commonly occurs in patients with low-level plasma HIV RNA. As noted earlier, if plasma HIV RNA is persistently less than 200 copies/mL the optimal strategy is unknown and many clinicians follow the current therapy while addressing potential obstacles to adherence and/or possible drug-drug or drug-food interactions. Once these potential reasons for low-level viremia are addressed the person should be monitored and have repeat resistance testing performed if levels increase. In patients with plasma HIV RNA persistently more than 200 copies/mL, consideration should be given to modifying therapy with a new regimen that includes 3 fully active agents, or, in select cases, 2 agents if one is an active pharmacologically boosted PI.

Clinical scenario: drug resistance testing shows no significant mutations
This is a common finding in clinical practice and in randomized controlled trials, and most frequently reflects poor adherence, which should be addressed before consideration of a therapeutic switch. A recent review of outcomes for individuals experiencing protocol-defined virologic failure on NRTIs plus a ritonavir-boosted PI showed similar outcomes for patients who remained on, versus patients who modified, their treatment regimens.[27] Although not a randomized study, it is consistent with the likelihood that enhanced adherence to interventions is sufficient to result in suppression in the absence of a therapeutic change. It is important to diligently assess regimen intolerance as a cause for the poor adherence, and, if intolerance is identified, a regimen switch should be considered.

Clinical scenario: individuals with a history of suboptimal virologic response who have been off therapy for months
This situation occurs frequently as individuals find themselves moving from provider to provider. Every effort should be made to obtain detailed medical records and get as comprehensive a history of previous treatment as possible. However, such detailed information is often difficult to obtain, particularly for individuals presenting with advanced HIV disease when there is some urgency to reinitiate ART. There are no studies to guide the optimal management in this setting. If patients state that their plasma HIV RNA was undetectable on their most recent regimens, it is reasonable to reinitiate such therapy with close follow-up. If they are not aware of their response to previous therapy, several options can be considered along with close follow-up.

- If individuals are able to say with confidence that they have not previously been treated with an unboosted PI or an InSTI, it is reasonable to assume that they do not have resistance to these drugs and could be initiated on such a combination along with NRTIs.
- If individuals are able to state what regimen they were most recently taking, it is reasonable to restart this drug combination with close follow-up and perhaps genotypic drug resistance testing performed when it is clear that there is inadequate virologic response, or at 4 to 8 weeks to better assess the extent of drug resistance previously selected.
- If there is no reliable history to work from, a prudent option is to initiate dual NRTIs plus a pharmacologically boosted PI with careful monitoring of response and early genotypic drug resistance testing to characterize the extent of resistance to the drugs in these classes with subsequent modification of the regimen.

ART-EXPERIENCED INDIVIDUALS WITH VIROLOGIC SUPPRESSION

Individuals may be considering a modification in their ART while virologically suppressed. Because any treatment modification can be associated with risk for virologic failure or new toxicity, there should be good justification for making a change, such as to reduce toxicity, enhance convenience, or to avoid drug-drug or drug-food interactions. Before any change is made there should be a careful review of each individual's treatment history and laboratory data.

Patients with no history of drug-resistant virus can be switched to any regimen that has been shown in treatment-naive individuals to be highly effective.[1,2] When switching to a non–pharmacologically boosted PI-based regimen the new combination should have at least 3 fully active drugs included.[1] If there was transmitted resistance or the possibility of previous virologic failure with potential or documented emergent drug resistance in the past, a switch from a pharmacologically boosted PI-based regimen should be made with caution.[24,61] Guidance for ART switches based on which drug or drugs are to be modified is provided later.

Switching NRTIs

The most common reasons for considering a change in NRTI(s) is because of emerging toxicity, or concerns about the emergence of toxicity. In this setting there are direct and indirect data suggesting that the strategies discussed later can be used under specific circumstances:

- Switch one NRTI to another (if there is susceptibility to the new agent)
- If there is susceptibility to the pharmacologically boosted PI:
  - Stop NRTIs and maintain the pharmacologically boosted PI
  - Stop select NRTIs and maintain the pharmacologically boosted PI plus either lamivudine or emtricitabine
  - Stop NRTIs and maintain the pharmacologically boosted PI plus an InSTI

NRTI-related toxicity was common with the widespread use of thymidine analogues such as zidovudine and stavudine. This toxicity led to several studies switching patients on stable suppressive therapy from thymidine analogues to alternative NRTIs. These studies showed that in the absence of NRTI resistance such switches resulted in sustained suppression and some reversal of many adverse events, including lipoatrophy.[62–64]

Although thymidine analogues are now rarely used as first-line therapy, tolerability remains the most common reason for considering a NRTI switch, typically from tenofovir disoproxil fumarate (DF) or abacavir. Management of these situations could include switching between these NRTIs, which has been formally studied with switches from abacavir to tenofovir DF with improvement in lipids.[65,66] Fewer data are available for switches from tenofovir DF to abacavir, but retrospective studies have shown improvement in renal markers while maintaining good viral suppression.[67]

An alternative strategy to switching from one NRTI to another is to switch to an NRTI-sparing regimen. The most data available for such a strategy come from studies of maintenance therapy with ritonavir-boosted PIs as monotherapy. These studies have shown sustained virologic suppression with modest increased risk of persistent low-level viremia, which in virtually all cases was not associated with emergence of drug resistance and usually responded to reintroduction of NRTIs.[68–70] Although switch studies are limited, there are data in treatment-naive individuals showing that viral suppression can be achieved in most cases with ritonavir-boosted PI plus an InSTI, such as in the European AIDS Treatment Network (NEAT001) / National Agency for AIDS Research (ANRS143) study with ritonavir-boosted darunavir plus raltegravir,[71] or with ritonavir-boosted lopinavir plus lamivudine as evaluated in the Global AntiRetroviral Design Encompassing Lopinavir/r and Lamivudine vs. LPV/r based standard therapy (GARDEL) study.[72] Although it is likely that these data from studies of treatment-naive individuals can be used as a strategy in patients without underlying drug-resistant virus, alternative ritonavir-boosted PIs or InSTIs would used in the absence of data.

Switching NNRTIs

A typical NNRTI-based regimen includes the use of 2 NRTIs. The most common reason for considering a change is toxicity or treatment simplification. Based on general principles and/or studies, the following strategies can be considered:

- Switch one susceptible NNRTI to another
- Switch the NNRTI to a susceptible InSTI

- Switch the NNRTI-based regimen to a susceptible pharmacologically boosted PI with either 2 NRTIs, lamivudine or emtricitabine alone, or with an InSTI

Until recently the most commonly used first-line NNRTIs were efavirenz and nevirapine. Both have been shown to be highly effective and convenient, with the main side effects associated with nevirapine being rash and hepatotoxicity, whereas central nervous system symptoms are the most common efavirenz toxicities. Efavirenz has a convenience advantage because it can be given as part of a single-tablet regimen with tenofovir DF and emtricitabine. There are studies showing that switches from efavirenz-based regimens can be made to other NNRTIs, including nevirapine, etravirine, and rilpivirine, with reduction in adverse events.[73–75] Several studies have shown that patients virologically suppressed on NRTIs plus efavirenz can also have the latter drug switched to an InSTI such as raltegravir or elvitegravir plus cobicistat with sustained viral control and a reduction in central nervous system–related adverse events.[76,77]

Although data are limited, a toxicity-inducing NNRTI could be switched to a susceptible pharmacologically boosted PI. With the limitations outlined earlier for the options for NRTI switches, there is indirect evidence that viral suppression is also maintained using one of several novel pharmacologically boosted PI-based regimens, including as monotherapy,[68–70] with lamivudine or emtricitabine alone,[72] or with an InSTI.[71] Switching a NNRTI to a CCR5 antagonist–based regimen is not recommended in virologically suppressed individuals because of the inability to assess whether the individual harbors CXCR4-using virus. Although tropism testing can be performed on proviral DNA, this approach has not been fully validated.

There are some highly treatment-experienced patients using a second-generation NNRTI, such as etravirine, as part of a regimen developed based on assessment of underlying resistance. In this case, a decision to stop or switch this drug to an alternative agent is complex and must be done with caution, as discussed later.

Switching a Pharmacologically Boosted PI

In the current era, PIs are almost exclusively used with pharmacologic boosting. A typical PI-based regimen in first-line, or often second-line, therapy includes 2 NRTIs, although in highly treatment-experienced patients this class can be used with more complex regimens. For patients virologically suppressed on a PI-containing regimen the most common reasons for considering a switch are because of toxicity, drug-drug interactions, or for treatment simplification. In this setting it is critical to determine whether there is underlying resistance to the NRTIs in the regimen. If so, there is considerable risk of virologic failure if the pharmacologically boosted PI is switched to any drugs with a lower genetic barrier to resistance, such as a pharmacologically unboosted PI, NNRTIs, or InSTIs. If there is any underlying PI resistance it is important to consider whether there is cross-resistance to any alternative PI being considered. In contrast, in first-line or second-line regimens in which the NRTIs are thought to be fully active and there is little PI resistance, based on general principles and/or available studies the following strategies should be effective:

- Switch to an alternative pharmacologically boosted PI
- Switch from a pharmacologically boosted to unboosted PI
- Switch the PI to a susceptible NNRTI
- Switch the PI to a susceptible InSTI

In the absence of PI resistance it is likely that any pharmacologically boosted PI could be switched to an alternative preferred PI regardless of whether the patient is minimally or highly treatment experienced. For example, in patients with limited drug resistance, atazanavir combined with ritonavir has been shown to maintain virologic suppression in patients switching from a ritonavir plus lopinavir–based regimen.[78] If there are concerns about tolerability with low-dose ritonavir used as a pharmacologic booster, there are several studies showing that in the absence of underlying resistance patients suppressed on atazanavir plus ritonavir can maintain suppression when switched to therapeutically dosed atazanavir (400 mg once daily) without ritonavir.[79–81] Although the removal of ritonavir reduces pill burden and potential side effects it must be noted that drug-drug interactions may change, including the inability to use tenofovir DF and possibly dosing around acid-reducing agents.

Virologically suppressed individuals without underlying drug-resistant virus can switch a pharmacologically boosted PI to an NNRTI with the potential for enhanced convenience and improved tolerability.[82] Again, there is an increased risk of virologic failure in this setting if there is preexisting NRTI resistance.[61] Switching a PI to an InSTI has also been shown to be a viable option with improvement in lipids and gastrointestinal toxicity,[83,84] as long as there is no evidence of underlying NRTI resistance.[24]

Modification of boosted PI to a CCR5 antagonist–based regimen is not routinely advised because in virologically suppressed individuals it is not possible to assess whether there are CXCR4-using viruses present in plasma. Although a tropism test can be performed on proviral DNA, such an approach has not been fully validated.

Switching from an InSTI

InSTIs are commonly used as first-line therapy with dual NRTIs either as separate agents or as a single-tablet regimen with elvitegravir plus cobicistat. They are also widely used in treatment-experienced individuals with multidrug-resistant virus. For patients virologically suppressed on an InSTI-containing regimen with minimal underlying drug resistance the most common reasons for considering a switch are for convenience if not on a single-tablet regimen, to eliminate drug-drug interactions if on cobicistat plus elvitegravir, or for tolerability. In considering a switch from an InSTI it is critical to determine whether there is underlying resistance to the non-InSTI agents in the regimen. If not, switching to an alternative InSTI or any other fully active agent is likely to maintain viral suppression. If underlying resistance is present, switches to an alternative fully active InSTI is likely to be effective, but other switches would need to be done with great caution.

Switching ART in Patients Virologically Suppressed with Underlying Multidrug Resistance

General principles outlined earlier apply in this setting. The new regimen should include at least 3 fully active agents, with the exception of when the regimen includes a fully active pharmacologically boosted PI if less active drugs might be sufficient. Switches in this setting are complicated and should be done with expert consultation, recognizing that these individuals may be at particularly high risk for virologic failure and selection of additional drug resistance mutations. One situation in which there are good data supporting a switch is going from enfuvirtide to an InSTI in patients who have never been previously treated with a drug in this class.[85]

Monitoring After Antiretroviral Switch

After any change in a fully suppressive regimen careful follow-up is needed to assess clinical and laboratory tolerability as well as to ensure maintenance of virologic suppression. Although there are no studies to define optimal follow-up, it is reasonable to do a clinical and laboratory assessment at a minimum of 2 to 6 weeks after the switch, and then as appropriate based on the type of switch and the potential for new adverse events.

SUMMARY/DISCUSSION

This article has focused on ART-experienced individuals who are being assessed for modification in therapy because of suboptimal virologic response or while virologically suppressed, typically to enhance convenience, improve tolerability, or reduce drug-drug or drug-food interactions. Regardless of the reason for an ART switch, the goal is to achieve or maintain virologic suppression. Each case is unique and requires a thorough assessment of past ART use, tolerability, and resistance testing. In complicated cases, consultation with a treatment expert is highly recommended.

REFERENCES

1. Panel on antiretroviral guidelines for adults and adolescents. Guidelines for the use of antiretroviral agents in HIV-1-infected adults and adolescents. Department of Health and Human Services. Available at: http://aidsinfo.nih.gov/contentFiles/adultandadolescentGL.pdf. Accessed May 4, 2014.
2. Thompson MA, Aberg JA, Hoy JF, et al. Antiretroviral treatment of adult HIV infection: 2012 recommendations of the International Antiviral Society-USA panel. JAMA 2012;308:387–402.
3. Swenson LC, Min JE, Woods CK, et al. HIV drug resistance detected during low-level viraemia is associated with subsequent virologic failure. AIDS 2014. [Epub ahead of print].
4. Delaugerre C, Gallien S, Flandre P, et al. Impact of low-level-viremia on HIV-1 drug-resistance evolution among antiretroviral treated-patients. PLoS One 2012;7:e36673.
5. Ribaudo H, Lennox J, Currier J, et al. Virologic failure endpoint definition in clinical trials: is using HIV-RNA threshold <200 copies/mL better than <50 copies/mL? An analysis of ACTG studies. 16th Conference on Retroviruses and Opportunistic Infections. Monteal (Canada), February 8–11, 2009.
6. Mocroft A, Ruiz L, Reiss P, et al. Virological rebound after suppression on highly active antiretroviral therapy. AIDS 2003;17:1741–51.
7. Bosch RJ, Bennett K, Collier AC, et al, Group for the AIDS Clinical Trials. Pre-treatment factors associated with 3-year (144-week) virologic and immunologic responses to potent antiretroviral therapy. J Acquir Immune Defic Syndr 2007; 44:268–77.
8. Lodwick R, Costagliola D, Reiss P, et al. Triple-class virologic failure in HIV-infected patients undergoing antiretroviral therapy for up to 10 years. Arch Intern Med 2010;170:410–9.
9. Phillips AN, Staszewski S, Weber R, et al. HIV viral load response to antiretroviral therapy according to the baseline CD4 cell count and viral load. JAMA 2001; 286:2560–7.
10. Gonzalez-Serna A, Min JE, Woods C, et al. Performance of HIV-1 drug resistance testing at low level viraemia and its ability to predict future virologic outcomes and viral evolution in treatment-naive individuals. Clin Infect Dis 2014;58:1165–73.
11. Petersen ML, van der Laan MJ, Napravnik S, et al. Long-term consequences of the delay between virologic failure of highly active antiretroviral therapy and regimen modification. AIDS 2008;22:2097–106.
12. Mocroft A, Phillips AN, Miller V, et al. The use of and response to second-line protease inhibitor regimens: results from the EuroSIDA study. AIDS 2001;15:201–9.

13. Clotet B, Bellos N, Molina JM, et al. Efficacy and safety of darunavir-ritonavir at week 48 in treatment-experienced patients with HIV-1 infection in POWER 1 and 2: a pooled subgroup analysis of data from two randomised trials. Lancet 2007; 369:1169–78.

14. Katlama C, Haubrich R, Lalezari J, et al. Efficacy and safety of etravirine in treatment-experienced, HIV-1 patients: pooled 48 week analysis of two randomized, controlled trials. AIDS 2009;23:2289–300.

15. Daar ES, Tierney C, Fischl MA, et al. Atazanavir plus ritonavir or efavirenz as part of a 3-drug regimen for initial treatment of HIV-1. Ann Intern Med 2011;154: 445–56.

16. Molina JM, Cahn P, Grinsztejn B, et al. Rilpivirine versus efavirenz with tenofovir and emtricitabine in treatment-naive adults infected with HIV-1 (ECHO): a phase 3 randomised double-blind active-controlled trial. Lancet 2011;378:238–46.

17. Bunupuradah T, Chetchotisakd P, Ananworanich J, et al. A randomized comparison of second-line lopinavir/ritonavir monotherapy versus tenofovir/lamivudine/lopinavir/ritonavir in patients failing NNRTI regimens: the HIV STAR study. Antivir Ther 2012;17:1351–61.

18. Boyd MA, Kumarasamy N, Moore CL, et al. Ritonavir-boosted lopinavir plus nucleoside or nucleotide reverse transcriptase inhibitors versus ritonavir-boosted lopinavir plus raltegravir for treatment of HIV-1 infection in adults with virological failure of a standard first-line ART regimen (SECOND-LINE): a randomised, open-label, non-inferiority study. Lancet 2013;381:2091–9.

19. Paton N, Kityo C, Hoppe A, et al. A pragmatic randomised controlled strategy trial of three second-line treatment options for use in public health rollout programme settings: the Europe-Africa Research Network for Evaluation of Second-line Therapy (EARNEST) trial. 7th International AIDS Society Conference on HIV Pathogenesis, Treatment and Prevention. Kuala Lumpur (Malaysia), June 30-July 3, 2013.

20. Waters L, Bansi L, Asboe D, et al. Second-line protease inhibitor-based antiretroviral therapy after non-nucleoside reverse transcriptase inhibitor failure: the effect of a nucleoside backbone. Antivir Ther 2013;18:213–9.

21. World Health Organization. Consolidated guidelines on the use of antiretroviral drugs for treating and preventing HIV infection. 2013.

22. Ruxrungtham K, Pedro RJ, Latiff GH, et al. Impact of reverse transcriptase resistance on the efficacy of TMC125 (etravirine) with two nucleoside reverse transcriptase inhibitors in protease inhibitor-naive, nonnucleoside reverse transcriptase inhibitor-experienced patients: study TMC125-C227. HIV Med 2008;9:883–96.

23. Sax PE, DeJesus E, Mills A, et al. Co-formulated elvitegravir, cobicistat, emtricitabine, and tenofovir versus co-formulated efavirenz, emtricitabine, and tenofovir for initial treatment of HIV-1 infection: a randomised, double-blind, phase 3 trial, analysis of results after 48 weeks. Lancet 2012;379:2439–48.

24. Eron JJ, Young B, Cooper DA, et al. Switch to a raltegravir-based regimen versus continuation of a lopinavir-ritonavir-based regimen in stable HIV-infected patients with suppressed viraemia (SWITCHMRK 1 and 2): two multicentre, double-blind, randomised controlled trials. Lancet 2010;375:396–407.

25. Mills AM, Nelson M, Jayaweera D, et al. Once-daily darunavir/ritonavir vs. lopinavir/ritonavir in treatment-naive, HIV-1-infected patients: 96-week analysis. AIDS 2009;23:1679–88.

26. Molina JM, Andrade-Villanueva J, Echevarria J, et al. Once-daily atazanavir/ritonavir compared with twice-daily lopinavir/ritonavir, each in combination with

tenofovir and emtricitabine, for management of antiretroviral-naive HIV-1-infected patients: 96-week efficacy and safety results of the CASTLE Study. J Acquir Immune Defic Syndr 2010;53:323–32.

27. Zheng Y, Hughes MD, Lockman S, et al. Antiretroviral therapy and efficacy after virologic failure on first-line boosted protease inhibitor regimens. Clin Infect Dis 2014. [Epub ahead of print].

28. Molina JM, Lamarca A, Andrade-Villanueva J, et al. Efficacy and safety of once daily elvitegravir versus twice daily raltegravir in treatment-experienced patients with HIV-1 receiving a ritonavir-boosted protease inhibitor: randomised, double-blind, phase 3, non-inferiority study. Lancet Infect Dis 2012;12:27–35.

29. DeJesus E, Rockstroh JK, Henry K, et al. Co-formulated elvitegravir, cobicistat, emtricitabine, and tenofovir disoproxil fumarate versus ritonavir-boosted atazanavir plus co-formulated emtricitabine and tenofovir disoproxil fumarate for initial treatment of HIV-1 infection: a randomised, double-blind, phase 3, non-inferiority trial. Lancet 2012;379:2429–38.

30. Lennox JL, DeJesus E, Lazzarin A, et al. Safety and efficacy of raltegravir-based versus efavirenz-based combination therapy in treatment-naive patients with HIV-1 infection: a multicentre, double-blind randomised controlled trial. Lancet 2009;374:796–806.

31. Clotet B, Feinberg J, van Lunzen J, et al. Once-daily dolutegravir versus darunavir plus ritonavir in antiretroviral-naive adults with HIV-1 infection (FLAMINGO): 48 week results from the randomised open-label phase 3b study. Lancet 2014. [Epub ahead of print].

32. Walmsley SL, Antela A, Clumeck N, et al. Dolutegravir plus abacavir-lamivudine for the treatment of HIV-1 infection. N Engl J Med 2013;369:1807–18.

33. Raffi F, Jaeger H, Quiros-Roldan E, et al. Once-daily dolutegravir versus twice-daily raltegravir in antiretroviral-naive adults with HIV-1 infection (SPRING-2 study): 96 week results from a randomised, double-blind, non-inferiority trial. Lancet Infect Dis 2013;13:927–35.

34. Yazdanpanah Y, Fagard C, Descamps D, et al. High rate of virologic suppression with raltegravir plus etravirine and darunavir/ritonavir among treatment-experienced patients infected with multidrug-resistant HIV: results of the ANRS 139 TRIO trial. Clin Infect Dis 2009;49:1441–9.

35. Eron JJ, Cooper DA, Steigbigel RT, et al. Efficacy and safety of raltegravir for treatment of HIV for 5 years in the BENCHMRK studies: final results of two randomised, placebo-controlled trials. Lancet Infect Dis 2013;13:587–96.

36. Capetti A, Landonio S, Meraviglia P, et al. 96 Week follow-up of HIV-infected patients in rescue with raltegravir plus optimized backbone regimens: a multicentre Italian experience. PLoS One 2012;7:e39222.

37. Steigbigel RT, Cooper DA, Kumar PN, et al. Raltegravir with optimized background therapy for resistant HIV-1 infection. N Engl J Med 2008;359: 339–54.

38. Gulick RM, Lalezari J, Goodrich J, et al. Maraviroc for previously treated patients with R5 HIV-1 infection. N Engl J Med 2008;359:1429–41.

39. Lalezari JP, Henry K, O'Hearn M, et al. Enfuvirtide, an HIV-1 fusion inhibitor, for drug-resistant HIV infection in North and South America. N Engl J Med 2003; 348:2175–85.

40. Elion R, Molina JM, Ramon Arribas Lopez J, et al. A randomized phase 3 study comparing once-daily elvitegravir with twice-daily raltegravir in treatment-experienced subjects with HIV-1 infection: 96-week results. J Acquir Immune Defic Syndr 2013;63:494–7.

41. Cahn P, Pozniak AL, Mingrone H, et al. Dolutegravir versus raltegravir in antiretroviral-experienced, integrase-inhibitor-naive adults with HIV: week 48 results from the randomised, double-blind, non-inferiority SAILING study. Lancet 2013;382:700–8.

42. Cooper DA, Steigbigel RT, Gatell JM, et al. Subgroup and resistance analyses of raltegravir for resistant HIV-1 infection. N Engl J Med 2008;359:355–65.

43. Hicks CB, Cahn P, Cooper DA, et al. Durable efficacy of tipranavir-ritonavir in combination with an optimised background regimen of antiretroviral drugs for treatment-experienced HIV-1-infected patients at 48 weeks in the randomized evaluation of strategic intervention in multi-drug resistant patients with Tipranavir (RESIST) studies: an analysis of combined data from two randomised open-label trials. Lancet 2006;368:466–75.

44. Molina JM, Cohen C, Katlama C, et al. Safety and efficacy of darunavir (TMC114) with low-dose ritonavir in treatment-experienced patients: 24-week results of POWER 3. J Acquir Immune Defic Syndr 2007;46:24–31.

45. Castagna A, Maggiolo F, Penco G, et al. Dolutegravir in antiretroviral-experienced patients with raltegravir- and/or elvitegravir-resistant HIV-1: 24-week results of the Phase III VIKING-3 Study. J Infect Dis 2014. [Epub ahead of print].

46. Eron JJ, Clotet B, Durant J, et al. Safety and efficacy of dolutegravir in treatment-experienced subjects with raltegravir-resistant HIV type 1 infection: 24-week results of the VIKING Study. J Infect Dis 2013;207:740–8.

47. Vingerhoets J, Azijn H, Fransen E, et al. TMC125 displays a high genetic barrier to the development of resistance: evidence from in vitro selection experiments. J Virol 2005;79:12773–82.

48. Madruga JV, Cahn P, Grinsztejn B, et al. Efficacy and safety of TMC125 (etravirine) in treatment-experienced HIV-1-infected patients in DUET-1: 24-week results from a randomised, double-blind, placebo-controlled trial. Lancet 2007; 370:29–38.

49. Lazzarin A, Campbell T, Clotet B, et al. Efficacy and safety of TMC125 (etravirine) in treatment-experienced HIV-1-infected patients in DUET-2: 24-week results from a randomised, double-blind, placebo-controlled trial. Lancet 2007; 370:39–48.

50. Vingerhoets J, Tambuyzer L, Azijn H, et al. Resistance profile of etravirine: combined analysis of baseline genotypic and phenotypic data from the randomized, controlled phase III clinical studies. AIDS 2010;24:503–14.

51. Naeger LK, Struble KA. Food and drug administration analysis of tipranavir clinical resistance in HIV-1-infected treatment-experienced patients. AIDS 2007;21: 179–85.

52. Katlama C, Esposito R, Gatell JM, et al. Efficacy and safety of TMC114/ritonavir in treatment-experienced HIV patients: 24-week results of POWER 1. AIDS 2007;21:395–402.

53. Madruga JV, Berger D, McMurchie M, et al. Efficacy and safety of darunavir-ritonavir compared with that of lopinavir-ritonavir at 48 weeks in treatment-experienced, HIV-infected patients in TITAN: a randomised controlled phase III trial. Lancet 2007;370:49–58.

54. de Meyer S, Vangeneugden T, van Baelen B, et al. Resistance profile of darunavir: combined 24-week results from the POWER trials. AIDS Res Hum Retroviruses 2008;24:379–88.

55. Cahn P, Fourie J, Grinsztejn B, et al. Week 48 analysis of once-daily vs. twice-daily darunavir/ritonavir in treatment-experienced HIV-1-infected patients. AIDS 2011;25:929–39.

56. Coakley E, Chappey C, Benhamida J, et al. Defining the upper and lower phenotypic clinical cut-offs for darunavir/ritonavir by the PhenoSense assay. 14th Conference on Retroviruses and Opportunistic Infections. Los Angeles, February 25–28, 2007.

57. Winters BH, Vermeiren E, Van Craenenbroeck P, et al. Development of Virco®TYPE resistance analysis, including clinical cut-offs, for TMC114. Antivir Ther 2006;11:S180.

58. Raffanti SP, Fusco JS, Sherrill BH, et al. Effect of persistent moderate viremia on disease progression during HIV therapy. J Acquir Immune Defic Syndr 2004;37: 1147–54.

59. Ledergerber B, Lundgren JD, Walker AS, et al. Predictors of trend in CD4-positive T-cell count and mortality among HIV-1-infected individuals with virological failure to all three antiretroviral-drug classes. Lancet 2004;364:51–62.

60. Deeks SG, Hoh R, Neilands TB, et al. Interruption of treatment with individual therapeutic drug classes in adults with multidrug-resistant HIV-1 infection. J Infect Dis 2005;192:1537–44.

61. Martínez E, Arnaiz JA, Podzamczer D, et al. Substitution of nevirapine, efavirenz, or abacavir for protease inhibitors in patients with human immunodeficiency virus infection. N Engl J Med 2003;349:1036–46.

62. Martin A, Smith DE, Carr A, et al. Reversibility of lipoatrophy in HIV-infected patients 2 years after switching from a thymidine analogue to abacavir: the MITOX Extension Study. AIDS 2004;18:1029–36.

63. Ribera E, Larrousse M, Curran A, et al. Impact of switching from zidovudine/lamivudine to tenofovir/emtricitabine on lipoatrophy: the RECOMB study. HIV Med 2013;14:327–36.

64. Moyle GJ, Sabin CA, Cartledge J, et al. A randomized comparative trial of tenofovir DF or abacavir as replacement for a thymidine analogue in persons with lipoatrophy. AIDS 2006;20:2043–50.

65. Behrens G, Maserati R, Rieger A, et al. Switching to tenofovir/emtricitabine from abacavir/lamivudine in HIV-infected adults with raised cholesterol: effect on lipid profiles. Antivir Ther 2012;17:1011–20.

66. Campo R, DeJesus E, Bredeek UF, et al. SWIFT: prospective 48 week study to evaluate efficacy and safety of switching to emtricitabine/tenofovir from lamivudine/abacavir in virologically suppressed HIV-1 infected patients on a boosted protease inhibitor containing antiretroviral regimen. Clin Infect Dis 2013;56:1637–45.

67. Harris M, Guillemi S, Chan K, et al. Effects on renal function of a switch from tenofovir (TDF)- to abacavir (ABC)-based highly active antiretroviral therapy (HAART), with or without atazanavir. 7th International AIDS Symposium Conference on HIV Pathogenesis, Treatment and Prevention. Kuala Lumpur (Malaysia), June 30-July 3, 2013.

68. Katlama C, Valentin MA, Algarte-Genin G, et al. Efficacy of darunavir/ritonavir maintenance monotherapy in patients with HIV-1 viral suppression: a randomized open-label, noninferiority trial, MONOI-ANRS 136. AIDS 2010;24: 2365–74.

69. Arribas JR, Delgado R, Arranz A, et al. Lopinavir-ritonavir monotherapy versus lopinavir-ritonavir and 2 nucleosides for maintenance therapy of HIV: 96-week analysis. J Acquir Immune Defic Syndr 2009;51:147–52.

70. Arribas J, Horban A, Gerstoft J, et al. The MONET trial: darunavir/ritonavir with or without nucleoside analogues, for patients with HIV RNA below 50 copies/mL. AIDS 2010;24:223–30.

71. Raffi F, Babiker AG, Richert L, et al. First-line RAL + DRV/r is non-inferior to TDF/FTC + DRV/r: The NEAT001/ANRS143 Randomised Trial. 21st Conference on Retroviruses and Opportunistic Infections. Boston, March 3–6, 2014.

72. Cahn P, Andrade-Villanueva J, Arribas JR, et al. Dual therapy with lopinavir and ritonavir plus lamivudine versus triple therapy with lopinavir and ritonavir plus two nucleoside reverse transcriptase inhibitors in antiretroviral-therapy-naive adults with HIV-1 infection: 48 week results of the randomised, open label, non-inferiority GARDEL trial. Lancet Infect Dis 2014;14:572–80.

73. Schouten JT, Krambrink A, Ribaudo HJ, et al. Substitution of nevirapine because of efavirenz toxicity in AIDS Clinical Trials Group A5095. Clin Infect Dis 2010;50: 787–91.

74. Waters L, Fisher M, Winston A, et al. A phase IV, double-blind, multicentre, randomized, placebo-controlled, pilot study to assess the feasibility of switching individuals receiving efavirenz with continuing central nervous system adverse events to etravirine. AIDS 2011;25:65–71.

75. Mills AM, Cohen C, Dejesus E, et al. Efficacy and safety 48 weeks after switching from efavirenz to rilpivirine using emtricitabine/tenofovir disoproxil fumarate-based single-tablet regimens. HIV Clin Trials 2013;14:216–23.

76. Nguyen A, Calmy A, Delhumeau C, et al. A randomized cross-over study to compare raltegravir and efavirenz (SWITCH-ER study). AIDS 2011;25:1481–7.

77. Pozniak A, Markowitz M, Mills A, et al. Switching to coformulated elvitegravir, cobicistat, emtricitabine, and tenofovir versus continuation of non-nucleoside reverse transcriptase inhibitor with emtricitabine and tenofovir in virologically suppressed adults with HIV (STRATEGY-NNRTI): 48 week results of a randomised, open-label, phase 3b non-inferiority trial. Lancet Infect Dis 2014;14: 590–9.

78. Mallolas J, Podzamczer D, Milinkovic A, et al. Efficacy and safety of switching from boosted lopinavir to boosted atazanavir in patients with virologic suppression receiving a LPV/r-containing HAART: the ATAZIP study. J Acquir Immune Defic Syndr 2009;51:29–36.

79. Squires KE, Young B, DeJesus E, et al. ARIES 144 week results: durable virologic suppression in HIV-infected patients simplified to unboosted atazanavir/abacavir/lamivudine. HIV Clin Trials 2012;13:233–44.

80. Ghosn J, Carosi G, Moreno S, et al. Unboosted atazanavir-based therapy maintains control of HIV type-1 replication as effectively as a ritonavir-boosted regimen. Antivir Ther 2010;15:993–1002.

81. Gatell J, Salmon-Ceron D, Lazzarin A, et al. Efficacy and safety of atazanavir-based highly active antiretroviral therapy in patients with virologic suppression switched from a stable, boosted or unboosted protease inhibitor treatment regimen: the SWAN Study (AI424-097) 48-week results. Clin Infect Dis 2007; 44:1484–92.

82. Palella FJ Jr, Fisher M, Tebas P, et al. Simplification to rilpivirine/emtricitabine/tenofovir disoproxil fumarate from ritonavir-boosted protease inhibitor antiretroviral therapy in a randomized trial of HIV-1 RNA-suppressed participants. AIDS 2014; 28:335–44.

83. Martinez E, Larrousse M, Llibre JM, et al. Substitution of raltegravir for ritonavir-boosted protease inhibitors in HIV-infected patients: the SPIRAL study. AIDS 2010;24:1697–707.

84. Arribas JR, Pialoux G, Gathe J, et al. Simplification to coformulated elvitegravir, cobicistat, emtricitabine, and tenofovir versus continuation of ritonavir-boosted protease inhibitor with emtricitabine and tenofovir in adults with virologically

suppressed HIV (STRATEGY-PI): 48 week results of a randomised, open-label, phase 3b, non-inferiority trial. Lancet Infect Dis 2014;14:581–9.

85. De Castro N, Braun J, Charreau I, et al. Switch from enfuvirtide to raltegravir in virologically suppressed multidrug-resistant HIV-1-infected patients: a randomized open-label trial. Clin Infect Dis 2009;49:1259–67.

HIV-Related Metabolic Comorbidities in the Current ART Era

Amy H. Warriner, MD, Greer A. Burkholder, MD, Edgar Turner Overton, MD*

KEYWORDS

- HIV • Aging • Comorbidity • Multimorbidity • Inflammation • Immune activation

KEY POINTS

- As a consequence of earlier diagnosis and better treatment, HIV-infected persons are living longer but are also frequently exposed to effective antiretroviral therapy (ART) for longer duration.
- As patients age, they are challenged not only by HIV but also age-related diseases that may be affected by both the underlying HIV infection and ART.
- Persistent low-level inflammation likely plays a significant role in the accelerated appearance of these age-related diseases.
- Because of this complex interplay of HIV infection, ART-related factors, and traditional risk factors, HIV-infected patients are at increased risk for chronic conditions, such as cardiovascular disease, renal disease, bone disease, and diabetes mellitus, compared with uninfected persons, and may have onset of these conditions at an earlier age.

INTRODUCTION

The widespread use of potent combination antiretroviral therapy (ART) has produced significant gains in survival,[1–4] resulting in an aging HIV-infected population in developed countries.[5,6] In the United States, it is estimated that more than one-half of HIV-infected persons will be over age 50 years by 2015.[5] This demographic shift to an older population has been accompanied by changing morbidity and mortality patterns, with a decline in the morbidity and mortality owing to AIDS and concomitant rise in the proportion owing to non–AIDS-related diseases.[2–4,7–12]

Disclosure: The authors have nothing to disclose.
These authors contributed equally to this work.
Department of Medicine, University of Alabama at Birmingham School of Medicine, 908 20th Street South, CCB Room 330A, Birmingham, AL 35294, USA
* Corresponding author.
E-mail address: toverton@uab.edu

Infect Dis Clin N Am 28 (2014) 457–476
http://dx.doi.org/10.1016/j.idc.2014.05.003
0891-5520/14/$ – see front matter © 2014 Elsevier Inc. All rights reserved.

id.theclinics.com

Aging and persistent inflammation place patients at increasing risk for many comorbidities, including cardiovascular disease (CVD), renal disease, diabetes, and low bone mineral density (BMD).[13–16] Obesity and traditional risk factors, especially smoking, also play a role.[17–23] Despite advances in ART, adverse effects and toxicities continue to affect long-term health, particularly with regard to dyslipidemia, insulin resistance (IR), bone loss, and renal dysfunction.[24–28]

A disproportionate number of HIV-infected patients are ethnic minorities or of lower socioeconomic status, groups known to experience significant health disparities and greater risk for chronic disease.[29,30] Higher rates of substance abuse may also contribute.[9,31] Finally, chronic hepatitis C virus (HCV) coinfection is common among HIV-infected patients and can increase risk for diabetes mellitus, atherosclerosis, renal disease, and bone disease (**Fig. 1**).[32–37]

Although further study is needed, the synergistic effect of the these factors seems to result in accentuated aging, in which HIV-infected patients are at increased risk for CVD, renal disease, diabetes mellitus, and low BMD compared with uninfected persons of a similar age.[14,38] In addition, multimorbidity is highly prevalent among HIV-infected patients, affecting up to 65%.[39–42] HIV-infected patients also seem to experience accelerated aging, in which they are risk for multimorbidity and frailty earlier in life.[14,38,43]

Given the aging of the HIV-infected population, increasing morbidity and mortality owing to non–AIDS-related conditions, and the high prevalence of multimorbidity, HIV providers are increasingly called upon to balance treatment of HIV with prevention and treatment of other major chronic diseases. This paper reviews the epidemiology, pathophysiology, prevention, and treatment of important age-related comorbidities in HIV-infected patients, including atherosclerotic CVD, renal disease, obesity, diabetes mellitus, and bone disease.

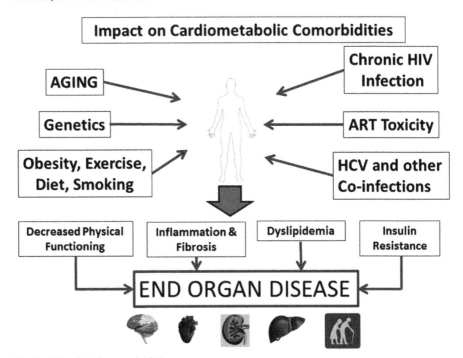

Fig. 1. HIV-related comorbidities.

CVD
Epidemiology

Atherosclerosis is a chronic inflammatory disease in which plaque formation is triggered by arterial wall injury, lipoprotein deposition, endothelial activation, and proinflammatory molecules, and in HIV-infected patients is likely owing to the complex interplay of HIV- and ART-related factors with traditional risk factors, although the pathophysiology is incompletely understood.[44,45] CVD is a major cause of mortality among HIV-infected patients, responsible for up to 15% of deaths.[3,4,9-12] HIV-infected patients are disproportionately impacted by CVD with increased carotid artery intima medial thickening, subclinical coronary artery atherosclerosis, endothelial dysfunction, and silent ischemic heart disease compared with uninfected controls.[46-50] Atherosclerotic plaques in HIV-infected patients are more likely to have morphologic features associated with higher risk for rupture.[51] Risk for acute myocardial infarction among HIV-infected patients is 1.5- to 2-fold greater than uninfected persons, and increased risk of cerebrovascular events has also been reported.[52-57]

HIV-Related Factors

HIV-related chronic immune activation and inflammation contribute to increased risk for CVD. Patterns of T-cell activation, as well as markers of monocyte and macrophage activation (soluble CD14 and CD163), have been linked to subclinical atherosclerosis.[58-64] In the Strategies for Management of Antiretroviral Therapy (SMART) study, HIV-infected patients randomized to episodic rather than continuous ART had increased risk for CVD events (hazard ratio, 1.6; 95% CI, 1.0–2.5; $P = .05$), suggesting HIV replication is an important contributor.[65] The SMART investigators subsequently demonstrated an association between elevated plasma HIV-1 RNA and interleukin-6 (IL-6), a proinflammatory cytokine involved in atherosclerotic plaque formation, and D-dimer, a biomarker of coagulation, as well as an independent association between incident CVD events and baseline markers of inflammation and coagulation (IL-6, high-sensitivity C-reactive protein, and D-dimer).[45,66,67] In participants not taking ART, they observed an increase in serum procoagulants and decrease in anticoagulants compared with those on ART.[68] These data indicate a relationship between HIV replication, inflammation, and CVD. In addition, there is evidence for an association between elevated plasma HIV-1 RNA and endothelial dysfunction with clear improvement in endothelial function after ART initiation.[69-72]

Immune activation is noted even among HIV-infected patients on ART, and although inflammatory markers decrease after ART initiation, some markers remain elevated compared with uninfected controls, indicating factors beyond HIV replication are involved.[58-64] Reactivation of viral infections such as cytomegalovirus has been linked with subclinical atherosclerosis in HIV-infected patients.[73-75] Early in HIV infection, there is massive depletion of CD4 cells in gut-associated lymphoid tissue, leading to increased microbial translocation, a process driving immune activation.[76-78] In chronically infected patients, there is incomplete recovery of these cells after ART initiation.[76] Thus, even HIV-infected patients with viral suppression on ART have significantly increased markers of microbial translocation compared with uninfected controls.[79] Both lipopolysaccharide and soluble CD14 (sCD14), a lipopolysaccharide scavenger receptor on monocytes, have been associated with subclinical carotid artery atherosclerosis among HIV-infected patients.[62] Lipopolysaccharide has been associated with elevated triglycerides, elevated low-density lipoprotein cholesterol, decreased insulin sensitivity, and higher Framingham risk score in HIV-infected patients.[79]

Finally, HIV itself is associated with dyslipidemia; a proatherogenic pattern of decreased high-density lipoprotein cholesterol, elevated triglycerides, and very low-density lipoprotein cholesterol is observed in ART-naïve patients.[80]

Traditional Risk Factors

Traditional risk factors such as age, smoking, dyslipidemia, hypertension, and diabetes mellitus must not be overlooked in the discussion of CVD.[3,81–88] Up to 50% to 70% of HIV-infected patients are current cigarette smokers compared with 20% of the general population.[20] In the Data Collection on Adverse Events of Anti-HIV Drugs (D:A:D) cohort, smoking cessation was associated with a greater than 1.5-fold decline in adjusted incidence rate ratio of CVD events between the first year and more than 3 years after quitting.[89] Another study on acute coronary syndrome reported a population attributable risk of 54% for smoking among HIV-infected patients as opposed to 17% in uninfected controls.[90] As noted, dyslipidemia prevalence is higher with HIV than in uninfected patients, likely related to HIV and ART.[40,52] Overweight/obesity is now common in the HIV-infected population and also increases risk for dyslipidemia, hypertension, and diabetes mellitus.[16,91]

Prevention

Two mainstays of CVD prevention among HIV-infected patients are treatment with ART to reduce HIV-related immune activation and inflammation and aggressive prevention and control of modifiable risk factors.[65,92] The most recent antiretroviral guidelines recommend treatment of all HIV-infected patients with ART, regardless of CD4 count.[93] Owing to the metabolic side effects of ART, all HIV-infected patients should be screened for dyslipidemia and diabetes mellitus at baseline and, thereafter, per HIV-specific guidelines.[94] Routine HIV care should include counseling and pharmacotherapy for smoking cessation, counseling on physical activity, healthy dietary practices, weight loss in overweight/obese patients, and management of dyslipidemia, hypertension, and diabetes mellitus according to general population guidelines.[95–97] In patients with baseline CVD risk factors or a prior history of CVD, providers should consider avoiding ART agents, which convey increased risk for dyslipidemia and IR. Whether there is a role for the anti-inflammatory effects of statins regardless of low-density lipoprotein cholesterol level is currently under study.[98] As a consequence of guideline-driven care, polypharmacy is an all-too-common problem for HIV-infected persons and an area of concern as we try to balance disease prevention and medication toxicity for our aging population.[14]

RENAL
Epidemiology

The incidence of HIV-associated nephropathy, renal failure, and end-stage renal disease have declined thanks to improved virologic suppression with ART.[99–103] Results from the SMART Study confirm the detrimental effects of uncontrolled viremia on renal function.[65] Subjects who followed the treatment interruption strategy were at greater risk of developing fatal or nonfatal renal disease compared with patients randomized to continuous ART. In subsequent analyses from the same trial, treatment interruption was also associated with elevated inflammatory biomarkers, suggesting a relationship between viremia, inflammation, and renal disease.[66]

Despite controlled viremia, up to 30% of HIV-infected patients have prevalent renal dysfunction.[15] One recent cohort identified 40% of HIV-infected patients with Stage 1 kidney disease (estimated glomerular filtration rate, <90 mL/min/1.73 m^2) but only

3% with stage 2 or greater disease (estimated glomerular filtration rate, <60 mL/min/1.73 m^2).[104] Furthermore, ART-related renal toxicities have been identified: Proteinuria, renal tubular damage, interstitial nephritis, and nephrolithiasis.[105] Other comorbidities, specifically hypertension, obesity and type 2 diabetes mellitus, are increasingly prevalent and likely increase the risk for renal disease.[17,105–107]

Numerous antiretrovirals (ARVs) have been associated with renal dysfunction, including crystal deposition from drugs like indinavir and atazanavir.[108] Tenofovir has been implicated to cause proximal tubular damage via mitochondrial toxicity, preventing reabsorption of filtered phosphorus, potassium, amino acids, and glucose.[109] Tenofovir is widely recommended as a component of first-line therapy for HIV and seems to induce a modest amount of renal dysfunction in HIV-infected persons.[93,110] The risk seems greatest in those who are coadministered ritonavir-boosted PIs.[111] The administration of boosted protease inhibitors can lead to decreased flux of tenofovir out of renal tubular epithelial cells and augment this tubulopathy.[112] One study evaluated 964 patients initiating tenofovir-containing ART and 683 tenofovir-sparing ART. Exposure to tenofovir caused significantly greater glomerular filtration rate decline over 4 years.[113] Evidence of proximal tubule dysfunction was also more prevalent among tenofovir-treated patients. The focus on tenofovir toxicity is particularly warranted given the expanding use of tenofovir for the treatment of hepatitis B infection and as a component of pre-exposure prophylaxis for HIV infection.[114,115] A recent analysis from the iPREX study confirmed that creatinine clearance significantly declined among seronegative men who have sex with men who received emtricitabine/tenofovir for pre-exposure prophylaxis, although the decline was very modest and did not progress.[116]

Prevention

Updated guidelines for screening and treating renal disease in HIV-infected persons by the HIV Medical Association of the Infectious Diseases Society of America recommend that all HIV-infected patients be screened annually for proteinuria and renal function through assessment of estimated glomerular filtration rate.[15] Creatinine-based equations are helpful to identify persons with kidney disease, but serum creatinine may be affected by factors other than glomerular filtration, notably muscle mass, liver disease, dietary intake, age, race/ethnicity, and gender.[117] Although the calculated equations account for some of the effects of muscle mass, age, race/ethnicity, and gender, they overestimate glomerular function for persons with lower creatinine intake or production, as can occur in persons with liver disease and possibly advanced HIV infection.[117]

Recent data illustrate that formulae utilizing cystatin C, a small nonglycosylated protein, provide glomerular filtration rate estimates equivalent to serum creatinine-based measures that are not affected by muscle mass or decreased creatinine production.[118–121] Several studies have examined cystatin C as a marker of kidney function in the setting of comorbidity and HIV-infected persons, and demonstrated that both creatinine and cystatin C were good markers of renal function[104,122–126]; however, cystatin C was significantly associated with mortality endpoints.[127] The authors concluded that serum cystatin C levels better reflected renal function independent of confounding factors, such as systemic inflammation or weight. Further research is needed to clarify whether cystatin C should be used to measure renal function in the setting of HIV.

Urine dipsticks and spot urine microalbumin quantification, which are used extensively in the management of diabetes mellitus, can also provide the HIV practitioner a means to monitor renal function and screen for preclinical dysfunction related to

HIV infection, its treatment, or concomitant comorbidities such as hypertension or diabetes mellitus. In 1 large cohort study, 13% of HIV-infected persons had at least trace proteinuria by urinary dipstick and 11% had urine microalbumin greater than 30 mg/dL.[104] Considering the relatively inexpensive cost of spot urine microalbumin quantification, its integration into the routine care of HIV warrants further evaluation.

BONE DISEASE
Epidemiology

BMD, as measured by dual-energy x-ray absorptiometry (DXA) scans, serves as a surrogate marker of fracture risk and provides data to categorize persons with osteoporosis (T-score ≤ -2.5) and osteopenia (T-score ≤ -1.0) based on World Health Organization criteria.[128] Similar to the data discussed for other non-AIDS comorbidities, low BMD, specifically osteoporosis and consequent fragility fractures, occur at an earlier age than is expected in HIV-infected persons. There is evidence that persons with HIV are at greater risk of having low BMD compared with non–HIV-infected persons[129–133] and this change is associated with an increased risk of fracture.[134,135] These findings were summarized nicely in a metaanalysis in which HIV-infected men and women, when compared with uninfected controls, had a 3.7-fold increased risk of osteoporosis (T-score ≤ -2.5) and 6.4-fold increased risk of low BMD (T-score < -1.0).[16] Effort is being taken to understand the etiology of bone loss, persons most at risk of developing fractures, and appropriate prevention and treatment strategies in HIV-infected persons. A recently published study evaluating BMD in HIV-infected adolescents and matched seronegative adolescents reported that there were striking reductions not only in BMD, as measured by DXA, but also bone strength or quality, as assessed by high-resolution computed tomography at the distal radius and tibia.[136] This study has implications regarding long-term risk for fragility fractures for individuals who are infected early in life and fail to reach peak BMD.

Risk Factors for Low BMD

Common risk factors for osteoporosis in the general population are similarly associated with low BMD among HIV-infected persons and include older age,[137–139] lower BMI,[137–140] and menopausal state.[140] In contrast with the general population, male sex has been associated with a greater risk of low BMD among HIV-infected cohorts.[139,140] HCV coinfection and drug use are also associated with lower BMD and these risk factors are more common among HIV-infected persons.[140]

The specific effects of individual ARVs is often challenging because combination therapy is the standard of care. That being said, there seems to be a catabolic window during the first 48 to 96 weeks after ART initiation in which HIV-infected individuals are particularly susceptible to bone loss, regardless of the ARVs selected, with subsequent stabilization of BMD by 96 weeks.[141] In a recent metaanalysis comparing ART-naïve, HIV-infected persons with a group on ART, the ART-treated cohort had a 2.5-fold greater risk of low BMD, largely osteoporosis.[16] However, there was no adjustment for potential confounders. In other studies, longer ART duration has been associated with lower BMD.[137,142,143] In the SMART study, loss of BMD was greater among patients receiving continuous ART when compared with patients on intermittent ART.[144] Furthermore, markers of bone turnover were increased among subjects receiving continuous ART, and intermittent ART was associated with an initial decrease in bone turnover followed by stabilization.[145] This latter stabilization occurred despite an increase in inflammatory markers and increased bone resorption cytokines. These findings support an ART-related bone toxicity.

Tenofovir is frequently implicated as a cause of bone toxicity owing to its effect at the proximal tubule leading to a Fanconi-like syndrome with phosphate wasting.[146] Treatment with tenofovir led to significant reductions in BMD of children that were reversed with tenofovir cessation.[147] Notably, longitudinal studies have confirmed that longer tenofovir duration is associated with greater loss of BMD.[139] Data from pre-exposure prophylaxis studies in seronegative adults confirm the relationship between tenofovir and BMD loss.[148]

A captivating ARV agent has recently piqued the interest among bone mavens in the HIV field: Tenofovir alafenamide fumarate (TAF), an investigational tenofovir prodrug. Data regarding changes in BMD comparing TAF versus tenofovir in combination with the same additional ARVs have confirmed the superiority of TAF over tenofovir at both total hip (−0.6% vs −2.4%; $P<.001$) and lumbar spine (−1.0% vs −3.4%; $P<.001$) BMD changes after 48 weeks of therapy.[149]

The relationship between exposure to protease inhibitors and bone loss is also intriguing. In recently published work by Hernandez-Vallejo and colleagues,[150] osteoblast precursor cells exposed to ritonavir boosted protease inhibitors lost proliferative capacity, demonstrated increased oxidative stress and markers of senescence and failed to differentiate into osteoblasts. These in vitro data suggest that the balance between osteoblast bone formation and osteoclast bone resorption is dysregulated by protease inhibitors, leading to excessive bone loss. The mechanism by which protease inhibitors induces loss of BMD remains unclear. Clearly, we will have numerous alternative ARV options to consider in the future.

Fracture Risk

The updated guidelines from the National Osteoporosis Foundation now recognize both HIV infection and ART as risk factors for osteoporosis and fragility fractures.[151] This addition reflects the growing data on fractures and HIV.[135,152,153] For instance, a 3-fold increased risk of incident fracture was identified among HIV-infected subjects in the HIV Outpatient Study (HOPS) when compared with a representative sample of the US population at large, with a striking increased risk among young (ages 25–54) HIV-infected persons.[154] A similar 3-fold increased risk of any fracture was seen among HIV-infected persons in a Danish cohort.[155] Another study evaluating fracture risk derived from US Medicare data, including 13,000 HIV-infected and 2.5 million seronegative persons, demonstrated a 50% increased risk of fracture among the HIV-infected cohort.[156] As with low BMD, fracture risk has been reported to be increased within the catabolic window, an early period after ART initiation.[153] Furthermore, certain ARVs have been associated with incident fractures, with exposure to tenofovir and protease inhibitors being reported most commonly.[157,158] HCV has also been implicated in fracture incidence. Recently reported Medicaid data from five states demonstrated a 2-fold increase in fracture rate among HCV monoinfected, a 1.5-fold increase in fracture rate among HIV-infected, and an additive effect for coinfected persons compared with uninfected individuals.[33] These data were confirmed in 2 other cohort studies, although data from the Veterans Aging Cohort Study failed to confirm the association of fracture with HCV.[152,159,160] Of note, the authors of the latter study conjectured that, by controlling for fibrosis, they had mitigated the effects of HCV infection.

Screening for Low BMD

The appropriate time to initiate osteoporosis screening using DXA in HIV-infected persons is still slightly unclear, but current recommendations are to screen all HIV-infected postmenopausal women, HIV-infected men 50 years and older, and younger HIV-infected persons with a recent fracture.[141] A retrospective analysis of HIV-infected patients in Spain also helps us to understand how DXA findings may progress.[161] In this study of mainly men with a median age of 39 and an average of 4 DXA scans, the median time to progression from normal BMD to osteopenia range was 6.7 years and occurred in approximately one-third of those with normal BMD at baseline. However, among those with a baseline T-score between −0.6 and −1.0, time to progression to osteopenia was only 1.7 years. Among those with osteopenia-range T-scores at baseline, time to progression to osteoporosis was more than 8.5 years among the 25% that progressed, shorter in those who were older (>40 years old) and with lower T-scores (<−1.8).[161] These findings emphasize the importance of considering osteoporosis risk factors in determining overall screening rates and fracture risk. Other methods of assessing fracture risk in HIV-infected patients have been minimally evaluated. In 2 studies utilizing the World Health Organization's FRAX calculator, fracture risk was underestimated in HIV-infected persons.[162,163] However, the combined use of FRAX and the Aging Male Symptoms scale may be useful in HIV-infected men.[163]

DIABETES MELLITUS
Epidemiology

Several cohorts of HIV-infected individuals in North America have demonstrated an high prevalence of diabetes mellitus (14%) as well as IR, a precursor for diabetes mellitus.[23,29,164] This prevalence is similar to that demonstrated by data from the 2005 to 2006 National Health and Nutrition Examination Survey, where the crude prevalence for diabetes mellitus among the general US population was 13% and for prediabetes mellitus is 30% (either impaired fasting glucose or impaired glucose tolerance).[165] Traditional risk factors, such as sedentary lifestyle, unhealthy diet, and obesity, were significantly associated with diabetes mellitus.

In the Multicenter AIDS Cohort Study, HIV-infected men had a greater odds of IR than HIV-negative men, regardless of ART exposure,[166] and diabetes mellitus incidence was 4 times higher among HIV-infected men on ART compared with uninfected men.[23] Furthermore, each additional year of nucleoside reverse transcriptase use (NRTI) increased the odds of hyperinsulinemia.[166] A recent analysis evaluating 752 HIV-infected women enrolled in the Study to Understand the Natural History of HIV/AIDS in the Era of Effective Therapy and the HOPS reported that diabetes mellitus was present in 14.2% of the women.[29] Similarly, the Women's Interagency HIV Study demonstrated that HIV-infected women prescribed ART had greater IR as quantified by the Homeostatic Model Assessment (HOMA-IR) compared with HIV-negative women.[164] Of note, the latter study reported that longer cumulative NRTI exposure was associated with greater HOMA-IR values.

Risk Factors

There have been many proposed etiologies for this increased risk for IR among HIV-infected persons, including ART. IR has been reported in HIV-negative subjects after brief exposure to ARVs, indicating that even short-term exposure to some, but not all, ARVs, may induce IR.[167–170] Multiple studies of long-term ART exposure, specifically cumulative NRTI use, have shown an association between these medications and an increased risk of IR and diabetes mellitus.[91,164,166] Protease inhibitors, such as ritonavir, may act directly on mediators of glucose uptake, affecting glucose regulation.[171] However, several studies in HIV-negative populations taking short-term, ritonavir-boosted lopinavir or unboosted atazanavir have reported conflicting findings regarding insulin metabolism, indicating that the causative pathway may be more complex and multifactorial.[167–170]

Increased body mass index has a consistent association with IR. Although HIV disease is traditionally thought of as a wasting illness, patients engaged in care and treated with ART typically experience significant weight gain. A recent study illustrated that 60% of HIV-infected patients gain weight once they engage in care.[172] In a recent study of 681 HIV-infected adults, 44% were overweight or obese (BMI >25.0 kg/m^2) and over 24 months, 20% moved from normal to over-weight/obese BMI categories.[18] These data confirm the findings of other HIV cohort studies and likely reflect the obesity epidemic affecting the population as a whole in Western, industrialized nations.[173] Clinicians should recognize the risk for both obesity and IR among their HIV-infected patients and develop preventive strategies.

IR and diabetes mellitus have been previously associated with HCV infection, likely mediated through impairment of hepatic glucose clearance.[34] In a recent study investigating risk factors for HCV treatment failure among HIV-infected persons, IR was the strongest predictor of failure to achieve a sustained virologic response; the highest sustained virologic response rate (35%) was in patients with an HOMA-IR of less than 2.[174] IR has been shown to reduce treatment effectiveness in patients with HCV monoinfection, as well.[175] Furthermore, IR is associated with steatosis and liver stiffness and possibly even increased risk of hepatocellular carcinoma, which may further complicate the management of liver disease in HIV-infected patients.[34,176,177] Thus, the strong association between HCV and IR has ramifications for treatment and long-term outcomes of both HIV and HCV infection.

Inflammation has been identified as a key player in the development of IR in the general population.[178,179] A recent study in HIV-infected persons initiating ART reported that higher levels of the inflammatory markers high-sensitivity C-reactive protein, sTNFR1 and sTNFR2 were associated with an increased risk for diabetes mellitus despite suppressive ART.[180] These data suggest that the inflammatory milieu of HIV infection may also contribute to development of IR. Inflammatory biomarkers are affected by other factors identified as independently associated with IR, most notably obesity and chronic HCV infection.[37,181] Longer-term follow-up from prospective longitudinal cohorts will further elucidate the complex relationship between HIV-related chronic inflammation, ARV use, and IR.

Obesity and HIV

Before the availability of ART, AIDS wasting was a common AIDS-defining condition. However, the US obesity epidemic has spread into HIV clinics, as well. Up to two-thirds of the HIV populations in US and African populations have been found to be overweight or obese.[18,172,182–187] In a rural South African population, obesity was more than 6-fold more common among HIV-infected women than men, but men were more likely to have hypertension associated with obesity.[184] In a US population followed for 12 months after the initiation of ART, more weight gain occurred among women than men (8.6 vs 3.6 kg; $P = .04$); among those started on PI-containing ART regimen than non–PI-containing ART regimen (9.0 vs 2.7 kg; $P = .001$) and among those with lower CD4 counts (<200 cells/mm^3) than those with CD4 counts above 200 cells/mm^3 (8.9 vs 0.3 kg; $P<.0001$).[187] These findings are supported by similar results from another US population in which HIV-infected persons with lower baseline CD4 counts (<50 cells/mm^3) and those treated with a ritonavir-boosted PI regimen had the greatest increases in BMI.[18] With the comorbidities associated with obesity, including diabetes mellitus, CVD, obstructive sleep apnea, and urinary incontinence, efforts to better understand and manage the weight gain and obesity after virologic suppression are needed.

SUMMARY

In the current ART era, the AIDS defining complications can be minimized with engagement in care and adherence to ART, yet the success of treatment has created new challenges. Particularly, the recognition of cardiometabolic comorbidities that seem to occur at an accelerated rate owing to persistent inflammation of HIV, ART toxicity, and preexisting health disparities for many HIV-infected persons. Future research will balance the aggressive guideline approach to these comorbidities with the potential complications of polypharmacy, quality-of-life issues, and alternative strategies such as exercise and dietary interventions. The next decade will see a brave, new world in the field of HIV.

REFERENCES

1. Antiretroviral Therapy Cohort Collaboration. Life expectancy of individuals on combination antiretroviral therapy in high-income countries: a collaborative analysis of 14 cohort studies. Lancet 2008;372:293–9.
2. Weber R, Ruppik M, Rickenbach M, et al. Decreasing mortality and changing patterns of causes of death in the Swiss HIV Cohort Study. HIV Med 2013;14: 195–207.
3. Data Collection on Adverse Events of Anti-HIV drugs (D:A:D) Study Group. Factors associated with specific causes of death amongst HIV-positive individuals in the D:A:D Study. AIDS 2010;24:1537–48.
4. Palella FJ Jr, Baker RK, Moorman AC, et al. Mortality in the highly active antiretroviral therapy era: changing causes of death and disease in the HIV outpatient study. J Acquir Immune Defic Syndr 2006;43:27–34.
5. Effros RB, Fletcher CV, Gebo K, et al. Aging and infectious diseases: workshop on HIV infection and aging: what is known and future research directions. Clin Infect Dis 2008;47:542–53.
6. High KP, Brennan-Ing M, Clifford DB, et al. HIV and aging: state of knowledge and areas of critical need for research. A report to the NIH Office of AIDS Research by the HIV and Aging Working Group. J Acquir Immune Defic Syndr 2012;60(Suppl 1):S1–18.
7. Wada N, Jacobson LP, Cohen M, et al. Cause-specific life expectancies after 35 years of age for human immunodeficiency syndrome-infected and human immunodeficiency syndrome-negative individuals followed simultaneously in long-term cohort studies, 1984-2008. Am J Epidemiol 2013;177:116–25.
8. Neuhaus J, Angus B, Kowalska JD, et al. Risk of all-cause mortality associated with nonfatal AIDS and serious non-AIDS events among adults infected with HIV. AIDS 2010;24(5):697–706.
9. Antiretroviral Therapy Cohort Collaboration. Causes of death in HIV-1-infected patients treated with antiretroviral therapy, 1996-2006: collaborative analysis of 13 HIV cohort studies. Clin Infect Dis 2010;50:1387–96.
10. Marin B, Thiébaut R, Bucher HC, et al. Non-AIDS-defining deaths and immunodeficiency in the era of combination antiretroviral therapy. AIDS 2009;23: 1743–53.
11. French AL, Gawel SH, Hershow R, et al. Trends in mortality and causes of death among women with HIV in the United States: a 10-year study. J Acquir Immune Defic Syndr 2009;51:399–406.

12. Lewden C, May T, Rosenthal E, et al. Changes in causes of death among adults infected by HIV between 2000 and 2005: the "Mortalité 2000 and 2005" surveys (ANRS EN19 and Mortavic). J Acquir Immune Defic Syndr 2008;48:590–8.
13. Neuhaus J, Jacobs DR Jr, Baker JV, et al. Markers of inflammation, coagulation, and renal function are elevated in adults with HIV infection. J Infect Dis 2010; 201:1788–95.
14. Pathai S, Bajillan H, Landay AL, et al. Is HIV a model of accelerated or accentuated aging? J Gerontol A Biol Sci Med Sci 2014;69(7):833–42. http://dx.doi.org/10.1093/Gerona/glt168.
15. Gupta SK, Eustace JA, Winston JA, et al. Guidelines for the management of chronic kidney disease in HIV-infected patients: recommendations of the HIV Medicine Association of the Infectious Diseases Society of America. Clin Infect Dis 2005;40:1559–85.
16. Brown TT, Qaqish RB. Antiretroviral therapy and the prevalence of osteopenia and osteoporosis: a meta-analytic review. AIDS 2006;20:2165–74.
17. Crum-Cianflone N, Tejidor R, Medina S, et al. Obesity among patients with HIV: the latest epidemic. AIDS Patient Care STDS 2008;22:925–30.
18. Tate T, Willig AL, Willig JH, et al. HIV infection and obesity: where did all the wasting go? Antivir Ther 2012;17(7):1281–9.
19. Thompson-Paul A, Wei S, Mattson C, et al. Prevalence of obesity in a nationally representative sample of HIV+ adults receiving medical care in the US: Medical Monitoring Project, 2009. 20th Conference on Retroviruses and Opportunistic Infections [abstract: 777]. Atlanta, March 3–6, 2013.
20. Nahvi S, Cooperman NA. Review: the need for smoking cessation among HIV-positive smokers. AIDS Educ Prev 2009;21(Suppl 3):14–27.
21. Khalsa A, Karim R, Mack WJ, et al. Correlates of prevalent hypertension in a large cohort of HIV-infected women: Women's Interagency HIV Study. AIDS 2007;21: 2539–41.
22. Medina-Torne S, Ganesan A, Barahona I, et al. Hypertension is common among HIV-infected persons, but not associated with HAART. J Int Assoc Physicians AIDS Care (Chic) 2012;11:20–5.
23. Brown TT, Cole SR, Li X, et al. Antiretroviral therapy and the prevalence and incidence of diabetes mellitus in the multicenter AIDS cohort study. Arch Intern Med 2005;165:1179–84.
24. Grunfeld C. Dyslipidemia and its treatment in HIV infection. Top HIV Med 2010; 18(3):112–8.
25. Feeney ER, Mallon PW. Insulin resistance in treated HIV infection. Best Pract Res Clin Endocrinol Metab 2011;25:443–58.
26. Schafer JJ, Manlangit K, Squires KE. Bone health and human immunodeficiency virus infection. Pharmacotherapy 2013;33:665–82.
27. Ryom L, Mocroft A, Kirk O, et al. Association between antiretroviral exposure and renal impairment among HIV-positive persons with normal baseline renal function: the D:A:D study. J Infect Dis 2013;207:1359–69.
28. Kalayjian RC, Lau B, Mechekano RN, et al. Risk factors for chronic kidney disease in a large cohort of HIV-1 infected individuals initiating antiretroviral therapy in routine care. AIDS 2012;26:1907–15.
29. Buchacz K, Baker RK, Palella FJ Jr, et al. Disparities in prevalence of key chronic diseases by gender and race/ethnicity among antiretroviral-treated HIV-infected adults in the US. Antivir Ther 2013;18:65–75.
30. Centers for Disease Control and Prevention. CDC Health Disparities and Inequalities Report—United States, 2011. MMWR Surveill Summ 2011;60(Suppl):1–113.

31. Green TC, Kershaw T, Lin H, et al. Patterns of drug use and abuse among aging adults with and without HIV: a latent class analysis of a US Veteran cohort. Drug Alcohol Depend 2010;110(3):208–20.

32. Lucas GM, Jing Y, Sulkowski M, et al. Hepatitis C viremia and the risk of chronic kidney disease in HIV-infected individuals. J Infect Dis 2013;208:1240–9.

33. Lo Re V 3rd, Volk J, Newcomb CW, et al. Risk of hip fracture associated with hepatitis C virus infection and hepatitis C/human immunodeficiency virus coinfection. Hepatology 2012;56:1688–98.

34. Moucari R, Asselah T, Cazals-Hatem D, et al. Insulin resistance in chronic hepatitis C: association with genotypes 1 and 4, serum HCV RNA level, and liver fibrosis. Gastroenterology 2008;134:416–23.

35. Jain MK, Aragaki C, Fischbach L, et al. Hepatitis C is associated with type 2 diabetes mellitus in HIV-infected persons without traditional risk factors. HIV Med 2007;8:491–7.

36. Gillis J, Smieja M, Cescon A, et al. Risk of cardiovascular disease associated with HCV and HBV co-infection among antiretroviral-treated HIV-infected individuals. Antivir Ther 2014;19(3):309–17. http://dx.doi.org/10.3851/IMP2724.

37. Adinolfi LE, Restivo L, Zampino R, et al. Chronic HCV infection is a risk of atherosclerosis. Role of HCV and HCV-related steatosis. Atherosclerosis 2012;221:496–502.

38. Guaraldi G, Orlando G, Zona S, et al. Premature age-related comorbidities among HIV-infected persons compared with the general population. Clin Infect Dis 2011;53:1120–6.

39. Kim DJ, Westfall AO, Chamot E, et al. Multimorbidity patterns in HIV-infected patients: the role of obesity in chronic disease clustering. J Acquir Immune Defic Syndr 2012;61:600–5.

40. Goulet JL, Fultz SL, Rimland D, et al. Aging and infectious diseases: do patterns of comorbidity vary by HIV status, age, and HIV severity? Clin Infect Dis 2007; 45:1593–601.

41. Salter ML, Lau B, Go VF, et al. HIV infection, immune suppression, and uncontrolled viremia are associated with increased multimorbidity among aging injection drug users. Clin Infect Dis 2011;53:1256–64.

42. Hasse B, Ledergerber B, Furrer H, et al. Morbidity and aging in HIV-infected persons: the Swiss HIV cohort study. Clin Infect Dis 2011;53:1130–9.

43. Desquilbet L, Jacobson LP, Fried LP, et al. HIV-1 infection is associated with an earlier occurrence of a phenotype related to frailty. J Gerontol A Biol Sci Med Sci 2007;62:1279–86.

44. Libby P, Ridker PM, Hansson GK. Progress and challenges in translating the biology of atherosclerosis. Nature 2011;473:317–25.

45. Shrestha S, Irvin MR, Grunfeld C, et al. HIV, inflammation, and calcium in atherosclerosis. Arterioscler Thromb Vasc Biol 2014;34:244–50.

46. Grunfeld C, Delaney JA, Wanke C, et al. Preclinical atherosclerosis due to HIV infection: carotid intima-medial thickness measurements from the FRAM study. AIDS 2009;23:1841–9.

47. Hsue PY, Lo JC, Franklin A, et al. Progression of atherosclerosis as assessed by carotid intima-media thickness in patients with HIV infection. Circulation 2004; 109:1603–8.

48. Lo J, Abbara S, Shturman L, et al. Increased prevalence of subclinical coronary atherosclerosis detected by coronary computed tomography angiography in HIV-infected men. AIDS 2010;24:243–53.

49. Solages A, Vita JA, Thornton DJ, et al. Endothelial function in HIV-infected persons. Clin Infect Dis 2006;42:1325–32.

50. Kristoffersen US, Lebech AM, Wiinberg N, et al. Silent ischemic heart disease and pericardial fat volume in HIV-infected patients: a case-control myocardial perfusion scintigraphy study. PLoS One 2013;8(8):e72066. http://dx.doi.org/10.1371/journal.pone.0072066.

51. Zanni MV, Abbara S, Lo J, et al. Increased coronary atherosclerotic plaque vulnerability by coronary computed tomography angiography in HIV-infected men. AIDS 2013;27:1263–72.

52. Triant VA, Lee H, Hadigan C, et al. Increased acute myocardial infarction rates and cardiovascular risk factors among patients with human immunodeficiency virus disease. J Clin Endocrinol Metab 2007;92:2506–12.

53. Freiberg MS, Chang CC, Kuller LH, et al. HIV infection and the risk of acute myocardial infarction. JAMA Intern Med 2013;173:614–22.

54. Durand M, Sheehy O, Baril JG, et al. Association between HIV infection, antiretroviral therapy, and risk of acute myocardial infarction: a cohort and nested case-control study using Québec's public health insurance database. J Acquir Immune Defic Syndr 2011;57:245–53.

55. Chow FC, Regan S, Feske S, et al. Comparison of ischemic stroke incidence in HIV-infected and non-HIV-infected patients in a US health care system. J Acquir Immune Defic Syndr 2012;60:351–8.

56. Vinikoor MJ, Napravnik S, Floris-Moore M, et al. Incidence and clinical features of cerebrovascular disease among HIV-infected adults in the Southeastern United States. AIDS Res Hum Retroviruses 2013;29:1068–74.

57. Rasmussen LD, Engsig FN, Christensen H, et al. Risk of cerebrovascular events in persons with and without HIV: a Danish nationwide population-based cohort study. AIDS 2011;25:1637–46.

58. Kaplan RC, Sinclair E, Landay AL, et al. T cell activation and senescence predict subclinical carotid artery disease in HIV-infected women. J Infect Dis 2011;203:452–63.

59. Kaplan RC, Sinclair E, Landay AL, et al. T cell activation predicts carotid artery stiffness among HIV-infected women. Atherosclerosis 2011;217:207–13.

60. Merlini E, Luzi K, Suardi E, et al. T-cell phenotypes, apoptosis and inflammation in HIV+ patients on virologically effective cART with early atherosclerosis. PLoS One 2012;7(9):e46073. http://dx.doi.org/10.1371/journal.pone.0046073.

61. Longenecker CT, Funderburg NT, Jiang Y, et al. Markers of inflammation and CD8 T-cell activation, but not monocyte activation, are associated with subclinical carotid artery disease in HIV-infected individuals. HIV Med 2013;14:385–90.

62. Kelesidis T, Kendall MA, Yang OO, et al. Biomarkers of microbial translocation and macrophage activation: association with progression of subclinical atherosclerosis in HIV-1 infection. J Infect Dis 2012;206:1558–67.

63. Burdo TH, Lo J, Abbara S, et al. Soluble CD163, a novel marker of activated macrophages, is elevated and associated with noncalcified coronary plaque in HIV-infected patients. J Infect Dis 2011;204:1227–36.

64. Subramanian S, Tawakol A, Burdo TH, et al. Arterial inflammation in patients with HIV. JAMA 2012;308:379–86.

65. Strategies for Management of Antiretroviral Therapy (SMART) Study Group. CD4+ count-guided interruption of antiretroviral treatment. N Engl J Med 2006;355:2283–96.

66. Kuller LH, Tracy R, Belloso W, et al. Inflammatory and coagulation biomarkers and mortality in patients with HIV infection. PLoS Med 2008;5(10):e203. http://dx.doi.org/10.1371/journal.pmed.0050203.

67. Duprez DA, Neuhaus J, Kuller LH, et al. Inflammation, coagulation and cardiovascular disease in HIV-infected individuals. PLoS One 2012;7(9):e44454. http://dx.doi.org/10.1371/journal.pone.0044454.
68. Baker JV, Brummel-Ziedins K, Neuhaus J, et al. HIV replication alters the composition of extrinsic pathway coagulation factors and increases thrombin generation. J Am Heart Assoc 2013;2(4):e000264.
69. Blum A, Hadas V, Burke M, et al. Viral load of the human immunodeficiency virus could be an independent risk factor for endothelial dysfunction. Clin Cardiol 2005;28:149–53.
70. Oliviero U, Bonadies G, Apuzzi V, et al. Human immunodeficiency virus per se exerts atherogenic effects. Atherosclerosis 2009;204:586–9.
71. Baker JV, Neuhaus J, Duprez D, et al. HIV replication, inflammation, and the effect of starting antiretroviral therapy on plasma asymmetric dimethylarginine, a novel marker of endothelial dysfunction. J Acquir Immune Defic Syndr 2012; 60:128–34.
72. Torriani FJ, Komarow L, Parker RA, et al. Endothelial function in human immunodeficiency virus-infected antiretroviral-naive subjects before and after starting potent antiretroviral therapy: The ACTG (AIDS Clinical Trials Group) Study 5152s. J Am Coll Cardiol 2008;52(7):569–76.
73. Hsue PY, Hunt PW, Sinclair E, et al. Increased carotid intima-media thickness in HIV patients is associated with increased cytomegalovirus-specific T-cell responses. AIDS 2006;20:2275–83.
74. Parrinello CM, Sinclair E, Landay AL, et al. Cytomegalovirus immunoglobulin G antibody is associated with subclinical carotid artery disease among HIV-infected women. J Infect Dis 2012;205:1788.
75. Masiá M, Robledano C, Ortiz de la Tabla V, et al. Increased carotid intima-media thickness associated with antibody responses to varicella-zoster virus and cytomegalovirus in HIV-infected patients. PLoS One 2013;8(5):e64327. http://dx.doi.org/10.1371/journal.pone.0064327.
76. Guadalupe M, Reay E, Sankaran S, et al. Severe CD4+ T-cell depletion in gut lymphoid tissue during primary human immunodeficiency virus type 1 infection and substantial delay in restoration following highly active antiretroviral therapy. J Virol 2003;77:11708–17.
77. Sankaran S, George MD, Reay E, et al. Rapid onset of intestinal epithelial barrier dysfunction in primary human immunodeficiency virus infection is driven by imbalance between immune response and mucosal repair and regeneration. J Virol 2008;82:538–45.
78. Brenchley JM, Price DA, Schacker TW, et al. Microbial translocation is a cause of systemic immune activation in chronic HIV infection. Nat Med 2006;12:1365–71.
79. Pedersen KK, Pedersen M, Trøseid M, et al. Microbial translocation in HIV infection is associated with dyslipidemia, insulin resistance, and risk of myocardial infarction. J Acquir Immune Defic Syndr 2013;64:425–33.
80. El-Sadr WM, Mullin CM, Carr A, et al. Effects of HIV disease on lipid, glucose and insulin levels: results from a large antiretroviral-naive cohort. HIV Med 2005;6(2):114–21.
81. Kwong GP, Ghani AC, Rode RA, et al. Comparison of the risks of atherosclerotic events versus death from other causes associated with antiretroviral use. AIDS 2006;20:1941–50.
82. Lichtenstein KA, Armon C, Buchacz K, et al. Low CD4+ T cell count is a risk factor for cardiovascular disease events in the HIV outpatient study. Clin Infect Dis 2010;51:435–47.

83. Jung O, Bickel M, Ditting T, et al. Hypertension in HIV-1-infected patients and its impact on renal and cardiovascular integrity. Nephrol Dial Transplant 2004;19: 2250–8.

84. Savès M, Chêne G, Ducimetière P, et al. Risk factors for coronary heart disease in patients treated for human immunodeficiency virus infection compared with the general population. Clin Infect Dis 2003;37:292–8.

85. Lifson AR, Neuhaus J, Arribas JR, et al. Smoking-related health risks among persons with HIV in the strategies for management of antiretroviral therapy clinical trial. Am J Public Health 2010;100:1896–903.

86. Worm SW, De Wit S, Weber R, et al. Diabetes mellitus, preexisting coronary heart disease, and the risk of subsequent coronary heart disease events in patients infected with human immunodeficiency virus: the Data Collection on Adverse Events of Anti-HIV Drugs (D:A:D Study). Circulation 2009;119: 805–11.

87. Oh JY, Greene K, He H, et al. Population-based study of risk factors for coronary heart disease among HIV-infected persons. Open AIDS J 2012;6:177–80.

88. Nüesch R, Wang Q, Elzi L, et al. Risk of cardiovascular events and blood pressure control in hypertensive HIV-infected patients: Swiss HIV Cohort Study (SHCS). J Acquir Immune Defic Syndr 2013;62:396–404.

89. Petoumenos K, Worm S, Reiss P, et al. Rates of cardiovascular disease following smoking cessation in patients with HIV infection: results from the D:A:D study. HIV Med 2011;12:412–21.

90. Calvo-Sánchez M, Perelló R, Pérez I, et al. Differences between HIV-infected and uninfected adults in the contributions of smoking, diabetes and hypertension to acute coronary syndrome: two parallel case-control studies. HIV Med 2013;14:40–8.

91. Ledergerber B, Furrer H, Rickenbach M, et al. Factors associated with the incidence of type 2 diabetes mellitus in HIV-infected participants in the Swiss HIV Cohort Study. Clin Infect Dis 2007;45:111–9.

92. Grinspoon SK, Grunfeld C, Kotler DP, et al. State of the science conference: initiative to decrease cardiovascular risk and increase quality of care for patients living with HIV/AIDS: executive summary. Circulation 2008;118(2): 198–210.

93. Panel on Antiretroviral Guidelines for Adults and Adolescents. Guidelines for the use of antiretroviral agents in HIV-1-infected adults and adolescents. Department of Health and Human Services. Available at: http://aidsinfo.nih.gov/ContentFiles/AdultandAdolescentGL.pdf. Accessed March 3, 2013.

94. Aberg JA, Gallant JE, Ghanem KG, et al. Primary care guidelines for the management of persons infected with HIV: 2013 update by the HIV Medicine Association of the Infectious Diseases Society of America. Clin Infect Dis 2014;58(1): 1–10.

95. James PA, Oparil S, Carter BL, et al. 2014 evidence-based guideline for the management of high blood pressure in adults: report from the panel members appointed to the Eighth Joint National Committee (JNC 8). JAMA 2014;311: 507–20.

96. Stone NJ, Robinson JG, Lichtenstein AH, et al. Treatment of blood cholesterol to reduce atherosclerotic cardiovascular disease risk in adults: synopsis of the 2013 ACC/AHA cholesterol guideline. Ann Intern Med 2014;160(5):339–43. http://dx.doi.org/10.7326/M14-0126.

97. American Diabetes Association. Standards of medical care in diabetes–2014. Diabetes Care 2014;37(Suppl 1):S14–80.

98. Overton ET, Kitch D, Benson CA, et al. The effect of statin therapy in reducing the risk of serious non-AIDS-defining events and non-accidental death. Clin Infect Dis 2013;56(10):1471–9.

99. Lucas GM, Eustace JA, Sozio S, et al. Highly active antiretroviral therapy and the incidence of HIV-1-associated nephropathy and response to highly-active anti-retroviral therapy. Lancet 1998;352:783–4.

100. Ross MJ, Klotman PE. Recent progress in HIV-associated nephropathy. J Am Soc Nephrol 2002;13:2997–3004.

101. Jones R, Stebbing J, Nelson M, et al. Renal dysfunction with tenofovir disproxil fumarate-containing highly active antiretroviral therapy regimens is not observed more frequently: a cohort and case-control study. J Acquir Immune Defic Syndr 2004;37:1489–95.

102. Schwartz EJ, Szczech LA, Ross MJ, et al. Highly active antiretroviral therapy and the epidemic of HIV+ end-stage renal disease. J Am Soc Nephrol 2005; 16:2412–20.

103. Mocroft A, Kirk O, Gatell J, et al. Chronic renal failure among HIV-1-infected patients. AIDS 2007;21:1119–27.

104. Overton ET, Patel P, Mondy K, et al. Cystatin C and baseline renal function among HIV-infected persons in the SUN Study. AIDS Res Hum Retroviruses 2012;28(2):148–55.

105. Röling J, Schmid H, Fischereder M, et al. HIV-associated renal diseases and highly active antiretroviral therapy-induced nephropathy. Clin Infect Dis 2006; 42:1488–95.

106. Baekken M, Os I, Sandvik L, et al. Hypertension in an urban HIV-positive population compared with the general population: influence of combination antiretroviral therapy. J Hypertens 2008;26:2126–33.

107. Butt AA, McGinnis K, Rodriguez-Barradas MC, et al. HIV infection and the risk of diabetes mellitus. AIDS 2009;23:1227–34.

108. Jao M, Wyatt CM. Antiretroviral medications: adverse effects on the kidney. Adv Chronic Kidney Dis 2010;17:71–82.

109. Kohler JJ, Hosseini SH, Hoying-Brandt A, et al. Tenofovir renal toxicity targets mitochondria of renal proximal tubules. Lab Invest 2009;89:513–9.

110. Cooper RD, Wiebe N, Smith N, et al. Systematic review and meta-analysis: renal safety of tenofovir disoproxil fumarate in HIV-infected patients. Clin Infect Dis 2010;51:496–505.

111. Gallant J, Moore RD. Renal function with use of a tenofovir-containing initial antiretroviral regimen. AIDS 2009;23:1971–5.

112. Albini L, Cesana BM, Motta D, et al. A randomized, pilot trial to evaluate glomerular filtration rate by creatinine or cystatin C in naive HIV-infected patients after tenofovir/emtricitabine in combination with atazanavir/ritonavir or efavirenz. J Acquir Immune Defic Syndr 2012;59(1):18–30.

113. Horberg M, Tang B, Towner W, et al. Impact of tenofovir on renal function in HIV-infected, anti-retroviral naive patients. J Acquir Immune Defic Syndr 2010;53:62–9.

114. Jenh AM, Thio CL, Pham PA. Tenofovir for the treatment of hepatitis B virus. Pharmacotherapy 2009;29:1212–27.

115. Okwundu CI, Okoromah CA. Antiretroviral pre-exposure prophylaxis (PrEP) for preventing HIV in high-risk individuals. Cochrane Database Syst Rev 2009;(1):CD007189.

116. Solomon MM, Lama JR, Glidden DV, et al, for the iPrEx Study Team. Changes in renal function associated with oral emtricitabine/tenofovir disoproxil fumarate use for HIV pre-exposure prophylaxis. AIDS 2014;28(6):851–9.

117. Shemesh O, Golbetz H, Kriss JP, et al. Limitations of creatinine as a filtration marker in glomerulopathic patients. Kidney Int 1985;28:830–8.
118. Filler G, Bökenkamp A, Hofmann W, et al. Cystatin C as a marker of GFR-history, indications, and future research. Clin Biochem 2005;38:1–8.
119. Grubb A, Simonsen O, Sturfelt G, et al. Serum concentration of cystatin C, factor D and beta 2-microglobulin as a measure of glomerular filtration rate. Acta Med Scand 1985;218:499–503.
120. Simonsen O, Grubb A, Thysell H. The blood serum concentration of cystatin C (gamma-trace) as a measure of the glomerular filtration rate. Scand J Clin Lab Invest 1985;45:97–101.
121. Stevens LA, Coresh J, Schmid CH, et al. Estimating GFR using serum cystatin C alone and in combination with serum creatinine: a pooled analysis of 3,418 individuals with CKD. Am J Kidney Dis 2008;51:395–406.
122. Shlipak MG, Katz R, Kestenbaum B, et al. Rate of kidney function decline in older adults: a comparison using creatinine and cystatin C. Am J Nephrol 2009;30:171–8.
123. Odden MC, Chertow GM, Fried LF, et al. Cystatin C and measures of physical function in elderly adults: the Health, Aging, and Body Composition (HABC) Study. Am J Epidemiol 2006;164:1180–9.
124. Odden MC, Scherzer R, Bacchetti P, et al. Cystatin C level as a marker of kidney function in human immunodeficiency virus infection: the FRAM study. Arch Intern Med 2007;167:2213–9.
125. Jones CY, Jones CA, Wilson IB, et al. Cystatin C and creatinine in an HIV cohort: the nutrition for healthy living study. Am J Kidney Dis 2008;51:914–24.
126. Mocroft A, Wyatt C, Szczech L, et al. Interruption of antiretroviral therapy is associated with increased plasma cystatin C. AIDS 2009;23:71–82.
127. Menon V, Shlipak M, Wang X, et al. Cystatin C as a risk factor for outcomes in CKD. Ann Intern Med 2007;147:19–27.
128. Kanis JA, Melton LJ 3rd, Christiansen C, et al. The diagnosis of osteoporosis. J Bone Miner Res 1994;9(8):1137–41.
129. Brown TT, Ruppe MD, Kassner R, et al. Reduced bone mineral density in human immunodeficiency virus-infected patients and its association with increased central adiposity and postload hyperglycemia. J Clin Endocrinol Metab 2004; 89(3):1200–6.
130. Bruera D, Luna N, David DO, et al. Decreased bone mineral density in HIV-infected patients is independent of antiretroviral therapy. AIDS 2003;17(13):1917–23.
131. Mondy K, Yarasheski K, Powderly WG, et al. Longitudinal evolution of bone mineral density and bone markers in human immunodeficiency virus-infected individuals. Clin Infect Dis 2003;36(4):482–90.
132. Nolan D, Upton R, McKinnon E, et al. Stable or increasing bone mineral density in HIV-infected patients treated with nelfinavir or indinavir. AIDS 2001;15(10):1275–80.
133. Tebas P, Powderly WG, Claxton S, et al. Accelerated bone mineral loss in HIV-infected patients receiving potent antiretroviral therapy. AIDS 2000;14(4):F63–7.
134. Prior J, Burdge D, Maan E, et al. Fragility fractures and bone mineral density in HIV positive women: a case-control population-based study. Osteoporos Int 2007;18(10):1345–53.
135. Triant VA, Brown TT, Lee H, et al. Fracture prevalence among human immunodeficiency virus (HIV)-infected versus non-HIV-infected patients in a large U.S. healthcare system. J Clin Endocrinol Metab 2008;93(9):3499–504.
136. Yin MT, Lund E, Shah J, et al. Lower peak bone mass and abnormal trabecular and cortical microarchitecture in young men infected with HIV early in life. AIDS 2013;28(3):345–53.

137. Kim HS, Chin BS, Shin HS. Prevalence and risk factors of low bone mineral density in Korean HIV-infected patients: impact of abacavir and zidovudine. J Korean Med Sci 2013;28(6):827–32.

138. Li Vecchi V, Soresi M, Giannitrapani L, et al. Dairy calcium intake and lifestyle risk factors for bone loss in HIV-infected and uninfected Mediterranean subjects. BMC Infect Dis 2012;12:192.

139. Bonjoch A, Figueras M, Estany C, et al. High prevalence of and progression to low bone mineral density in HIV-infected patients: a longitudinal cohort study. AIDS 2010;24(18):2827–33.

140. Pinto Neto LF, Ragi-Eis S, Vieira NF, et al. Low bone mass prevalence, therapy type, and clinical risk factors in an HIV-infected Brazilian population. J Clin Densitom 2011;14(4):434–9.

141. McComsey GA, Tebas P, Shane E, et al. Bone Disease in HIV: a practical review and recommendations for HIV Providers. Clin Infect Dis 2010;51:937–46.

142. Aydin OA, Karaosmanoglu HK, Karahasanoglu R, et al. Prevalence and risk factors of osteopenia/osteoporosis in Turkish HIV/AIDS patients. Braz J Infect Dis 2013;17:707–11.

143. Short CE, Shaw SG, Fisher MJ, et al. Prevalence of and risk factors for osteoporosis and fracture among a male HIV-infected population in the UK. Int J STD AIDS 2014;25:113–21.

144. Grund B, Peng G, Gibert CL, et al. Continuous antiretroviral therapy decreases bone mineral density. AIDS 2009;23(12):1519–29.

145. Hoy J, Grund B, Roediger M, et al. Interruption or deferral of antiretroviral therapy reduces markers of bone turnover compared with continuous therapy: the SMART body composition substudy. J Bone Miner Res 2013;28(6):1264–74.

146. Woodward CL, Hall AM, Williams IG, et al. Tenofovir-associated renal and bone toxicity. HIV Med 2009;10(8):482–7.

147. Purdy JB, Gafni RI, Reynolds JC, et al. Decreased bone mineral density with off-label use of tenofovir in children and adolescents infected with human immunodeficiency virus. J Pediatr 2008;152(4):582–4.

148. Liu AY, Vittinghoff E, Sellmeyer DE, et al. Bone mineral density in HIV-negative men participating in a tenofovir pre-exposure prophylaxis randomized clinical trial in San Francisco. PLoS One 2011;6(8):e23688.

149. Sax P, Brar I, Elion R, et al. 48 Week Study of Tenofovir Alafenamide (TAF) vs. Tenofovir Disoproxil Fumarate (TDF), Each in a Single Tablet Regimen (STR) with Elvitegravir, Cobicistat, and Emtricitabine [E/C/F/TAF vs. E/C/F/TDF] for Initial HIV Treatment. 53rd Interscience Conference on Antimicrobial Agents and Chemotherapy (ICAAC) [abstract: H-1464d]. Denver, September 10–13, 2013.

150. Hernandez-Vallejo SJ, Beaupere C, Larghero J, et al. HIV protease inhibitors induce senescence and alter osteoblastic potential of human bone marrow mesenchymal stem cells: beneficial effect of pravastatin. Aging Cell 2013;12:955–65.

151. National Osteoporosis Foundation. 2013 Clinician's guide to prevention and treatment of osteoporosis. Available at: http://nof.org/files/nof/public/content/resource/913/files/580.pdf. Accessed February 15, 2014.

152. Womack JA, Goulet JL, Gibert C, et al, Veterans Aging Cohort Study Project Team. Physiologic frailty and fragility fracture in HIV-infected male veterans. Clin Infect Dis 2013;56(10):1498–504.

153. Yin MT, Kendall MA, Wu X, et al. Fractures after antiretroviral initiation. AIDS 2012;26(17):2175–84.

154. Young B, Dao CN, Buchacz K, et al, HIV Outpatient Study (HOPS) Investigators. Increased rates of bone fracture among HIV-infected persons in the HIV

Outpatient Study (HOPS) compared with the US general population, 2000-2006. Clin Infect Dis 2011;52(8):1061–8.

155. Prieto-Alhambra D, Guerri-Fernandez R, De Vries F, et al. HIV infection and its association with an excess risk of clinical fractures: a nation-wide case-control study. J Acquir Immune Defic Syndr 2014;66(1):90–5.

156. Warriner AH, Smith W, Curtis JR, et al. Fracture among older and younger HIV+ Medicare beneficiaries. 20th Conference on Retroviruses and Opportunistic Infections [abstract: 820]. Atlanta, March 3–6, 2013.

157. Battalora L, Buchacz K, Armon C, et al. Low bone mineral density is associated with increased risk of incident fracture in HIV-infected adults. 14th European AIDS Conference [abstract: PS1/4]. Brussels, October 16–19, 2013.

158. Bedimo R, Maalouf NM, Zhang S, et al. Osteoporotic fracture risk associated with cumulative exposure to tenofovir and other antiretroviral agents. AIDS 2012;26(7):825–31.

159. Hansen AB, Gerstoft J, Kronborg G, et al. Incidence of low and high-energy fractures in persons with and without HIV infection: a Danish population-based cohort study. AIDS 2012;26(3):285–93.

160. Maalouf N, Zhang S, Drechsler H, et al. Hepatitis C co-infection and severity of liver disease as risk factors for osteoporotic fractures among HIV-infected patients. J Bone Miner Res 2013;28:2577–83.

161. Negredo E, Bonjoch A, Gomez-Mateu M, et al. Time of progression to osteopenia/osteoporosis in chronically HIV-infected patients: screening DXA scan. PLoS One 2012;7(10):e46031.

162. Peters BS, Perry M, Wierzbicki AS, et al. A cross-sectional randomised study of fracture risk in people with HIV infection in the probono 1 study. PLoS One 2013; 8(10):e78048.

163. Pepe J, Isidori AM, Falciano M, et al. The combination of FRAX and ageing male symptoms scale better identifies treated HIV males at risk for major fracture. Clin Endocrinol 2012;77(5):672–8.

164. Tien PC, Schneider MF, Cole SR, et al. Antiretroviral therapy exposure and insulin resistance in the women's interagency HIV study. J Acquir Immune Defic Syndr 2008;49(4):369–76.

165. Cowie CC, Rust KF, Ford ES, et al. Full accounting of diabetes and pre-diabetes in the U.S. population in 1988-1994 and 2005-2006. Diabetes Care 2009;32(2):287–94.

166. Brown TT, Li X, Cole SR, et al. Cumulative exposure to nucleoside analogue reverse transcriptase inhibitors is associated with insulin resistance markers in the multicenter AIDS cohort study. AIDS 2005;19(13):1375–83.

167. Dubé MP, Shen C, Greenwald M, et al. No impairment of endothelial function or insulin sensitivity with 4 weeks of the HIV protease inhibitors atazanavir or lopinavir-ritonavir in healthy subjects without HIV infection: a placebo-controlled trial. Clin Infect Dis 2008;47(4):567–74.

168. Noor MA, Parker RA, O'Mara E, et al. The effects of HIV protease inhibitors atazanavir and lopinavir/ritonavir on insulin sensitivity in HIV-seronegative healthy adults. AIDS 2004;18(16):2137–44.

169. Schwarz J, Lee GA, Park S, et al. Indinavir increases glucose production in healthy HIV-negative men. AIDS 2004;18(13):1852–4.

170. Taylor SA, Lee GA, Pao VY, et al. Boosting dose ritonavir does not alter peripheral insulin sensitivity in healthy HIV-seronegative volunteers. J Acquir Immune Defic Syndr 2010;55(3):361–4.

171. Vyas AK, Koster JC, Tzekov A, et al. Effects of the HIV protease inhibitor ritonavir on GLUT4 knock-out mice. J Biol Chem 2010;285(47):36395–400.

172. Crum-Cianflone N, Roediger MP, Eberly L, et al, Infectious Disease Clinical Research Program HIV Working Group. Increasing rates of obesity among HIV-infected persons during the HIV epidemic. PLoS One 2010;5(4):e10106.

173. Vasan RS, Pencina MJ, Cobain M, et al. Estimated risks for developing obesity in the Framingham heart study. Ann Intern Med 2005;143(7):473–80.

174. Vachon MC, Factor SH, Branch AD, et al. Insulin resistance predicts re-treatment failure in an efficacy study of peginterferon-α-2a and ribavirin in HIV/HCV co-infected patients. J Hepatol 2011;54(1):41–7.

175. Dai C, Huang J, Hsieh M, et al. Insulin resistance predicts response to peginterferon-alpha/ribavirin combination therapy in chronic hepatitis C patients. J Hepatol 2009;50(4):712–8.

176. Lonardo A, Ballestri S, Adinolfi LE, et al. Hepatitis C virus-infected patients are 'spared' from the metabolic syndrome but not from insulin resistance. A comparative study of nonalcoholic fatty liver disease and hepatitis C virus-related steatosis. Can J Gastroenterol 2009;23(4):273–8.

177. Bani-Sadr F, Loko M, Winnock M, et al. Insulin resistance predicts hepatocarcinoma occurrence in HIV/HCV co-infected patients. 51st Interscience Conference on Antimicrobial Agents and Chemotherapy (ICAAC) [abstract: H3-814]. Chicago, September 17–20, 2011.

178. Hu G, Jousilahti P, Tuomilehto J, et al. Association of serum C-reactive protein level with sex-specific type 2 diabetes risk: a prospective Finnish study. J Clin Endocrinol Metab 2009;94(6):2099–105.

179. Pradhan AD, Manson JE, Rifai N, et al. C-reactive protein, interleukin 6, and risk of developing type 2 diabetes mellitus. JAMA 2001;286:327–34.

180. Brown TT, Tassiopoulos K, Bosch RJ, et al. Association between systemic inflammation and incident diabetes in HIV-infected patients after initiation of antiretroviral therapy. Diabetes Care 2010;33(10):2244–9.

181. de Heredia FP, Gómez-Martínez S, Marcos A. Obesity, inflammation and the immune system. Proc Nutr Soc 2012;71(2):332–8.

182. Amorosa V, Synnestvedt M, Gross R, et al. A tale of 2 epidemics: the intersection between obesity and HIV infection in Philadelphia. J Acquir Immune Defic Syndr 2005;39:557–61.

183. Wrottesley SV, Micklesfield LK, Hamill MM, et al. Dietary intake and body composition in HIV-positive and -negative South African women. Public Health Nutr 2014;17(7):1603–13.

184. Malaza A, Mossong J, Barnighausen T, et al. Hypertension and obesity in adults living in a high HIV prevalence rural area in South Africa. PLoS One 2012;7(10): e47761.

185. Frantz JM, Murenzi A. The physical activity levels among people living with human immunodeficiency virus/acquired immunodeficiency syndrome receiving high active antiretroviral therapy in Rwanda. SAHARA J 2013;10(3–4):113–8.

186. Taylor BS, Liang Y, Garduno LS, et al. High risk of obesity and weight gain for HIV-infected uninsured minorities. J Acquir Immune Defic Syndr 2014;65(2): e33–40.

187. Lakey W, Yang LY, Yancy W, et al. Short communication: from wasting to obesity: initial antiretroviral therapy and weight gain in HIV-infected persons. AIDS Res Hum Retroviruses 2013;29(3):435–40.

Human Immunodeficiency Virus and Coinfection with Hepatitis B and C

Lindsay A. Petty, MD[a],*, Jennifer L. Steinbeck, MD[a],
Kenneth Pursell, MD[a], Donald M. Jensen, MD[b]

KEYWORDS

- Hepatitis B virus • Hepatitis C virus • HIV • Coinfection • DAA

KEY POINTS

- In HIV-infected individuals, coinfection with HBV and/or HCV is common because of shared modes of transmission.
- HIV accelerates progression of liver disease because of HBV or HCV and results in increased morbidity and mortality associated with viral hepatitis.
- Treatment of HBV in coinfected patients can lead to anti-HBV or anti-HIV drug resistance if regimens are not carefully chosen.
- As the new direct-acting antivirals become available for HCV, treatment will become easier with less adverse effects, less drug-drug interactions, and dramatically increased rates of success.

BACKGROUND

A disproportionate number of people with human immunodeficiency virus (HIV) are affected by viral hepatitis compared with the general population, because they are at higher risk due to similar routes of transmission of these blood-borne pathogens, as well as chronic persistence of virus in most hosts.[1] Of all patients with HIV infection in the United States, about 10% are coinfected with hepatitis B virus (HBV) and 25% are coinfected with hepatitis C virus (HCV). Therefore, in total about one-third of the HIV population is affected by viral hepatitis.[2,3] In the era of highly active antiretroviral therapy (HAART), liver disease has become a leading cause of morbidity and mortality in HIV-infected persons and is the second leading cause of death in HIV-infected individuals, causing 9% of deaths.[4] Coinfection with viral hepatitis, caused by either

[a] Department of Infectious Diseases and Global Health, University of Chicago Medical Center, 5841 South Maryland Avenue, MC 5065, Chicago, IL 60637, USA; [b] Department of Medicine, Center for Liver Disease, University of Chicago Medical Center, 5841 South Maryland Avenue, MC 7120, Chicago, IL 60637, USA
* Corresponding author.
E-mail address: lindsay.petty@uchospitals.edu

Infect Dis Clin N Am 28 (2014) 477–499
http://dx.doi.org/10.1016/j.idc.2014.05.005
0891-5520/14/$ – see front matter © 2014 Elsevier Inc. All rights reserved.

id.theclinics.com

HBV or HCV, is the main cause of liver disease. Multiple issues arise, including the dual toxicities to the liver from both viral hepatitis and ART, as well as the potential need for altering the selection of antiretroviral therapy (ART) in the setting of potential treatment of viral hepatitis, possibly affecting both the timing and the choice of therapy. In the setting of the release of new direct-acting antiviral (DAA) agents, the treatment of HIV/HCV-coinfected patients is rapidly evolving and improving.

EPIDEMIOLOGY AND RISK FACTORS
HBV and HBV/HIV

Hepatitis B is a DNA virus that infects humans. Although there is a trend toward decreasing prevalence of HBV, this infection remains the leading cause of chronic liver disease globally with 2 billion individuals being exposed and 350 million people with chronic infection worldwide.[5,6] It is estimated that HBV is responsible for 30% of cirrhosis and 53% of hepatocellular carcinoma (HCC).[7] The prevalence of HBV varies with geographic location. In regions with the highest prevalence, including sub-Saharan Africa and East Asia, 5% to 10% of adults are chronically infected. In regions with the lowest prevalence, including Western Europe and North America, less than 1% of adults are chronically infected.[8]

HBV is highly contagious, more so than HIV or HCV. Given the shared modes of transmission between HIV and HBV, these infections occur together with relative frequency. Both are transmitted via perinatal, parenteral, and sexual contacts (**Table 1**).[9] HBV can be transmitted from infected blood or bodily fluids via injection, mucous membranes, or wounds.[10] HBV replicates to high titers in blood, but it can also be found in other bodily fluids, including semen, cervical secretions, and saliva.[8] As in HBV infection alone, the epidemiology of coinfection of HIV/HBV varies with geographic region. It is estimated that the prevalence of chronic hepatitis B in HIV-infected individuals is 5% to 20%.[11] Therefore, of the 35 million worldwide infected with HIV, 2 to 4 million are estimated to have chronic hepatitis B.[9] A study of more than 16,000 HIV-infected individuals in the United States found a prevalence of 7.8% of chronic HBV for unvaccinated subjects, which is significantly higher than the less than 1% prevalence of the general population.[8,12]

Table 1					
Transmission rates of HIV and viral hepatitis					
Mode	HIV	HBV	HBV/HIV	HCV	HCV/HIV
Perinatal	10%–20%	5%–90%[a]	10%–90%[a]	<2%–7%	10%–20%
Sex	<1%	Up to 90%[b]	Up to 90%[b]	<1%	<1%–3%[c]
Needle stick	0.30%	7%–30%	Unknown	1%–3%	Unknown

[a] Transmisison risk less than 10% if HBsAg positive and HBeAg negative increases to 70%–90% if HBsAg positive and HBeAg positive.
[b] Depends on level of HBV DNA.
[c] Values are based on data from HCV serodiscordant heterosexual couples.
Adapted from Lacombe K, Rockstroh JK. HIV and viral hepatitis co-infections: advances and challenges. Gut 2012;61(Suppl 1):i48; with permission; and *Additional data from* Germanaud J, Causse X, Dhumeaux D. Transmission of hepatitis C by accidental needlestick injuries. Evaluation of risk. Presse Med 1994;23(23):1078–82; and Mast EE, Margolis HS, Fiore AE, et al. A comprehensive immunization strategy to eliminate transmission of hepatitis B virus infection in the United States: recommendations of the Advisory Committee on Immunization Practices (ACIP) part 1: immunization of infants, children, and adolescents. MMWR Recomm Rep 2005;54(RR-16):1–31. Available at: Centers for Disease Control and Prevention. Accessed December 16, 2008.

HCV and HCV/HIV

Hepatitis C is an RNA flavivirus that infects humans.[5] About 3 to 4 million people in the United States are chronically infected with HCV, and 10,000 to 20,000 die each year from complications related to liver disease caused by HCV.[13] In the United States, a recent review of death certificate data suggests that deaths related to HCV now exceed those caused by HIV (15,106 vs 12,734).[14] The virus is most efficiently transmitted through parenteral means, including injection drug use (IDU) or contaminated blood or medical equipment.[15] Much less commonly, it can be transmitted through sexual contact or perinatal vertical transmission (see **Table 1**).[13,15–17] The predominant risk factors vary geographically. In the United States, IDU is the biggest risk factor, in particular since the initiation of blood product screening.[18] It is estimated that 75% of all HCV infections in the Unites States are in people born between 1945 and 1965.[3] The incidence of new infections in the United States has declined overall since blood product screening was instituted. However, the chronically HCV-infected population is aging, likely resulting in more cirrhosis seen in the coming years.

Given the similar routes of transmission, coinfection with HIV and HCV is common. IDU is a common means of transmitting both viruses, and 50% to 90% of injection drug users with HIV also have HCV.[3] In addition, cohorts have shown that there is an increased risk of transmission among certain subpopulations, in particular, HIV-positive men who have sex with men (MSM). An increased incidence of newly acquired HCV has been seen in multiple cohorts.[19–21] The precise cause of this increased incidence is unknown. Some studies have shown correlations with anal sex and mucosal damage, including sexually transmitted infections with genital ulcerations or certain sexual practices, and this mucosal breakdown has been hypothesized to increase risk of sexual transmission.[16,22] However, a recent Swiss cohort did not show increased incidence of HCV in MSM who are HIV-negative.[19] HIV also increases the rate of vertical transmission of HCV to newborns by 4 to 5 times.[17,23] Overall, there is a high rate of HIV/HCV coinfection due to shared avenues of transmission, as well as increased rates of HCV transmission in select HIV-positive populations.

GENOTYPES

HBV

There are 8 identified genotypes of HBV, with multiple subgenotypes as well. In contrast to HCV, the genotype has a significant implication on clinical outcomes and natural history but minimal relation to the response to therapy. Genotype C, in particular, is associated with the highest risk of HCC and cirrhosis.[24] The genotypes have characteristic geographic patterns.[25] In the United States, genotype B and C are found in Asian individuals; genotype A2 and D are found in those of European and Middle Eastern descent. The clinical significance, if any, of subgenotypes is not yet known and routine genotype testing is not routinely performed.[24]

HCV

There are 6 major HCV genotypes, with multiple subtypes and strains. Genotypes 1 to 3 are distributed globally, with 60% of worldwide infections caused by genotypes 1a and 1b. The different genotypes are geographically distributed, with genotype 1a mostly seen in Northern Europe and North America (genotype 1 constitutes 70% of US infections), and genotype 2 is less commonly seen, but more often in Europe than North America.[5,23,26] In regards to interferon (IFN)-based therapy, the genotypes do influence response to treatment, with genotype 1 associated with a poorer response compared with more favorable responses to genotypes 2 and 3.[27] With directly acting agents now available for INF-free regimens, however, the outcomes have become more similar across the genotypes. The specific genotype is still likely to be used to guide DAA treatment regimen decisions.

IL28B

A single nucleotide polymorphism (SNP) near the IL28B gene in the human host, which encodes INF-λ, has been identified, and this SNP appears to be a critical part of the innate immune system's defense against HCV. For INF-based therapies, monoinfected individuals with the CC genotype of the SNP were more than 3 times as likely to clear HCV RNA compared with individuals with CT and TT genotypes, and similar spontaneous clearance differences have been seen in the coinfected population.[28,29] Variations in IL28B are also associated with treatment outcomes, but mostly in genotypes 1 and 4. The influence of IL28B polymorphism on treatment outcome is attenuated but still present for regimens using the new DAA agents based on preliminary data.[30]

NATURAL HISTORY OF COINFECTED STATES
HBV in HIV

The course of HBV is both variable and complex, being influenced by multiple factors, including the host immune response, viral fitness, HBV genotype, age, alcohol consumption, and coinfection with HIV, HCV, or hepatitis D virus.[25] The natural history of chronic HBV includes 3 major phases of *immune tolerant*, *immune active*, and *inactive carrier*. Although infected individuals generally progress through these phases, some will reactivate and return from the *inactive carrier* state back to the *immune active* phase.[10] The *immune tolerant* phase is characterized by positive HBeAg, high levels of HBV DNA but normal alanine aminotransferase (ALT) levels and no or little liver fibrosis or inflammation on biopsy. There is no cytotoxic T-cell activity against the virus, because the immune system does not recognize the virus in this phase. The *immune tolerant* phase predominantly occurs in individuals infected at birth via perinatal transmission from mothers who are positive for HBeAg. It is uncommon in those infected after birth. Although this phase can last for decades, liver disease does not appear to progress during this time.

Most individuals infected with HBV eventually progress from the *immune tolerant* to the *immune active* phase. ALT levels increase and evidence of liver disease can be found on biopsy. HBV DNA levels are elevated but generally lower than the prior phase, and levels decrease while progressing through this phase. A weak cytotoxic T-cell response can occur, resulting in HBeAg seroconversion and possible suppression of HBV DNA.

Following seroconversion, there are 3 possible situations. The majority progress to the *inactive carrier* state. It is marked by normal ALT levels, low or frequently undetectable levels of HBV DNA, and HBeAg negative; HBsAg remains detectable. Liver inflammation and fibrosis improve and can even reverse. Although most who enter this state remain here long-term, a minority will achieve HBsAg clearance. Notably, an estimated 20% will reactivate to the immune active phase. In addition, despite seroconversion, the infected individual may sometimes remain in the *immune active* phase. Finally, one can revert back to HBeAg seropositivity. The latter is more common among genotypes C or F.[24,25]

HIV has a significant deleterious impact on the natural history and progression of HBV infection. The HIV/HBV-coinfected population has an increased rate of replication of HBV, as noted by higher HBV DNA levels and decreased rates of spontaneous clearance.[31–33] In a prospective cohort of men, 12% of the coinfected had loss of HBeAg at 5 years compared with 49% of HBV-monoinfected.[34] Not only does HIV increase the risk of developing chronic infection, but it also is associated with an increased rate of reactivation.[31,35]

In addition, HIV is thought to result in the accelerated progression of liver disease. The coinfected have faster rates of liver fibrosis, in addition to increased rates of cirrhosis, end-stage liver disease, HCC, and liver-related mortality.[32,33,36,37] A prospective study of 5293 MSM, including 326 who were positive for HBsAg, found that mortality due to liver disease was significantly higher in the coinfected (14.2/1000 person-years) compared with those with HBV alone (0.8/1000 person-years).[37] Notably, there is limited knowledge on the effect of adult acquired HIV when HBV infection has been established for many years, as in perinatal transmission, as most research has been conducted in locations where HBV is acquired in adulthood.[31]

Of the different phases, it is those in the *immune active* phase who are at the highest risk of developing HCC.[24] HIV coinfection further amplifies this association. Depending on the mode of transmission and the age of acquisition, the lifetime risk of HCC in chronic HBV ranges from 15% to 40%. In addition, several other factors have been found to have an increased risk of HCC in chronic HBV, including male sex, age over 40, family history, smoking, alcohol, and aflatoxin exposure.[24]

HIV with HBV

Although HIV has been found to have significant impact on the outcomes of HBV, the reverse has not been reliably demonstrated, and controversy exists regarding the effect of HBV on the natural history of HIV. A study of the EuroSIDA cohort found that chronic HBV had no impact on progression to AIDS or responses to HAART. Chronic HBV did significantly increase liver-related mortality in HIV-infected individuals.[38] Two prior longitudinal studies and one retrospective study also did not find any evidence of HBV leading to HIV/AIDS progression.[39–41]

Contrary to this, other observations have suggested that HBV is associated with a more rapidly progressive HIV course.[42] A retrospective analysis including 64 HIV/HBV-coinfected individuals with chronic HBV showed that the risk of AIDS or death was nearly 2-fold higher among coinfected chronic HBV individuals compared with HIV-monoinfected individuals.[43] An international study found that coinfected individuals had a lower baseline CD4 T-cell count with a median of 137 cells/mL compared with 159 cells/mL in HIV-monoinfected individuals before therapy.[11] A meta-analysis including data on greater than 12,000 patients found that coinfected patients had worsened overall mortality. This study did not support that this difference was due to increased AIDS progression but speculated that severe hepatic complications could explain the reduced survival.[41]

HCV in HIV

After transmission, the incubation period for HCV ranges from 2 weeks to 6 months (considered *acute infection*), with 80% of individuals experiencing no symptoms.[13,44] About 80% of patients infected with HCV will develop chronic infection, and approximately one-third of those will progress to cirrhosis.[13,45,46] In a recent study looking at the difference in all-cause mortality between patients with chronic HCV who achieve sustained HCV virologic response (SVR) to treatment versus those who do not, the 10-year cumulative incidence risk of liver-related mortality or transplantation was 1.9% versus 27.4%, respectively.[47] Of those who did not achieve SVR and died, 70% were due to liver-related causes.[47]

Individuals with HIV have overall worse outcomes associated with HCV than the HCV-monoinfected population. From the start, HIV-infected persons are less likely to clear HCV viremia following acute infection.[46,48] In the setting of acute HCV, clearance of HCV RNA of at least 2 log within 4 weeks of diagnosis was a strong predictor for spontaneous clearance. If not clear by 12 weeks, then the coinfected individual is likely to develop chronic HCV infection.[49] In addition, the coinfected population is more likely to have higher HCV RNA viral loads and set points.[46,48]

HIV increases the speed of progression to liver disease compared with monoinfected individuals.[46,50–52] Cirrhosis has been seen in coinfected individuals as early as 6 to 10 years after HCV infection, compared with 10 to 20 years in monoinfected individuals.[1] The risk of cirrhosis or decompensated liver disease in HIV/HCV-coinfected patients is 3 times more than monoinfected patients, regardless of CD4 count.[53,54] The exact mechanism of this acceleration of fibrosis is unclear. There have been multiple studies looking to explain this acceleration of fibrosis on the molecular level. Some studies have found a link to immunosuppression with low HCV-specific CD8+ T-cell responses, chronic immune activation, and increased circulation of proinflammatory cytokines.[55–57] In addition, there is an increased risk of HCC in coinfected compared with monoinfected individuals.[54]

In a meta-analysis in the HAART era, estimates of coinfected individuals with cirrhosis were found to be 21% (95% confidence interval [CI], 16%–28%) and 49% (40%–49%) after 20 and 30 years, respectively.[50] The overall risk of cirrhosis in the HAART era for coinfected compared with monoinfected individuals was slightly lower compared with a pre-HAART meta-analysis (relative risk: 2.11, 95% CI, 1.51–2.96 vs 2.92, 1.70–5.01).[50] HAART has not been shown in studies to fully correct the differences between the 2 populations.[50] However, initiation of ART on coinfected veterans recently showed a significant reduction in the rate of hepatic decompensation, by 28% to 41% on average.[58]

HIV with HCV

The effect that HCV has on HIV is controversial. One study showed impaired immune reconstitution with initiation of ART in coinfected patients.[59] However, one study looking at 5957 HIV-positive patients with approximately 33% HCV prevalence did not show that HCV serostatus affected the risk of HIV disease progression, or that there were any virologic or immunologic responses to HAART that were worsened.[2]

Although the overall progression of immunologic responses is debatable, there is significant concern regarding the extrahepatic manifestations of HCV, especially in a population already at higher risk for cardiovascular disease and renal disease because of their HIV infection. These extrahepatic manifestations are hypothesized to be due to persistent immune activation and inflammation.[60] Monoinfection with HIV infection increases the risk of cardiovascular disease and renal disease. The REVEAL-C study showed an increase in the rate of cardiovascular events, kidney disease, and some cancers in HIV-uninfected patients with chronic hepatitis C.[61] In coinfected populations, persistent HCV-RNA has also been associated with an increased risk of cardiovascular disease and renal disease compared with HIV monoinfected patients.[62–64]

Although coinfection with HCV or HBV has been shown to be an independent risk factor for ART-associated hepatotoxicity,[65] the number of patients this actually affects may be less significant, especially if certain antiretroviral agents are avoided and less hepatotoxic ones are used instead. The coinfected population is more likely to experience hepatotoxicity on ART, although more likely with nevarapine (NNRTI: nonnucleoside reverse transcriptase inhibitor), efavirenz (NNRTI), or high-dose ritonavir (PI: protease inhibitor) regimens.[66–68] High-dose ritonavir regimens are no longer used.

Ritonavir is now only used to boost another PI. Only about 10% of patients receiving boosted ritonavir develop severe hepatotoxicity, however, and most cases are asymptomatic and resolve whether ARV is modified or not; this may differ based on stage of fibrosis.[66,69] Stavudine (NRTI: nucleoside reverse transcriptase inhibitor) and didanosine (DDI; NRTI) are associated with increased risk of hepatotoxicity as well as substantial neurotoxicity and metabolic disorders, and thus, are no longer recommended for therapy.[70] Raltegravir (INSTI, integrase inhibitor) has shown good safety profiles in the coinfected population and thus is one of the preferred backbone agents for patients with viral liver disease.[71] Thus, there are multiple drug limitations in HIV/HCV-coinfected individuals based on increased risk of hepatotoxicity as well as drug-drug interactions. However, the overall risk of hepatotoxicity with ART is decreased after successful treatment of HCV infection.[72]

DIAGNOSIS AND SCREENING: IN THE HIV-INFECTED POPULATION

It is recommended that all HIV-infected individuals be screened for HBV as well as HCV.[3,18,73–75]

In regards to screening for HBV, initial testing for evidence of past or present HBV infection should be performed in all HIV-infected patients. This testing should include HBsAg, anti-HBc total, and anti-HBs.[9,76] Those who test negative should be immunized. The presence of HBsAg on 2 occasions at least 6 months apart defines chronic HBV infection.[31,76] These patients should undergo further evaluation with HBeAg, anti-HBe, HBV DNA testing as well as liver chemistries, complete blood count, and prothrombin time.[9,76] A low threshold to evaluate for HBV infection should exist in patients with HIV infection if unexplained liver disease occurs, as spontaneous reverse seroconversion with the disappearance of anti-HBs and the reappearance of HBsAg can develop.[31] The extent of liver fibrosis should also be monitored, which can be done with noninvasive testing such as transient elastometry. Indirect monitoring with ultrasound, fibrotests, and platelet counts is preferred, with biopsy helpful in the setting of discrepancies among these tests or the clinical picture. Chronic hepatitis B infection increases the risk for HCC. Thus, ultrasound should be performed every six months, plus or minus the measurement of serum α-fetoprotein.[9] The American Association of Study of Liver Disease (AASLD) does not recommend the routine use of AFP, but many practitioners use it as an adjunctive piece of data to make clinical decisions, although this is controversial.

In regards to screening for HCV infection, initial testing should involve anti-HCV detection using sensitive immunoassays. A positive result demonstrates exposure to HCV; it cannot distinguish acute versus chronic infection.[77] False negatives may occur in the severely immunosuppressed (CD4 $<100/mm^3$), and true negatives may occur in acute HCV (within 12 weeks of acquisition).[77,78] If a negative test result occurs in the setting of high suspicion based on risk factors (such as increased aminotransferases, high-risk sexual behavior, and IDU), then further testing should be performed for HCV RNA within 6 months to one year.[79] In addition, if HCV antibody testing is positive, then subsequent quantitative HCV RNA should be performed. Although a positive HCV RNA test is sufficient for the diagnosis of active hepatitis C, a negative cannot exclude active viremia because of transient declines, and a repeat test should be performed. When HCV RNA is positive, HCV genotype testing should be performed because it is the best predictor of response and also will guide treatment regimens.

Liver biopsy remains the gold standard for evaluation of HCV-related disease (stage of fibrosis), and many noninvasive imaging tests or predictive indexes are being developed and studied, and now biopsy is only used if the noninvasive modalities are not conclusive.[80–86] Biopsy is no longer required prior to initiating therapy for HCV infection. The utility of these studies in the coinfected population is less defined as treatment options improve, because earlier therapy is recommended given the more rapid progression of fibrosis in this population.

TREATMENT
HBV: Treatment of Monoinfection Compared with Coinfection: Limitations and Considerations

Patients with HIV infection who are also infected with HBV should be treated for both infections (**Table 2**). Ultimately, the treatment goal for both HBV-monoinfection and HIV/HBV-coinfection remains the same: to decrease the morbidity and mortality associated with HBV infection.[76] Given that multiple agents target both HIV and HBV, the treatment of these viruses is interconnected. Clinicians must be certain that the HIV regimen contains at least 2 HBV active drugs so that HBV resistance does not occur and so that HBV related immune reactivation syndrome does not occur.

The Department of Health and Human Services recommends that all coinfected patients receive ART with a dually active regimen against both HIV and HBV regardless of CD4 count.[87] In contrast, in HBV monoinfected patients, treatment is indicated for chronic HBV if the risk of liver-related morbidity and mortality in the near future and the likelihood of achieving a successful viral response are both high. Guidelines from the American Association of Study of Liver Disease (AASLD) provide further details on when to treat incorporating multiple factors, including ALT and HBV DNA levels and liver biopsy findings.[74]

Treatment of HBV Only

Treatment of HBV alone is not recommended. Such treatment in the coinfected patient can lead to resistance of both HBV and HIV if not managed carefully. If a patient refuses or is not taking ART, the options for HBV treatment are significantly limited due to the risk of creating HIV resistance if anti-HBV drugs that also have some anti-HIV activity are used.[88] Anti-HBV drugs, including tenofovir (TDF, NRTI), entecavir (ETV, NRTI), emtricitabine (FTC, NRTI), lamivudine (3TC, NRTI), adefovir (NRTI), and likely telbivudine (NRTI), all have some activity against HIV.[87] These drugs are all nucleoside or nucleotide analogues that target HBV DNA polymerase.[89] It is recommended that these agents not be given without the accompaniment of a fully suppressive ART regimen due to risk of inducing HIV resistance.[76] ETV and telbivudine have been

Table 2	
Treatment of HBV/HIV coinfection	
ART administered[a]	Preferred regimen: ART with 2 anti-HBV agents (TDF + FTC/3TC) Duration: indefinite
ART contraindicated/not utilized[b]	If HBV treatment indicated: PEG Duration: 48 wk *Do not administer without ART: TDF, ETV, FTC, 3TC, adefovir, telbivudine* If HBV treatment not indicated[b]: close monitoring

[a] Recommended that all receive ART regardless of CD4 count.
[b] If ART is not implemented, then decision to treat HBV is based on standards for HBV monoinfection.

associated with the selection of M184V and M204I mutation, respectively.[74,90,91] Adefovir and pegylated-INF-α-2a (PEG) are the only options for those not receiving ART, but there are limited data regarding the efficacy and safety of a regimen with one or both of these agents in the coinfected state. The former has limited value because it is less potent. If the HIV infection will not be treated, then the decision of when to initiate HBV therapy should follow the standards of HBV monoinfection.[76]

Treatment of Both HIV and HBV

For coinfected individuals, ART should include 2 agents with activity against HBV. The Department of Health and Human Services guidelines for treatment of HIV infection recommend TDF/FTC as the preferred NRTI backbone for ART-naive individuals.[87] These agents also have activity against HBV and it is thus also recommended for coinfected patients.[76] The AASLD practice guidelines recommend TDF/FTC or TDF/3TC as the preferred treatment of those planning to receive both HBV and HIV therapy.[74] TDF demonstrates activity against both wild-type and 3TC-resistant HBV and is suggested to decrease the rate of resistance to 3TC when combined with 3TC.[74,92–95] TDF resistance in HBV has not yet been reported.[76] TDF should be used with caution in those with renal dysfunction or at high risk for renal dysfunction. ETV, instead, can be added to a fully suppressive ART regimen.[76] Long-term use of 3TC or FTC alone should be avoided, as this can select for resistant HBV.[76,94,96] Resistance increases with increased duration of treatment.[76] There is approximately a 20% rate of development of 3TC resistance per year with this therapy alone in the coinfected; at 4 years, resistance is estimated to reach 90%.[94] Because 3TC-resistant HBV will have cross-resistance with other L-nucleosides, including telbivudine and FTC, this class of drugs should not be used if there is known 3TC-resistance.[76]

Treatment of HBV should be continued lifelong because there is a significant risk of relapse of hepatitis exists if therapy is discontinued.[76,89]

Monitoring Treatment of HBV in the Coinfected Patient

Appropriate monitoring is important to assess for treatment response, signs of developing resistance, or toxicity. HBV DNA and ALT levels should be monitored every 3 months; HBeAg should be checked every 3 to 6 months in HBeAg-positive individuals.[31,76] The HBV treatment endpoints include viral suppression and improved liver disease.[89] Viral suppression is defined as undetectable serum HBV DNA by polymerase chain reaction assay and loss of HBeAg (if previously positive). Improved liver disease is assessed by a decrease in ALT to within normal range. Complete response is defined as both biochemical and virological response, including loss of HBsAg. A response that persists while on therapy is a maintained response; a response that persists 6 or 12 months after discontinuation of therapy is a sustained response.[74] Other markers of favorable response include improved liver histology and development of anti-HBe.[76] In some HBV-monoinfected individuals, HBV therapy may be discontinued if multiple criteria are met, in particular including loss of HBeAg (if previously positive). However, in the HIV/HBV-coinfected patient on a stable ART regimen they are tolerating, therapy for HBV should continue lifelong.

Renal toxicity can be seen with TDF; therefore, serum creatinine and electrolytes should be checked at baseline and monitored every 3 to 6 months along with urinalysis every 6 months. If significant renal dysfunction occurs, TDF should be discontinued with alternative therapy chosen. If creatinine clearance is less than 10, then TDF should be discontinued as the pharmacokinetics have not been evaluated in nonhemodialysis patients with this level of renal dysfunction.[97] Providers should also consider holding TDF if there is a significant change from baseline while pursuing further work up to identify an etiology. Improvement of renal function can be seen.[76]

Lactic acidosis is an uncommon side effect of ETV use reported in treatment of monoinfected patients with advanced cirrhosis.[93] Telbivudine can result in creatinine phosphokinase (CPK) elevations and myopathy; therefore, CPK should be monitored at baseline, then every 3–6 months or sooner if symptoms develop.[76]

As mentioned, lifelong therapy is recommended in the coinfected state. A flare of hepatitis B in about 30% of cases, with possible decompensated liver disease, has been associated with early discontinuation of therapy.[95,98] Therefore, aminotransferases should be monitored every 6 weeks for 3 months and then every 3 months if therapy is prematurely stopped.[76] If there is a rise in aminotransferases, then it is recommended that therapy be re-started.

The presence of HBV has been associated with an increased risk of hepatotoxicity with ART, but clinically significant hepatotoxicity remains uncommon.[65,66,99,100] Thus, liver enzymes should be monitored monthly for the first 3–6 months after starting therapy and then every 3 months thereafter.[76]

It is also important to be aware of the risk of immune reconstitution inflammatory syndrome, which can be represented as a hepatitis flare in the coinfected patient within the first 6–12 weeks after starting ART.[31,76] Because the hepatic damage that occurs in HBV infection is predominantly a result of the immune response against infected hepatocytes, the immune reconstitution that occurs with ART can lead to worsened liver disease which is manifested by a rise in aminotransferases or a flare of hepatitis.[31] Such flares can be life-threatening and are part of the basis for recommending a regimen that treats HBV when administering ART. Utilizing two drugs active against HBV reduces the likelihood that IRIS will occur.[76] In general, a higher risk of IRIS has been seen in those who initiate therapy with a lower baseline CD4 count, especially when less than 50. Additionally, a higher baseline HIV-1 viral load and more rapid decline in viral load increases the risk for the development of IRIS.[101]

HCV: TREATMENT OF MONOINFECTION COMPARED WITH COINFECTION: LIMITATIONS AND CONSIDERATIONS

The primary goal of treatment is to achieve a sustained virologic response (SVR, defined as an undetectable HCV RNA 24 weeks after therapy completion). Some studies now use as an end point a shortened SVR period of 12 weeks because few monoinfected individuals rebound after this period.[49]

Coinfected patients who achieve SVR have lower rates of decompensated liver disease, HCC, and liver-related mortality compared with those patients who do not achieve SVR when followed for up to 10 years.[102,103]

Historically, the referral and initiation of HCV therapy in HIV/HCV-coinfected patients are low. This low amount is due to several factors, including lower response rates with PEG/ribavirin (RBV), medical comorbidities, neuropsychiatric comorbidities, perception of therapy, and adverse events associated with the IFN-based therapy.[104] The coinfected population has decreased response rates to HCV therapy compared with the monoinfected population. Coinfected patients may have increased HCV quasispecies (due to increased mutational rates), and therefore, decreased treatment responses.[105,106]

The newer DAAs, sofosbuvir (SOF) and simeprevir (SMV), have decreased drug interactions and adverse events, with high success in both monoinfected and coinfected individuals in early clinical trials.[107] This high success is changing the recommendations and attitudes for treatment in the coinfected population (**Table 3**).

PEG/RBV

PEG plus RBV was used extensively for treatment of HCV in the past. With the development of directly acting agents that are highly effective and well tolerated without being combined with IFN, and often without RBV, PEG and RBV will be less clinically relevant.

PEG/RBV combinations have been studied extensively in monoinfected individuals, but there have been only a few studies in the coinfected population. Both agents exhibit nonspecific antiviral activity. Interferon is an immunomodulatory agent that stimulates host antiviral genes, whereas the mechanism of action of RBV is poorly understood.[108] These studies are limited by fixed-dose RBV regimens and smaller sample sizes, but overall they show that coinfected patients have a decreased response to therapy in comparison with monoinfected groups (SVR is achieved in approximately 14%–35% vs 42%–46%).[109–112] In the past, RBV was shown to cause mitochondrial toxicity, so DDI (NRTI) was contraindicated in coinfected patients being treated with RBV-containing regimens.[113] Zidovudine (NRTI) is also contraindicated in combination with RBV because of increased rates of anemia.[114] Side effects of PEG and RBV include flulike symptoms, malaise, weight loss, anemia, neutropenia, and thrombocytopenia.[76,115] Contraindications to PEG/RBV therapy include a history of decompensated cirrhosis, pregnancy, inability to prevent pregnancy, uncontrolled depression, unstable cardiac or pulmonary conditions, and uncontrolled HIV with advanced immunosuppression.[76]

PROTEASE INHIBITOR + PEG/RBV (TELAPREVIR, BOCEPREVIR, SMV)

Telaprevir (TVR) and boceprevir (BOC) are NS3/4A protease inhibitors, as well as CYP3A inhibitors.[116] TVR as triple therapy (in combination with PEG/RBV) has been studied in coinfected patients, showing improved SVR rates compared with PEG/RBV (dual therapy) alone (74 vs 45%).[107] Also in the coinfected population, a study showed increased SVR rates in triple therapy including BOC compared with standard dual therapy (63% vs 29%).[117] Drawbacks remain in the use of these agents. First, both studies used extended courses of PEG/RBV, which is less ideal.

Table 3 Side effects of DAA				
Drug	**Abbrev.**	**Mechanism**	**CYP450 Complex**	**Side Effects**
Telaprevir	TVR	NS3/4A protease inhibitor	CYP3A inhibitor	Headache, rash, dysgeusia, GI disturbance, and anemia
Boceprevir	BOC	NS3/4A protease inhibitor	CYP3A inhibitor	Headache, dysgeusia, GI disturbance, and anemia
Simeprevir	SMV	NS3/4A protease inhibitor	Metabolized by CYP3A4	Pruritus, rash, photosensitivity, and increased bilirubin
Sofosbuvir	SOF	NS5B polymerase nucleotide analogue inhibitor	No interaction	Fatigue and headache
Ledipasvir	LDV	NS5A inhibitor	No interaction	Fatigue and headache

In addition, there is significant potential for drug-drug interactions between TVR/ BOC and multiple ARVs, although it is unclear how clinically significant these may be.[116,117] Finally, side effects continue to limit therapy for both protease inhibitors. Most common side effects of BOC include headache, dysgeusia, gastrointestinal (GI) disturbance, and anemia.[117] Most common side effects of TVR are rash and pruritus, GI disturbance, and anemia.[118] It seems likely that both BOC and TVR will have little role in the therapy for HCV if current results of more recently developed DAAs are confirmed by subsequent trials.

SMV is an NS3/4A protease inhibitor. It is metabolized primarily by cytochrome P450 3A4 (CYP3A4), so drug interactions remain a concern.[116] It provides pangenotypic activity in a once-daily pill, although it cannot be used as monotherapy. A phase III, open-label, single-arm study investigated SMV plus PEG/RBV in treatment-naive and treatment-experienced coinfected patients. Overall, 74% achieved SVR12, and 89% of patients met criteria allowing shortened therapy (24 weeks), with 78% achieving SVR12.[119] Virologic failures occurred, mostly because of emergence of mutations. In multiple studies, patients with Q80K mutations, a polymorphism found commonly (48% in the United States) in genotype 1a, showed a lower response to therapy, and therefore, baseline testing is recommended before using SMV.[119–121] In regards to drug-drug interactions with ARV, healthy controls demonstrated no significant interactions with TDF, rilpivirine (NNRTI), or raltegravir; however, there were alterations in SMV concentrations when dosed with EFV or darunavir/ritonavir (DRV/RTV, PI).[122] Adverse events include pruritus, rash, photosensitivity, and increased bilirubin.[119] Simepravir is likely to have a role in treating HCV when combined with other potent DAAs, but not with BOC or TVR.

NUCLEOTIDE INHIBITORS (SOF)

SOF is a nucleotide analogue inhibitor of the NS5B polymerase. It provides pangenotypic activity in a once-daily pill with high barrier to resistance and no clinically significant ART drug interactions.[118] It is not metabolized by the P450 enzyme complex. Preliminary data suggest that SOF + RBV treatment is safe with different ART regimens and may be equally safe and efficacious in patients that are coinfected compared with monoinfected, without HCV viral breakthrough.[118,123] Drug studies in healthy persons found no significant interactions with EFV, TDF, FTC, DRV/RTV, rilpivirine, and raltegravir.[116,124]

A 12-week triple therapy study looked at 23 coinfected patients treated with SOF in combination with PEG and weight-based RBV. In the setting of genotype 1 infection, 89% of the 19 coinfected patients who completed the trial achieved SVR12.[125] This achievement showed comparable efficacy to the larger trial of monoinfected individuals.[121] Phase III PHOTON-1 investigated SOF + RBV without INF and demonstrated achievement of SVR12 in 76%, 88%, and 67% of coinfected participants with HCV genotypes 1, 2, and 3, respectively.[123]

OTHER AGENTS IN DEVELOPMENT (COFORMULATIONS)

Newer coformulations of DAAs have demonstrated similar sustained response rates of greater than 90% in treatment-naïve and experienced patients. Recently submitted to the US Food and Drug Administration (FDA), a coformulation of ledipasvir (LDV), an NS5A inhibitor, with SOF, may soon be available.[126] This option shows promise with increased ease of use because of decreased pill burden as a fixed dose once-daily regimen, as well the first all oral regimen for HCV genotype 1. In the ELECTRON trial, LDV/SOF + RBV or GS-9699 was studied in the hard-to-treat population with advanced fibrosis or cirrhosis, and 100% achieved SVR12.[127] LDV/SOF has yet to be separately studied in the specifically coinfected population.

Another agent, an oral three DAA regimen plus RBV (Dasabuvir + RBV twice daily, ABT-450/ritonavir/Ombitasvir once daily), showed in SAPPHIRE-I and SAPPHIRE-II to have excellent outcomes in the HCV-monoinfected population, including the more difficult to treat genotype 1a.[128]

Studied also in the HIV/HCV-coinfected population, a new 2 DAA combination, MK-5172 and MK-8742, with or without RBV, has shown post-treatment sustained response rates above 90% for genotype 1 HCV patients, although this is still early data.[129]

Overall, there has been little studied of these newer combination agents thus far in the coinfected population, but the treatment of both the HCV-monoinfected and HIV/HCV-coinfected patient will continue to rapidly change in the near future as more data is obtained. All-oral, interferon free regimens are on the horizon for all genotypes.

CASE SELECTION FOR HCV THERAPY AND ART

Decision of when to start therapy for HCV depends on stage of disease, patient readiness, and comorbidities. Minimal disease can be monitored, but in the coinfected population, even mild disease may be appropriate for therapy given the acceleration of fibrosis in this population.[118]

ART is recommended for all coinfected patients, regardless of CD4 count. However, if the CD4 count is greater than 500, it may be reasonable to delay ART until treating their HCV to prevent drug interactions and risk of hepatotoxicity, as eradication of HCV with treatment may decrease the likelihood of drug-induced liver injury.[69,129]

PRACTICE GUIDELINES RECOMMENDATIONS

New guidelines were recently released by the AASLD and the Infectious Diseases Society of America to help guide the treatment of HCV in the setting of rapidly evolving therapy. Special attention was paid to the HIV/HCV-coinfected population. Because of its prolonged treatment course, adverse effects, and poor response rates, PEG/RBV alone or in combination with TVR or BOC is not recommended for the treatment of patients with HCV genotypes 1, 2, 3, or 4 who are coinfected with HIV. Triple-therapy recommendations for the treatment of HIV/HCV-coinfected individuals are based on genotype, IFN-eligibility, Q80K polymorphism in genotype 1a, and prior treatment response. The mainstay of therapy still includes PEG/RBV, but now typically with the addition of SOF or SMV. Interferon-based therapies will likely be falling out of therapy in the United States within the next 6–12 months. In addition, these recommendations help guide ART choice (**Table 4**).[121] Treatment of acute HCV has been shown to improve SVR rates, but the ideal treatment regimen has yet to be defined.[76]

MONITORING TREATMENT OUTCOME AND MANAGING ADVERSE EVENTS

When using IFN-based therapies, HCV RNA levels should be monitored at baseline, week 4, week 12, week 24 or end of treatment, and 24 weeks after treatment.[76] Additionally, CBC, CMP, and depression should be monitored every 2 weeks for the first month, then every month thereafter. SOF and RBV without PEG, in contrast, require less monitoring, and the FDA has endorsed SVR12 as an endpoint. Standard laboratory tests, including a complete blood count and comprehensive metabolic panel, should be monitored at 2, 4, 8, 12, 16, 20, and 24 weeks, to help identify

Table 4
HCV treatment recommendations in the setting of HIV/HCV coinfection

Genotype	Recommended	Alternative	Allowable ART
1	Treatment-naive and prior PEG/RBV relapsers IFN eligible: SOF + PEG/RBV × 12 wk IFN ineligible: SOF + RBV × 24 wk OR SOF + SMV ± RBV × 12 wk Treatment experienced (prior PEG/RBV nonresponders): SOF + SMV ± RBV × 12 wk	Treatment-naive and prior PEG/RBV relapsers IFN eligible: SMV × 12 wk + PEG/RBV × 24 wk IFN ineligible: None Treatment experienced (prior PEG/RBV nonresponders): IFN eligible: SOF + PEG/RBV × 12 wk IFN ineligible: SOF + RBV × 24 wk	For SOF use: ALL except DDI, AZT For SMV use: Limited to RAL, rilpivirine, maraviroc, enfuvirtide, TDF, FTC, 3TC, ABC
2 or 3	SOF + RBV × 12 wk	Treatment-naive and prior PEG/RBV relapsers: None Treatment experienced (prior PEG/RBV nonresponders): IFN eligible: SOF + PEG/RBV × 12 wk IFN ineligible: None	ALL except DDI and AZT
4	IFN eligible: SOF + PEG/RBV × 12 wk IFN ineligible: SOF + RBV × 24 wk	None	ALL except DDI and AZT
5 or 6	SOF + PEG/RBV × 12 wk	None	ALL except DDI and AZT

Abbreviations: ABC, abacavir; RAL, raltegravir.
Data from http://hcvguidelines.org/full-report/unique-patient-populations-hivhcv-coinfection-box-recommendations-hivhcv-coinfected. Accessed February 10, 2014.

expected adverse events. Additionally, TSH should be monitored every 3 months. Coinfected women experience a higher rate of adverse events than coinfected men, and pregnant women should not undergo therapy with PEG/RBV.[130] Anemia is one of the most significant adverse effects of RBV,[131] with dose-reduction still the recommended initial strategy, although some recommend the use of epoeitin or transfusions.[76,115] Thrombocytopenia and leukopenia are significant adverse effects of PEG, and dose reduction remains the initial strategy, although other management options, including eltrombopag and filgastram, are sometimes used.[76] Depression is another significant adverse effect of PEG, which can be managed with the use of antidepressants or mood stabilizers.[76]

OTHER ISSUES
Cost and Access to Care

There is significant concern that with the improved but costly therapies now available for HCV, certain populations will get treatment more easily than others. In resource-poor nations, HCV treatment will likely remain difficult. In developed nations, HCV may become a disease of those with difficult access to care and/or more difficult to treat, requiring PEG/RBV, such as those likely to be coinfected (homeless, active injection drug users, alcoholics, and illegal immigrants).[132] Awareness and advocacy will become a complementary part of therapy, especially in the coinfected population. Payers are currently reviewing indications for treatment based on disease severity which may be less relevant in the coinfected population given the more rapid progression of disease.

Primary and Secondary Prevention

Both the World Health Organization and the Advisory Committee on Immunization Practices advise universal infant HBV vaccination.[133] All individuals with HIV should be vaccinated against HBV if they do not have evidence of immunity or prior infection as defined by the presence of anti-HBsAb.[134] All patients should be assessed for response by obtaining anti-HBs titers at one month after series completion.[76] HIV-positive individuals tend to have lower response rates and durability to vaccination.[135,136] While immunocompetent patients respond to hepatitis B vaccination at rates greater than 90%, HIV-infected patients have been found to respond at rates of 24–56%.[137] Low CD4 counts and high viral loads are associated with decreased immunization success.[76,138,139] It is generally recommended that a standard vaccination schedule be initially followed. All who present to care should receive vaccination regardless of CD4 count as a response can be seen even with a low CD4. Anti-HBs titers should be obtained 1 month after completing the series.[76] If immunity is not achieved, as defined by the development of anti-HBsAb, revaccination using a double dose and/or 3 to 4 doses can be used.[140] At our institution, if there is no response to the initial vaccine series, then we are in the habit of repeating the vaccination series at a double dose. Although vaccination is important, patients should also be educated about transmission risks and avoidance of high risk behaviors.[76]

In contrast, there is no vaccine for hepatitis C. Preventing the spread of HCV involves avoiding unnecessary or unsafe injections, contaminated needles, or blood products, use of injection drugs or needle-sharing, unprotected sex, sharing sharp personal products that may be contaminated with blood, and tattoos or piercings with contaminated needles.[15] In addition, education and prevention to help prevent first infections, as well as recurrent HCV infections in high-risk groups, should be a mainstay of therapy in the HIV population.[107]

If an HIV-infected patient is found to be coinfected with HCV, they should have hepatitis A and B vaccination to prevent other hepatotoxic viruses. Those coinfected with HBV should receive hepatitis A vaccination as well. In addition, they should be regularly monitored for chronic liver disease every 6 months with a CMP, CBC, and INR. According to the AASLD, individuals with cirrhosis should be screened for HCC with an ultrasound every 6 to 12 months, and while controversial some practitioners also use AFP.

SUMMARY

In HIV-infected individuals, coinfection with HBV and/or HCV is common due to shared modes of transmission. It is known that HIV accelerates progression of liver disease and results in increased morbidity and mortality associated with viral hepatitis, but it is less clear if viral hepatitis has a direct effect on HIV. Treatment of viral hepatitis improves outcomes and should be considered in all HIV patients. Treatment of HBV without HIV is not advised because resistance can occur in both viruses. As the new DAAs for HCV become available, treatment will become easier with less adverse effects, less drug-drug interactions, and dramatically increased rates of success expected. There will still remain complications in the treatment of HCV in the coinfected population because of the need for continued PEG/RBV regimens when possible, and issues with cost and access to care.

REFERENCES

1. Verucchi G, Calza L, Manfredi R, et al. Human immunodeficiency virus and hepatitis C virus coinfection: epidemiology, natural history, therapeutic options and clinical management. Infection 2004;32:33–46.
2. Rockstroh JK, Mocroft A, Soriano V, et al. Influence of hepatitis C virus infection on HIV-1 disease progression and response to highly active antiretroviral therapy. J Infect Dis 2005;192:992–1002.
3. HIV and Viral Hepatitis. 2013. Available at: http://www.cdc.gov/hepatitis/Populations/PDFs/HIVandHep-FactSheet.pdf. Accessed January 15, 2014.
4. Weber R, Sabin CA, Friis-Moller N, et al. Liver-related deaths in persons infected with the human immunodeficiency virus: the D: A:D study. Arch Intern Med 2006;166:1632–41.
5. Te HS, Jensen DM. Epidemiology of Hepatitis B and C Viruses: a global overview. Clin Liver Dis 2010;14:1–21.
6. Lee WM. Hepatitis B virus infection. N Engl J Med 1997;337:1733–45.
7. Perz JF, Armstrong GL, Farrington LA, et al. The contributions of hepatitis B virus and hepatitis C virus infections to cirrhosis and primary liver cancer worldwide. J Hepatol 2006;45:529–38.
8. Hepatitis B. Revised 2013. Available at: http://www.who.int/mediacentre/factsheets/fs204/en/index.html. Accessed January 15, 2014.
9. Jimenez-Sousa MA, Berenguer J, Rallon N, et al. IL28RA polymorphism is associated with early hepatitis C virus (HCV) treatment failure in human immunodeficiency virus-/HCV-coinfected patients. J Viral Hepat 2013;20:358–66.
10. NIH Consensus Development Conference Statement on Management of Hepatitis B. Bethesda, October 20–22, 2008.
11. Thio CL, Smeaton L, Saulynas M, et al. Characterization of HIV-HBV coinfection in a multinational HIV-infected cohort. AIDS 2013;27:191–201.
12. Kellerman SE, Hanson DL, McNaghten AD, et al. Prevalence of chronic hepatitis B and incidence of acute hepatitis B infection in human immunodeficiency virus-infected subjects. J Infect Dis 2003;188:571–7.
13. Hepatitis C. Revised 2013. Available at: http://www.who.int/mediacentre/factsheets/fs164/en/index.html. Accessed January 26, 2014.
14. Ly KN, Xing J, Klevens RM, et al. The increasing burden of mortality from viral hepatitis in the United States between 1999 and 2007. Ann Intern Med 2012;156:271–8.
15. Recommendations for prevention and control of hepatitis C virus (HCV) infection and HCV related chronic disease. MMWR Recomm Rep 1998;47:1–39.
16. Tohme RA, Holmberg SD. Is sexual contact a major mode of hepatitis C virus transmission? Hepatology 2010;52:1497–505.
17. Thomas DL, Villano SA, Riester KA, et al. Perinatal transmission of hepatitis C virus from human immunodeficiency virus type 1-infected mothers. Women and Infants Transmission Study. J Infect Dis 1998;177:1480–8.
18. Screening for hepatitis C virus infection in adults: US Preventive Services Task Force recommendation statement. Available at: http://www.uspreventiveservicestaskforce.org/uspstf12/hepc/hepcfinalrs.htm. Accessed January 26, 2014.

19. Schmidt AJ, Falcato L, Zahno B, et al. Prevalence of hepatitis C in a Swiss sample of men who have sex with men: whom to screen for HCV infection? BMC Public Health 2014;14:3.
20. Wandeler G, Gsponer T, Bregenzer A, et al. Hepatitis C virus infections in the Swiss HIV Cohort Study: a rapidly evolving epidemic. Clin Infect Dis 2012;55:1408–16.
21. van der Helm JJ, Prins M, del Amo J, et al. The hepatitis C epidemic among HIV-positive MSM: incidence estimates from 1990 to 2007. AIDS 2011;25:1083–91.
22. van de Laar TJ, van der Bij AK, Prins M, et al. Increase in HCV incidence among men who have sex with men in Amsterdam most likely caused by sexual transmission. J Infect Dis 2007;196:230–8.
23. Alter MJ. Epidemiology of hepatitis C virus infection. World J Gastroenterol 2007;13:2436–41.
24. McMahon BJ. Natural history of chronic hepatitis B. Clin Liver Dis 2010;14:381–96.
25. Ghany MG, Doo EC. Assessment and management of chronic hepatitis B. Infect Dis Clin North Am 2006;20:63–79.
26. Houghton M. Hepatitis C viruses. 3rd edition. Philidelphia: Lipincott-Raven; 1996.
27. Mondelli MU, Silini E. Clinical significance of hepatitis C virus genotypes. J Hepatol 1999;31(Suppl 1):65–70.
28. Clausen LN, Weis N, Astvad K, et al. Interleukin-28B polymorphisms are associated with hepatitis C virus clearance and viral load in a HIV-1-infected cohort. J Viral Hepat 2011;18:e66–74.
29. Thomas DL, Thio CL, Martin MP, et al. Genetic variation in IL28B and spontaneous clearance of hepatitis C virus. Nature 2009;461:798–801.
30. Lange CM, Zeuzem S. IL28B single nucleotide polymorphisms in the treatment of hepatitis C. J Hepatol 2011;55:692–701.
31. Thio CL. Hepatitis B and human immunodeficiency virus coinfection. Hepatology 2009;49:S138–45.
32. Colin JF, Cazals-Hatem D, Loriot MA, et al. Influence of human immunodeficiency virus infection on chronic hepatitis B in homosexual men. Hepatology 1999;29:1306–10.
33. Puoti M, Torti C, Bruno R, et al. Natural history of chronic hepatitis B in co-infected patients. J Hepatol 2006;44:S65–70.
34. Gilson RJ, Hawkins AE, Beecham MR, et al. Interactions between HIV and hepatitis B virus in homosexual men: effects on the natural history of infection. AIDS 1997;11:597–606.
35. Bodsworth NJ, Cooper DA, Donovan B. The influence of human immunodeficiency virus type 1 infection on the development of the hepatitis B virus carrier state. J Infect Dis 1991;163:1138–40.
36. Di Martino V, Thevenot T, Colin JF, et al. Influence of HIV infection on the response to interferon therapy and the long-term outcome of chronic hepatitis B. Gastroenterology 2002;123:1812–22.
37. Thio CL, Seaberg EC, Skolasky R, et al. HIV-1, hepatitis B virus, and risk of liver-related mortality in the Multicenter Cohort Study (MACS). Lancet 2002;360:1921–6.
38. Konopnicki D, Mocroft A, de Wit S, et al. Hepatitis B and HIV: prevalence, AIDS progression, response to highly active antiretroviral therapy and increased mortality in the EuroSIDA cohort. AIDS 2005;19:593–601.

39. Scharschmidt BF, Held MJ, Hollander HH, et al. Hepatitis B in patients with HIV infection: relationship to AIDS and patient survival. Ann Intern Med 1992;117: 837–8.

40. Sinicco A, Raiteri R, Sciandra M, et al. Coinfection and superinfection of hepatitis B virus in patients infected with human immunodeficiency virus: no evidence of faster progression to AIDS. Scand J Infect Dis 1997;29:111–5.

41. Nikolopoulos GK, Paraskevis D, Hatzitheodorou E, et al. Impact of hepatitis B virus infection on the progression of AIDS and mortality in HIV-infected individuals: a cohort study and meta-analysis. Clin Infect Dis 2009;48:1763–71.

42. Eskild A, Magnus P, Petersen G, et al. Hepatitis B antibodies in HIV-infected homosexual men are associated with more rapid progression to AIDS. AIDS 1992;6:571–4.

43. Chun HM, Roediger MP, Hullsiek KH, et al. Hepatitis B virus coinfection negatively impacts HIV outcomes in HIV seroconverters. J Infect Dis 2012;205: 185–93.

44. Boesecke C, Wedemeyer H, Rockstroh JK. Diagnosis and treatment of acute hepatitis C virus infection. Infect Dis Clin North Am 2012;26:995–1010.

45. Alter MJ, Margolis HS, Krawczynski K, et al. The natural history of community-acquired hepatitis C in the United States. The Sentinel Counties Chronic non-A, non-B Hepatitis Study Team. N Engl J Med 1992;327:1899–905.

46. Thomas DL, Astemborski J, Rai RM, et al. The natural history of hepatitis C virus infection: host, viral, and environmental factors. JAMA 2000;284:450–6.

47. van der Meer AJ, Veldt BJ, Feld JJ, et al. Association between sustained virological response and all-cause mortality among patients with chronic hepatitis C and advanced hepatic fibrosis. JAMA 2012;308:2584–93.

48. Daar ES, Lynn H, Donfield S, et al. Relation between HIV-1 and hepatitis C viral load in patients with hemophilia. J Acquir Immune Defic Syndr 2001;26:466–72.

49. Boesecke C, Vogel M. HIV and hepatitis C co-infection: acute HCV therapy. Curr Opin HIV AIDS 2011;6:459–64.

50. Thein HH, Yi Q, Dore GJ, et al. Natural history of hepatitis C virus infection in HIV-infected individuals and the impact of HIV in the era of highly active antiretroviral therapy: a meta-analysis. AIDS 2008;22:1979–91.

51. Martin-Carbonero L, Benhamou Y, Puoti M, et al. Incidence and predictors of severe liver fibrosis in human immunodeficiency virus-infected patients with chronic hepatitis C: a European collaborative study. Clin Infect Dis 2004;38: 128–33.

52. Benhamou Y, Bochet M, Di Martino V, et al. Liver fibrosis progression in human immunodeficiency virus and hepatitis C virus coinfected patients. The Multivirc Group. Hepatology 1999;30:1054–8.

53. Graham CS, Baden LR, Yu E, et al. Influence of human immunodeficiency virus infection on the course of hepatitis C virus infection: a meta-analysis. Clin Infect Dis 2001;33:562–9.

54. Monga HK, Rodriguez-Barradas MC, Breaux K, et al. Hepatitis C virus infection-related morbidity and mortality among patients with human immunodeficiency virus infection. Clin Infect Dis 2001;33:240–7.

55. Kim AY, Lauer GM, Ouchi K, et al. The magnitude and breadth of hepatitis C virus-specific CD8+ T cells depend on absolute CD4+ T-cell count in individuals coinfected with HIV-1. Blood 2005;105:1170–8.

56. Balagopal A, Philp FH, Astemborski J, et al. Human immunodeficiency virus-related microbial translocation and progression of hepatitis C. Gastroenterology 2008;135:226–33.

57. Allison RD, Katsounas A, Koziol DE, et al. Association of interleukin-15-induced peripheral immune activation with hepatic stellate cell activation in persons coinfected with hepatitis C virus and HIV. J Infect Dis 2009;200:619–23.
58. Anderson JP, Tchetgen Tchetgen EJ, Lo Re V 3rd, et al. Antiretroviral therapy reduces the rate of hepatic decompensation among HIV- and hepatitis C virus-coinfected veterans. Clin Infect Dis 2014;58:719–27.
59. Greub G, Ledergerber B, Battegay M, et al. Clinical progression, survival, and immune recovery during antiretroviral therapy in patients with HIV-1 and hepatitis C virus coinfection: the Swiss HIV Cohort Study. Lancet 2000;356:1800–5.
60. Hansson GK. Inflammation, atherosclerosis, and coronary artery disease. N Engl J Med 2005;352:1685–95.
61. Lee MH, Yang HI, Lu SN, et al. Chronic hepatitis C virus infection increases mortality from hepatic and extrahepatic diseases: a community-based long-term prospective study. J Infect Dis 2012;206:469–77.
62. Gillis J, Smieja M, Cescon A, et al. Risk of cardiovascular disease associated with HCV and HBV co-infection among antiretroviral-treated HIV-infected individuals. Antivir Ther 2014;19(3):309–17.
63. Tsui JI, Vittinghoff E, Shlipak MG, et al. Association of hepatitis C seropositivity with increased risk for developing end-stage renal disease. Arch Intern Med 2007;167:1271–6.
64. Daghestani L, Pomeroy C. Renal manifestations of hepatitis C infection. Am J Med 1999;106:347–54.
65. Sulkowski MS, Thomas DL, Chaisson RE, et al. Hepatotoxicity associated with antiretroviral therapy in adults infected with human immunodeficiency virus and the role of hepatitis C or B virus infection. JAMA 2000;283:74–80.
66. Wit FW, Weverling GJ, Weel J, et al. Incidence of and risk factors for severe hepatotoxicity associated with antiretroviral combination therapy. J Infect Dis 2002;186:23–31.
67. Vispo E, Fernandez-Montero JV, Labarga P, et al. Low risk of liver toxicity using the most recently approved antiretroviral agents but still increased in HIV-hepatitis C virus coinfected patients. AIDS 2013;27:1187–8.
68. Sulkowski MS, Thomas DL, Mehta SH, et al. Hepatotoxicity associated with nevirapine or efavirenz-containing antiretroviral therapy: role of hepatitis C and B infections. Hepatology 2002;35:182–9.
69. Aranzabal L, Casado JL, Moya J, et al. Influence of liver fibrosis on highly active antiretroviral therapy-associated hepatotoxicity in patients with HIV and hepatitis C virus coinfection. Clin Infect Dis 2005;40:588–93.
70. Bonfanti P, Landonio S, Ricci E, et al. Risk factors for hepatotoxicity in patients treated with highly active antiretroviral therapy. J Acquir Immune Defic Syndr 2001;27:316–8.
71. Rockstroh J, Teppler H, Zhao J, et al. Safety and efficacy of raltegravir in patients with HIV-1 and hepatitis B and/or C virus coinfection. HIV Med 2012;13:127–31.
72. Labarga P, Soriano V, Vispo ME, et al. Hepatotoxicity of antiretroviral drugs is reduced after successful treatment of chronic hepatitis C in HIV-infected patients. J Infect Dis 2007;196:670–6.
73. Kaplan JE, Benson C, Holmes KK, et al. Guidelines for prevention and treatment of opportunistic infections in HIV-infected adults and adolescents: recommendations from CDC, the National Institutes of Health, and the HIV Medicine Association of the Infectious Diseases Society of America. MMWR Recomm Rep 2009;58:1–207 [quiz: CE1–4].

74. Lok AS, McMahon BJ. Chronic hepatitis B: update 2009. Hepatology 2009;50: 661–2.

75. Soriano V, Puoti M, Sulkowski M, et al. Care of patients coinfected with HIV and hepatitis C virus: 2007 updated recommendations from the HCV-HIV International Panel. AIDS 2007;21:1073–89.

76. Guidelines for the prevention and treatment of opportunistic infections in HIV-infected adults and adolescents: recommendations from the Centers for Disease Control and Prevention, the National Institutes of Health, and the HIV Medicine Association of the Infectious Diseases Society of America. Available at: http://aidsinfo. nih.gov/contentfiles/lvguidelines/adult_oi.pdf. Accessed February 3, 2014.

77. Pawlotsky JM. Use and interpretation of virological tests for hepatitis C. Hepatology 2002;36:S65–73.

78. Hadlich E, Alvares-Da-Silva MR, Dal Molin RK, et al. Hepatitis C virus (HCV) viremia in HIV-infected patients without HCV antibodies detectable by third-generation enzyme immunoassay. J Gastroenterol Hepatol 2007;22:1506–9.

79. Sulkowski MS, Moore RD, Mehta SH, et al. Hepatitis C and progression of HIV disease. JAMA 2002;288:199–206.

80. Moreno S, Garcia-Samaniego J, Moreno A, et al. Noninvasive diagnosis of liver fibrosis in patients with HIV infection and HCV/HBV co-infection. J Viral Hepat 2009;16:249–58.

81. Sterling RK, Lissen E, Clumeck N, et al. Development of a simple noninvasive index to predict significant fibrosis in patients with HIV/HCV coinfection. Hepatology 2006;43:1317–25.

82. Wilson LE, Torbenson M, Astemborski J, et al. Progression of liver fibrosis among injection drug users with chronic hepatitis C. Hepatology 2006;43:788–95.

83. Myers RP, Benhamou Y, Imbert-Bismut F, et al. Serum biochemical markers accurately predict liver fibrosis in HIV and hepatitis C virus co-infected patients. AIDS 2003;17:721–5.

84. Nunes D, Fleming C, Offner G, et al. HIV infection does not affect the performance of noninvasive markers of fibrosis for the diagnosis of hepatitis C virus-related liver disease. J Acquir Immune Defic Syndr 2005;40:538–44.

85. de Ledinghen V, Douvin C, Kettaneh A, et al. Diagnosis of hepatic fibrosis and cirrhosis by transient elastography in HIV/hepatitis C virus-coinfected patients. J Acquir Immune Defic Syndr 2006;41:175–9.

86. Kelleher TB, Mehta SH, Bhaskar R, et al. Prediction of hepatic fibrosis in HIV/ HCV co-infected patients using serum fibrosis markers: the SHASTA index. J Hepatol 2005;43:78–84.

87. Guidelines for the use of antiretroviral agents in HIV-1-infected adults and adolescents. Department of Health and Human Services. Available at: http:// aidsinfo.nih.gov/contentfiles/lvguidelines/AdultandAdolescentGL.pdf. Accessed February 4, 2014.

88. Wongprasit P, Manosuthi W, Kiertiburanakul S, et al. Hepatitis B virus drug resistance in HIV-1-infected patients taking lamivudine-containing antiretroviral therapy. AIDS Patient Care STDS 2010;24:205–9.

89. Koziel MJ, Peters MG. Viral hepatitis in HIV infection. N Engl J Med 2007;356: 1445–54.

90. McMahon MA, Jilek BL, Brennan TP, et al. The HBV drug entecavir - effects on HIV-1 replication and resistance. N Engl J Med 2007;356:2614–21.

91. Sasadeusz J, Audsley J, Mijch A, et al. The anti-HIV activity of entecavir: a multi-centre evaluation of lamivudine-experienced and lamivudine-naive patients. AIDS 2008;22:947–55.

92. Benhamou Y, Fleury H, Trimoulet P, et al. Anti-hepatitis B virus efficacy of teno-fovir disoproxil fumarate in HIV-infected patients. Hepatology 2006;43:548–55.
93. Lange CM, Bojunga J, Hofmann WP, et al. Severe lactic acidosis during treatment of chronic hepatitis B with entecavir in patients with impaired liver function. Hepatology 2009;50:2001–6.
94. Benhamou Y, Bochet M, Thibault V, et al. Long-term incidence of hepatitis B virus resistance to lamivudine in human immunodeficiency virus-infected patients. Hepatology 1999;30:1302–6.
95. Bellini C, Keiser O, Chave JP, et al. Liver enzyme elevation after lamivudine withdrawal in HIV-hepatitis B virus co-infected patients: the Swiss HIV Cohort Study. HIV Med 2009;10:12–8.
96. Pillay D, Cane PA, Ratcliffe D, et al. Evolution of lamivudine-resistant hepatitis B virus and HIV-1 in co-infected individuals: an analysis of the CAESAR study. CAESAR co-ordinating committee. AIDS 2000;14:1111–6.
97. Viread [package insert]. Gilead Sciences, Inc., Foster City, CA; 2013.
98. Dore GJ, Soriano V, Rockstroh J, et al. Frequent hepatitis B virus rebound among HIV-hepatitis B virus-coinfected patients following antiretroviral therapy interruption. AIDS 2010;24:857–65.
99. den Brinker M, Wit FW, Wertheim-van Dillen PM, et al. Hepatitis B and C virus co-infection and the risk for hepatotoxicity of highly active antiretroviral therapy in HIV-1 infection. AIDS 2000;14:2895–902.
100. Dore G. Antiretroviral therapy-related hepatotoxicity: predictors and clinical management. J HIV Ther 2003;8:96–100.
101. Lawn SD, Meintjes G. Pathogenesis and prevention of immune reconstitution disease during antiretroviral therapy. Expert Rev Anti Infect Ther 2011;9:415–30.
102. Berenguer J, Alvarez-Pellicer J, Martin PM, et al. Sustained virological response to interferon plus ribavirin reduces liver-related complications and mortality in patients coinfected with human immunodeficiency virus and hepatitis C virus. Hepatology 2009;50:407–13.
103. Mira JA, Rivero-Juarez A, Lopez-Cortes LF, et al. Benefits from sustained virologic response to pegylated interferon plus ribavirin in HIV/hepatitis C virus-coinfected patients with compensated cirrhosis. Clin Infect Dis 2013;56:1646–53.
104. Mehta SH, Genberg BL, Astemborski J, et al. Limited uptake of hepatitis C treatment among injection drug users. J Community Health 2008;33:126–33.
105. Sherman KE, Andreatta C, O'Brien J, et al. Hepatitis C in human immunodeficiency virus-coinfected patients: increased variability in the hypervariable envelope coding domain. Hepatology 1996;23:688–94.
106. Sherman KE, Rouster SD, Stanford S, et al. Hepatitis C virus (HCV) quasispecies complexity and selection in HCV/HIV-coinfected subjects treated with interferon-based regimens. J Infect Dis 2010;201:712–9.
107. Sulkowski MS, Sherman KE, Dieterich DT, et al. Combination therapy with telaprevir for chronic hepatitis C virus genotype 1 infection in patients with HIV: a randomized trial. Ann Intern Med 2013;159:86–96.
108. Feld JJ, Hoofnagle JH. Mechanism of action of interferon and ribavirin in treatment of hepatitis C. Nature 2005;436:967–72.
109. Chung RT, Andersen J, Volberding P, et al. Peginterferon Alfa-2a plus ribavirin versus interferon alfa-2a plus ribavirin for chronic hepatitis C in HIV-coinfected persons. N Engl J Med 2004;351:451–9.
110. Carrat F, Bani-Sadr F, Pol S, et al. Pegylated interferon alfa-2b vs standard interferon alfa-2b, plus ribavirin, for chronic hepatitis C in HIV-infected patients: a randomized controlled trial. JAMA 2004;292:2839–48.

111. Torriani FJ, Rodriguez-Torres M, Rockstroh JK, et al. Peginterferon Alfa-2a plus ribavirin for chronic hepatitis C virus infection in HIV-infected patients. N Engl J Med 2004;351:438–50.

112. Nunez M, Marino A, Miralles C, et al. Baseline serum hepatitis C virus (HCV) RNA level and response at week 4 are the best predictors of relapse after treatment with pegylated interferon plus ribavirin in HIV/HCV-coinfected patients. J Acquir Immune Defic Syndr 2007;45:439–44.

113. Lafeuillade A, Hittinger G, Chadapaud S. Increased mitochondrial toxicity with ribavirin in HIV/HCV coinfection. Lancet 2001;357:280–1.

114. Alvarez D, Dieterich DT, Brau N, et al. Zidovudine use but not weight-based ribavirin dosing impacts anaemia during HCV treatment in HIV-infected persons. J Viral Hepat 2006;13:683–9.

115. Behler CM, Vittinghoff E, Lin F, et al. Hematologic toxicity associated with interferon-based hepatitis C therapy in HIV type 1-coinfected subjects. Clin Infect Dis 2007;44:1375–83.

116. Karageorgopoulos DE, El-Sherif O, Bhagani S, et al. Drug interactions between antiretrovirals and new or emerging direct-acting antivirals in HIV/hepatitis C virus coinfection. Curr Opin Infect Dis 2014;27:36–45.

117. Sulkowski M, Pol S, Mallolas J, et al. Boceprevir versus placebo with pegylated interferon alfa-2b and ribavirin for treatment of hepatitis C virus genotype 1 in patients with HIV: a randomised, double-blind, controlled phase 2 trial. Lancet Infect Dis 2013;13:597–605.

118. Chastain CA, Naggie S. Treatment of genotype 1 HCV infection in the HIV coinfected patient in 2014. Curr HIV/AIDS Rep 2013;10:408–19.

119. Dieterich D, Rockstroh J, Orkin C, et al. Simeprevir (TMC435) plus peginterferon/ribavirin in patients co-infected with HCV genotype-1 and HIV-1: primary analysis of C212 study [abstract LBPS9/50]. 14th European AIDS Conference. Brussels, Belgium, October 16-19, 2013.

120. Lawitz E, Forns X, Zeuzem S, et al. Simeprevir (TMC435) with peginteron/ribavirin for treatment of chronic HCV genotype 1 infection in patients who relapsed after previous interferon-based therapy: results from PROMISE, a phase III trial. Digestive Disease Week 2013. Orlando, FL, May 18-21, 2013.

121. Unique patient populations: patients with HIV/HCV coinfection. Available at: http://www.hcvguidelines.org/full-report/unique-patient-populations. Accessed February 3, 2014.

122. Ouwerkerk-Mahadevan S, Sekar V, Simion A, et al. The pharmacokinetic interactions of the HCV protease inhibitor simeprevir (TMC435) with HIV antiretroviral agents in healthy volunteers (abstract). IDWeek 2012. San Diego, CA, October 17-21, 2012.

123. Sulkowski M, Rodriguez-Torres TM, Lalezari JP, et al. All-oral therapy with sofosbuvir plus ribavirin for the treatment of HCV genotype 1, 2, and 3 infection in patients co-infected with HIV (PHOTON-1). Hepatology 2013;58:313A–4A [abstract 212].

124. Kirby B, Mathias A, Rossi S, et al. No clinically significant pharmacokinetic interactions between sofosbuvir (GS-7977) and HIV antiretrovirals atripla, rilpivirine, darunavir/ritonavir, or raltegravir in healthy volunteers (abstract). 63rd Annual Meeting of the American Association of the Study of Liver Diseases. Boston, MA, November 9-13, 2012.

125. Rodriguez-Torres M, Rodriguez-Orengo J, Gaggar A, et al. Sofosbuvir and Peginterferon Alfa-2a/Ribavirin for Treatment-Naive Genotype 1-4 HCV-Infected Patients Who Are Coinfected With HIV. 53rd ICAAC 2013. Denver, CO, September 10-13, 2013.

126. Gilead Sciences I. Gilead Files for U.S. Approval of Ledipasvir/Sofosbuvir Fixed-Dose Combination Tablet for Genotype 1 Hepatitis C. 2014.

127. Gane EJ, Stedman CS, Hyland RH, et al. Once Daily Sofosbuvir/Ledipasvir Fixed Dose Combination with or without Ribavirin: the ELECTRON trial. 64th Annual Meeting of the American Association for the Study of Liver Diseases (AASLD 2013). Washington, DC, November 1-5, 2013.

128. Sulkowski M, Pol S, Hassanein T, et al. Efficacy and safety of the all-oral regimen, MK-5172/MK-8742 +/− RBV for 12 weeks in GT1 HCV/HIV co-infected patients: the C-WORTHY study. 49th European Association for the Study of the Liver International Liver Congress (EASL 2014) 2014.

129. Considerations for Antiretroviral Use in Patients with Coinfections: HIV/Hepatitis C Virus (HCV) Co-infection. Available at: http://aidsinfo.nih.gov/guidelines/html/1/adult-and-adolescent-arv-guidelines/26/hiv-hcv. Accessed January 28, 2014.

130. Bhattacharya D, Umbleja T, Carrat F, et al. Women experience higher rates of adverse events during hepatitis C virus therapy in HIV infection: a meta-analysis. J Acquir Immune Defic Syndr 2010;55:170–5.

131. Butt AA, Umbleja T, Andersen JW, et al. The incidence, predictors and management of anaemia and its association with virological response in HCV/HIV coinfected persons treated with long-term pegylated interferon alfa 2a and ribavirin. Aliment Pharmacol Ther 2011;33:1234–44.

132. Soriano V, Labarga P, Fernandez-Montero JV, et al. The changing face of hepatitis C in the new era of direct-acting antivirals. Antiviral Res 2013;97:36–40.

133. Mast EE, Margolis HS, Fiore AE, et al. A comprehensive immunization strategy to eliminate transmission of hepatitis B virus infection in the United States: recommendations of the Advisory Committee on Immunization Practices (ACIP) part 1: immunization of infants, children, and adolescents. MMWR Recomm Rep 2005;54:1–31.

134. Bridges CB, Coyne-Beasley T. Immunization Services Division NtCflaRD, C. D. C. Advisory committee on immunization practices recommended immunization schedule for adults aged 19 years or older - United States, 2014. MMWR Morb Mortal Wkly Rep 2014;63:110–2.

135. Loke RH, Murray-Lyon IM, Coleman JC, et al. Diminished response to recombinant hepatitis B vaccine in homosexual men with HIV antibody: an indicator of poor prognosis. J Med Virol 1990;31:109–11.

136. Bruguera M, Cremades M, Salinas R, et al. Impaired response to recombinant hepatitis B vaccine in HIV-infected persons. J Clin Gastroenterol 1992;14:27–30.

137. Bruguera M, Cremades M, Salinas R, et al. Impaired response to recombinant hepatitis B vaccine in HIV-infected persons. J Clin Gastroenterol 1992;14:27–30.

138. Tedaldi EM, Baker RK, Moorman AC, et al. Hepatitis A and B vaccination practices for ambulatory patients infected with HIV. Clin Infect Dis 2004;38:1478–84.

139. Overton ET, Sungkanuparph S, Powderly WG, et al. Undetectable plasma HIV RNA load predicts success after hepatitis B vaccination in HIV-infected persons. Clin Infect Dis 2005;41:1045–8.

140. Soriano V, Poveda E, Vispo E, et al. Hepatitis B in HIV-infected patients. Clin Liver Dis 2013;17:489–501.

Update on Opportunistic Infections in the Era of Effective Antiretroviral Therapy

Brian C. Zanoni, MD, MPH[a,b], Rajesh T. Gandhi, MD[b,c],*

KEYWORDS

- HIV • Opportunistic infections • Antiretroviral therapy • Diagnostics

KEY POINTS

- New diagnostic tests are improving the ability to detect tuberculosis (TB), cryptococcal meningitis (CM), and pneumocystis pneumonia (PCP) in human immunodeficiency virus (HIV)-infected patients.
- Randomized trials support early initiation of antiretroviral therapy (ART) in HIV-infected patients with TB; however, a slight delay in the initiation of ART in patients with CM may be warranted.
- Although new therapies have been tested in HIV-infected patients with progressive multifocal leukoencephalopathy (PML), ART is still the mainstay of therapy.
- Young HIV-infected males and females should receive the quadrivalent human papillomavirus (HPV) vaccine.
- Varicella vaccine is recommended for nonimmune HIV-infected individuals with CD4 cell count greater than $200/mm^3$. Zoster vaccine seems to be safe and immunogenic in HIV-infected patients with high CD4 cell counts on ART.

INTRODUCTION

Despite efforts to diagnose and treat HIV infection before patients develop advanced disease, opportunistic infections (OIs) continue to occur in the era of effective ART, particularly in those who have not yet been diagnosed with HIV and in those who are not receiving therapy. In the United States, approximately one-third of patients have a CD4 cell count less than $200/mm^3$ at the time of HIV diagnosis, placing them at risk for OIs.[1]

a Infectious Diseases Division, Massachusetts General Hospital, GRJ 504, 55 Fruit Street, Boston, MA 02114, USA; b Harvard Medical School, 25 Shattuck Street, Boston, MA 02115, USA; c Infectious Diseases Division and Ragon Institute, Massachusetts General Hospital, GRJ 504, 55 Fruit Street, Boston, MA 02114, USA
* Corresponding author. Infectious Diseases Division and Ragon Institute, Massachusetts General Hospital, GRJ 504, 55 Fruit Street, Boston, MA 02114.
E-mail address: RGANDHI@mgh.harvard.edu

Infect Dis Clin N Am 28 (2014) 501–518
http://dx.doi.org/10.1016/j.idc.2014.05.002
0891-5520/14/$ – see front matter © 2014 Elsevier Inc. All rights reserved.

id.theclinics.com

Although most OIs occur in patients with CD4 cell counts less than 200/mm^3, a small residual risk remains even in those with higher counts. A recent analysis of patients with CD4 cell counts greater than 200/mm^3 found that esophageal candidiasis, Kaposi sarcoma, and pulmonary TB were the most common opportunistic conditions in this population.[2] Factors associated with increased risk of acquired immunodeficiency syndrome (AIDS)-defining illness (ADI) in patients with a CD4 cell count greater than 500/mm^3 included injection drug use, older age, and having more than 10,000 copies/mL of HIV RNA.[2] The incidence of OIs seems to level off at a CD4 cell count of 750/mm^3, suggesting that immune reconstitution is near complete at this level.[2]

This review focuses on TB and cryptococcal infections, the most common OIs in patients living with HIV around the world, as well as on new developments in progressive multifocal leukoencephalopathy and PCP. In the sections on these conditions, updates on diagnosis, treatment, and complications, as well as information on when to start ART is provided. The article concludes with a discussion of new data on 2 vaccine-preventable OIs, HPV and varicella-zoster virus (VZV) infections. For information on other OIs, the readers may consult the recently updated US Department of Health and Human Services (DHHS) Guidelines for the Prevention and Treatment of Opportunistic Infection in HIV-Infected Adults and Adolescents, which provides a comprehensive review.[3]

TB in HIV-Infected Patients

Epidemiology
Since the widespread use of ART and intensive TB control efforts in the 1990s, TB incidence among HIV-infected individuals in the United States has declined; in fact, the decrease outpaces those seen in HIV-uninfected individuals.[4,5] In 2012, there were 9945 cases of TB in the United States, of whom 625 (7%) were coinfected with HIV.[4,5]

Latent TB infection
Patients should be tested for latent TB infection (LTBI) at the time of HIV diagnosis; if the result is negative, the test should be repeated if the patient is exposed to TB.[3] LTBI in HIV-infected individuals is defined as a tuberculin skin test (TST) with more than 5 mm of induration without clinical or radiographic evidence of active disease. However, a positive TST result is not completely specific for TB: patients who are infected with some nontuberculous mycobacteria or who have recently received BCG vaccination may have a false-positive result. A false-negative TST result may occur in patients with severe immunodeficiency; therefore, if the test result is negative when the patient's CD4 cell count is less than 200/mm^3, the test should be repeated after the patient receives ART and achieves immune reconstitution. Finally, the TST has several logistic disadvantages, including the need for a return visit for the test to be read and variability in how it is placed and interpreted.

Interferon gamma release assay (IGRA), a blood test, requires only a single visit and has higher specificity than the TST for diagnosis of LTBI. In HIV-uninfected individuals, there is good concordance (89%) between the IGRA and TST.[6] However, in HIV-infected individuals in low-TB-prevalence areas, the concordance between TST and IGRA results is not as good.[7] In addition, those with a CD4 cell count less than 200/mm^3 are more likely to have indeterminate results.[7] Nevertheless, both the TST and IGRA are considered appropriate tests for diagnosis of LTBI in HIV-infected patients.[8] Of note, although a recent study found that an IGRA had good sensitivity for active TB in HIV-infected patients,[7,8] other studies have found that the result of TST and IGRA may be negative in patients with TB; therefore, a negative result does not exclude active infection.[9]

Treatment of LTBI

Isoniazid (INH) daily for 9 months has been the standard therapy for patients with LTBI for many years.[10] The efficacy of INH monotherapy is 69% to 93%[11]; however, completion rates are low (30%–64%).[12,13] Recently, a study of once-weekly INH and rifapentine by directly observed therapy for 3 months was found to be as effective as 9 months of INH for preventing active TB and had a significantly higher completion rate (82% vs 69%).[14] However, this regimen is not recommended for HIV-infected individuals who are receiving ART because of the potential for drug interactions between rifapentine and ART.[3]

Diagnosis of Active TB

Typically, TB is diagnosed by detecting *Mycobacterium tuberculosis* in smear or culture from sputum or other samples (eg, in highly immunosuppressed patients, blood cultures may grow the organism). In patients with suspected pulmonary TB, sputum smears for acid-fast bacilli (AFB) should be performed, along with culture, which has higher sensitivity than smear. Culture of 3 sputum specimens should be considered because the second and third cultures increase the incremental AFB yield (by 17% and 10%, respectively).[15] In immunosuppressed patients, extrapulmonary TB is frequent; in this setting, the sputum AFB smear may yield a negative result. Fortunately, new diagnostic tests have been developed that are improving the ability to diagnose TB.

GeneXpert

Recent development of the GeneXpert MTB/RIF brings rapid point-of-care diagnostics to the field of TB. This automated nucleic-acid amplification test uses real-time polymerase chain reaction to amplify a TB-specific portion of the *rpoB* gene, which is then probed for mutations within the rifampin-resistance-determining region. This assay can provide results in a few hours compared with up to 6 weeks for mycobacterial culture. In a study of patients with suspected pulmonary TB conducted in Peru, Azerbaijan, South Africa, and India, the sensitivity of GeneXpert in smear-positive disease was 98%.[16] Among HIV-infected patients with pulmonary TB, the sensitivity was 94%. In smear-negative disease, the sensitivity for 1 GeneXpert test was 72.5%, for 2 tests was 85%, and for 3 tests was 90%.[16] The test also had high specificity (99%). When compared with phenotypic methods, the GeneXpert test correctly identified 98% of rifampin-resistant and rifampin-sensitive isolates.[16] (Other nucleic-acid-based genotypic methods can detect both INH and rifampin resistance).[17]

The GeneXpert test has now been tested in a variety of settings and on patients with pulmonary and extrapulmonary TB. A recent meta-analysis that analyzed 10,224 suspected specimens estimated a sensitivity of 90% (lower in smear-negative samples than in smear-positive sputa) and a specificity of 98% in diagnosing pulmonary TB.[18] The sensitivity for detecting rifampin resistance was 94% and the specificity was 97%. For extrapulmonary TB, the sensitivity was 80% and the specificity was 86%.[18]

At present, GeneXpert is approved for use on sputum only. Several studies evaluating the GeneXpert platform on extrapulmonary samples found variability in its sensitivity and specificity depending on the tissue and sample site.[19–22] Overall, the performance of the GeneXpert for extrapulmonary TB seems to improve with decreasing CD4 cell count.[19] Additional studies will be required to determine its effectiveness in diagnosing TB when used on samples other than sputum.

Lipopolysaccharide antigen lipoarabinomannan

The detection of the *M tuberculosis* cell wall lipopolysaccharide antigen lipoarabinomannan (LAM) in urine has been developed as a test to diagnose TB without regard to the specific anatomic site of infection. In a study of 199 patients with TB in South Africa, 16% of patients tested positive for LAM by enzyme-linked immunosorbent assay.[23] The sensitivity was highest in those with CD4 cell count less than 50/mm^3 (69%) and declined with increasing CD4 counts: 43% in those with CD4 counts between 50 and 99, 32% in those with CD4 counts between 100 and 199, and only 15% in those with CD4 counts greater than 200. Recently, a low-cost point-of-care lateral flow assay using a urine dipstick has been developed to detect LAM.[24,25]

Treatment of TB in HIV-infected patients

HIV-infected patients with TB should receive the same treatment as HIV-negative individuals. Particular attention should be given to drug interactions between antituberculous therapy and specific antiretroviral medications (**Table 1**). Daily therapy (5–7 d/wk), rather than intermittent dosing, is recommended during the intensive phase. During the continuation phase, daily or thrice-weekly dosing should be given; less frequent dosing has been associated with higher rates of treatment failure or relapse, perhaps because of malabsorption in HIV-TB coinfected patients with low CD4 cell counts.

When to start ART in an HIV-infected patient with TB

Sequential treatment, in which a course of therapy for TB is completed followed by ART initiation, has been shown to increase mortality in those with drug-sensitive or multidrug-resistant TB and is not recommended.[26,27] Several studies have demonstrated that integrated-treatment of HIV and TB improves survival, prevents other OIs, and may improve TB treatment outcomes.[26–29]

In the Starting Antiretroviral Therapy at Three Points in Tuberculosis (SAPIT) study, 642 HIV-infected South African adults with CD4 cell counts less than 500/mm^3 and smear-positive TB were randomized to start ART within 4 weeks after initiating TB therapy (early integrated therapy), within 4 weeks after completion of the intensive phase of TB treatment (late integrated therapy), or after TB treatment was completed (sequential therapy).[29] In all CD4 cell count strata, mortality was significantly higher in the sequential therapy group than in the combined integrated therapy groups.[26] The benefit of early integrated therapy was greatest in those with CD4 cell counts less than 50/mm^3.[29] Patients with higher CD4 cell counts who received late integrated therapy had a lower incidence of immune reconstitution inflammatory syndrome (IRIS) and adverse events requiring ART change compared with those who received early integrated therapy.[29]

The Cambodian Early versus Late Introduction of Antiretrovirals (CAMELIA) study randomized 661 HIV-infected Cambodian adults with TB and a median CD4 cell count of 25/mm^3 to start ART treatment at 2 or 8 weeks after initiation of TB therapy.[30] Although the incidence of IRIS was 2.5-fold higher in the 2-week ART group, this was outweighed by the mortality benefit: risk of death was significantly lower in the 2-week group (18%) than in the 8-week group (27%).

In the Immediate Versus Deferred Start of Anti-HIV Therapy in HIV-Infected Adults Being Treated for Tuberculosis (STRIDE) study (AIDS Clinical Trials Group, ACTG, trial A5221), 809 HIV-infected patients with suspected TB and a CD4 cell count of less than

Table 1
Drug interactions between antitubercular and antiretroviral medications

Anti-TB Drug	Antiretroviral Drug	Effects and Recommendations
Rifampin	Efavirenz	In patients weighing ≥60 kg, lower efavirenz C_{min} when administered with rifampin; no association between greater weight and reduced virologic suppression; no change in dose recommended[31]
	Elvitegravir/cobicistat/ tenofovir/emtricitabine	Cobicistat and elvitegravir levels may decrease—coadministration should be avoided
	Etravirine	Etravirine levels may decrease—coadministration should be avoided
	Maraviroc	Maraviroc level decreases—increase maraviroc to 600 mg twice daily or use alternative
	Nevirapine	Nevirapine level decreases—coadministration should be avoided if possible
	PI (with or without ritonavir)	PI level significantly decreases—coadministration should be avoided
	Raltegravir	Raltegravir level decreases—label advises increase in dose to 800 mg twice daily; monitor efficacy closely or switch rifampin to rifabutin
	Rilpivirine	Rilpivirine level decreases—coadministration should be avoided
	Zidovudine	Zidovudine level decreases—no dosage adjustments recommended; monitor efficacy
Rifabutin	Efavirenz	Rifabutin level decreases; efavirenz exposure unchanged—increase rifabutin to 450–600 mg daily
	Elvitegravir/cobicistat/ tenofovir/emtricitabine	Rifabutin metabolite level markedly increases; elvitegravir level decreases—coadministration should be avoided
	Etravirine	Etravirine and rifabutin levels decrease—no dosage adjustment recommended
	Maraviroc	May decrease maraviroc levels—if using with strong CYP3A4 inhibitor, maraviroc dosage should be 150 mg twice daily; if not, maraviroc dosage should be 300 mg twice daily
	Nevirapine	Rifabutin level increases; nevirapine level decreases—no dose adjustments recommended
	PI (with ritonavir boosting)	Rifabutin level significantly increases—use rifabutin 150 daily or 300 mg 3 times per week; consider monitoring levels and adjusting dose accordingly
	Rilpivirine	Rilpivirine level decreases—coadministration should be avoided

Abbreviation: PI, protease inhibitor.

Data from Panel on Opportunistic Infections in HIV-Infected Adults and Adolescents. Guidelines for the prevention and treatment of opportunistic infections in HIV-infected adults and adolescents: recommendations from the Centers for Disease Control and Prevention, the National Institutes of Health, and the HIV Medical Association of the Infectious Diseases Society of America. U.S. Department of Health and Human Services; 2013. Available at: http://aidsinfo.nih.gov/contentfiles/lvguidelines/adult_oi.pdf. Accessed February 15, 2014.

$250/mm^3$ were randomized to earlier ART (within 2 weeks of TB therapy initiation) or to later ART (between 8 and 12 weeks after starting TB therapy).[28] The earlier ART group had a lower rate of ADI or death than the later ART group (12.9% vs 16.1%), but the difference was not significant. In patients with a CD4 cell count less than $50/mm^3$, however, there was a significant decrease in new ADI or death in the earlier ART (15.5%) compared with the later ART group (26.6%). TB-IRIS occurred in 5% of patients in the earlier ART group and in 11% of those in the later ART group.[31]

Based on these findings, the World Health Organization recommends that ART should be started in all people with HIV and active TB regardless of the CD4 cell count and that TB treatment should be started first, followed by ART within the first 8 weeks of TB therapy.[32] The DHHS guidelines recommend ART for all HIV-infected individuals with TB. ART should be initiated within 2 weeks of TB therapy if the CD4 cell count is less than 50 cells/mm^3 and by 8 to 12 weeks if the CD4 cell count is higher (**Table 2**).[3]

TB meningitis
When ART should be started in patients with TB meningitis (TBM) is less certain. In a randomized study of 253 HIV-infected patients with TBM in Vietnam, there was no mortality benefit in patients who initiated ART immediately compared with those who deferred ART for 2 months after starting TB therapy. There were more severe adverse events in the immediate group than in the deferred group. The overall mortality was extremely high: 60% in the immediate ART group and 56% in the deferred ART group.[33] This study highlights the high mortality and severe complications associated with TBM.

Antiretroviral medication choice in patients with HIV/TB
Significant drug-drug interactions exist between TB therapy and several antiretroviral medications (see **Table 1**). Because rifampin markedly decreases levels of HIV protease inhibitors (PIs), nonnucleoside reverse transcriptase inhibitors, such as efavirenz, are often used in HIV/TB coinfected patients instead. Efavirenz-based regimens have been found to have lower rates of virologic failure than nevirapine-based ART in HIV/TB coinfected individuals.[34,35] In a study conducted in Thailand, there was no difference in virologic or immunologic outcomes with efavirenz, 600 mg daily, compared with 800 mg daily in HIV/TB coinfected individuals, supporting standard dosing of this drug in this population.[36] A recent pharmacokinetic evaluation of the STRIDE

Table 2 When to start antiretroviral therapy in patients with opportunistic infections (OIs)	
Opportunistic Infection	**When to Start ART**
• Cryptosporidiosis • Microsporidiosis • Progressive multifocal leukoencephalopathy	As part of initial therapy for the OI
• Pneumocystis pneumonia • Mycobacterium avium complex • Toxoplasmosis	Within ~2 wk of initiating OI treatment
• TB	• CD4 cell count <50/mm^3—within 2 wk after starting TB therapy • CD4 cell count >50/mm^3—within 8–12 wk after starting TB therapy
• Cryptococcal meningitis	~5 wk after starting antifungal therapy

Data from Refs.[3,54,56]

study found that coadministration of efavirenz and rifampin was associated with a trend toward higher, rather than lower, efavirenz C_{min} compared with efavirenz alone.[37] Those weighing 60 kg or more had lower efavirenz C_{min} than those weighing less than 60 kg but did not have lower viral suppression rates.

When an efavirenz-based regimen cannot be used, an HIV-PI-based regimen may be given with rifabutin, rather than rifampin-based TB therapy (rifabutin doses should be lowered because PIs increase its level). To overcome the PI-lowering effect of rifampin, high-dose ritonavir (the so-called superboosting) with lopinavir has been studied; although this regimen has favorable pharmacokinetic data when coadministered with rifampin, there have been unacceptably high rates of toxicity, intolerance, and treatment discontinuation.[38,39]

Levels of the HIV integrase inhibitor raltegravir are lowered when coadministered with rifampin. Doubling the standard raltegravir dose to 800 mg twice daily compensates for the effect of rifampin on raltegravir exposure but still results in low raltegravir trough concentrations.[40] In a randomized phase 2 trial of HIV-TB coinfected patients on rifampin-based therapy, standard dose raltegravir (400 mg twice daily) compared favorably to efavirenz and double-dose raltegravir (800 mg twice daily), but a larger phase 3 trial is needed to confirm these results.[41] In healthy HIV-negative volunteers, coadministration of rifabutin did not have a clinically meaningful effect on raltegravir pharmacokinetics.[42] Twice-daily dolutegravir with rifampin or once-daily dolutegravir with rifabutin seems to provide acceptable drug levels.[43] Although promising, more data are needed on the efficacy and toxicity of coadministration of HIV integrase inhibitors with TB therapy.

Cryptococcus

Epidemiology
The incidence of CM has decreased substantially in resource-rich settings during the era of effective ART. However, the global burden of cryptococcal infection is still substantial: in 2006, the number of cases was estimated to be 960,000 and the number of deaths due to CM was about 625,000.[44] This infection typically occurs in those with a CD4 cell count less than 100/mm³.

Diagnosis
In the United States, cryptococcal infection is usually diagnosed by serum or cerebrospinal fluid (CSF) cryptococcal antigen (CrAg) testing or by culture. Other testing methods, including India ink staining of CSF, are used in other parts of the world. In HIV-infected patients, the serum CrAg is usually positive in meningeal or nonmeningeal disease. Assays for detection of CrAg include latex agglutination (LA), enzyme immunoassay (EIA), or lateral flow assay (LFA). LA and EIA require laboratory expertise and infrastructure,[45] which are frequently not available in resource-limited settings.

CrAg LFA
The LFA is a dipstick immunochromatographic assay in which gold-conjugated, anti-cryptococcus antibodies deposited on the test strip membrane are used to detect CrAg in serum, plasma, CSF, or urine; if antigen is detected, a visible line appears. This easy, inexpensive, point-of-care test can be used for rapid diagnosis of cryptococcal infection without the need for significant laboratory infrastructure. A recent evaluation in 832 African patients with suspected meningitis reported a sensitivity and specificity for the LFA in CSF samples of 99.3% and 99.1%, respectively.[46] Notably, the LFA outperformed LA assays in terms of accuracy. In a recent study in 112 Ugandan patients with suspected meningitis, the CSF LFA titer at the time of

diagnosis correlated with fungal burden and mortality.[47] Near-perfect performance of LFA in patients with confirmed meningitis has also been demonstrated in plasma, serum, and urine specimens, with sensitivities greater than 95%.[46,48] However, more information is needed on the performance of the LFA in peripheral specimens in patients without meningitis. A study evaluating LFA accuracy among hospitalized patients in Thailand with respiratory illness found that, when compared with serum EIA, the sensitivity of LFA was 96% in serum and 70% in urine. Because of its ease of use and accuracy, the LFA may be used as a screening strategy for cryptococcal infection in patients with advanced HIV infection in areas of the world and populations in which there is a high prevalence of cryptococcal antigenemia, such as parts of sub-Saharan Africa.[49]

Treatment of CM: the induction phase
There have been many important clinical trials evaluating different treatment strategies for HIV-infected patients with CM.[49–51] In a recently published trial of induction therapy, 299 HIV-infected patients with CM were randomized to receive amphotericin B alone for 4 weeks, amphotericin B plus flucytosine for 2 weeks, or amphotericin B plus fluconazole, 400 mg twice daily for 2 weeks, all followed by fluconazole, 400 mg daily for 6 to 8 weeks.[52] The amphotericin B plus flucytosine group had a significantly lower mortality by day 70 than the amphotericin B alone group (hazard ratio [HR], 0.61); the amphotericin plus fluconazole group also had a lower mortality rate than the monotherapy group, but the difference was not significant (HR for death, 0.71; $P = .13$).

Historically, amphotericin B deoxycholate was the formulation used to treat CM; however, where available, lipid formulations of amphotericin B are now preferred because of improved tolerance.[53] Current US recommendations for the induction treatment of CM is with liposomal amphotericin B at 3 to 4 mg/kg/d in combination with flucytosine, 100 mg/kg divided into 4 equal doses daily for at least 2 weeks.[3]

Consolidation and maintenance therapy
After at least 2 weeks of induction therapy, if the patient has clinically responded and has a negative CSF culture, the patient may be switched to consolidation therapy with fluconazole, 400 mg daily for at least 8 weeks. The fluconazole dose may then be reduced to 200 mg daily; this maintenance phase of therapy should continue for at least 1 year. Therapy may be stopped in patients who have received at least 12 months of fluconazole maintenance therapy, who have CD4 cell counts of 100/mm^3 or more, and who have undetectable HIV RNA levels for 3 months or more on ART.[3]

When to start ART
Several studies have examined the optimal time to initiate ART in patients with CM. ACTG 5164, which randomized HIV-infected patients with acute OIs to receive early ART (within 14 days of OI diagnosis) or deferred ART (after OI therapy was completed) found that early ART improved outcomes[54]; however, only 35 subjects in this study had cryptococcal infection. A study from Zimbabwe that randomized 54 HIV-infected subjects with CM to receive early ART initiation (within 72 hours of CM diagnosis) or delayed ART initiation (after 10 weeks of treatment with fluconazole alone) found a nearly 3 times higher risk of mortality in the early ART arm.[55] Several features of this study limit its generalizability to resource-rich settings, including its use of fluconazole monotherapy and the inability to treat elevated intracranial pressure (ICP) with serial lumbar punctures; nevertheless, the trial highlighted the potential danger of early ART in patients with CM.

In the Cryptococcal Optimal ART Timing (COAT) study, HIV-infected patients who received induction therapy with amphotericin B plus fluconazole, 800 mg daily, were randomized to initiate early ART (within 48 hours of study entry, which was after 7–11 days of induction treatment) or deferred ART (4 weeks after randomization, approximately 5 weeks after initiation of antifungal therapy).[56] A Safety Monitoring Board stopped the study because of increased mortality in the early treatment group (40/88 [45%] vs 27/89 [30%], HR, 1.7; P = .03). The benefit of deferring ART was particularly evident in patients with CSF white blood cell count less than 5 cells/mm^3, or altered mental status. Based on the findings from this study, the optimal time to start ART may be approximately 5 weeks after initiation of antifungal therapy (see **Table 2**). In addition, effective management of increased ICP and complications, such as cryptococcal IRIS, are critical to achieving a successful outcome.

Cryptococcal IRIS

Cryptococcal IRIS presents as worsening clinical disease or new onset of symptoms of CM after initiation of ART.[57] Discerning risk factors for cryptococcal IRIS has been complicated by various reports with conflicting results.[58–60] Some risk factors include being ART naive, having higher HIV RNA levels, having persistent CSF fungal culture growth, having decreased levels of CSF protein, and having lower central nervous system (CNS) inflammation at the time of CM diagnosis.[59,61] There is limited evidence to guide treatment of cryptococcal IRIS. Recent guidelines suggest continuing antifungal therapy and ART and aggressive management of increased ICP, if present; some experts also recommend a brief steroid course.[3,57]

PML

PML is caused by John Cunningham Virus (JCV) infection of oligodendrocytes in the CNS, leading to focal demyelination. In the era of effective ART, the incidence of PML in HIV-infected individuals has decreased significantly.[62] Median survival has also improved, but mortality remains high; those who survive frequently have permanent neurologic deficits.[63] Although PML usually affects HIV-infected patients with low CD4 cell counts, there are reports of PML occurring in individuals with CD4 cell counts greater than 100/mm^3 as well as in HIV-uninfected patients receiving immunomodulatory antibodies as treatment of cancer or autoimmune disorders.[64,65]

Treatment of PML

At present, there is no effective antiviral agent against JC virus. In HIV-infected patients, treatment of PML consists of ART to reverse immunosuppression and restore anti–JC virus immunity. Although it has been proposed that ART with higher CNS penetration may prevent HIV-associated CNS diseases, such as PML, a cohort study of more than 22,000 HIV-infected individuals found that these CNS events were not significantly associated with the CNS penetration effectiveness (CPE) score of the antiretroviral regimen.[66] In addition, in the current era of effective ART, plasma HIV RNA level correlates with clinical outcomes in patients with neurologic AIDS-defining events, such as PML, whereas CPE does not.[63] In a patient with PML, a regimen should be chosen that has the highest likelihood of systemic suppression of HIV replication and immune restoration.

Several drugs with promising in vitro anti–JC activity have not been found to have clinical efficacy in patients with PML. Trials with cytarabine,[67] cidofovir,[68] and mefloquine[69] have been unsuccessful. It has recently been found that the serotonin receptor 5-hydroxytryptamine-2A can serve as a receptor for the JC virus; therefore, serotonin receptor inhibitors, such as mirtazapine, have been proposed as treatment of PML.[70] Several case reports suggested clinical benefit with mirtazapine in HIV-infected and noninfected individuals with PML; however, there have been no published randomized studies to date.[71–73]

PML-IRIS

Both unmasking of previously unrecognized PML and paradoxic worsening in patients with known PML have been observed after initiation of ART. Although steroids are sometimes used to treat PML-IRIS, their role is still controversial.[64,74] One of the postulated mechanisms of PML-IRIS is that CCR5+ immune cells mediate this complication. For this reason, maraviroc, a CCR5 antagonist, was given to an HIV-negative woman with multiple sclerosis who was at high risk for PML-IRIS after receiving natilizumab.[75] In this case report, maraviroc seemed to initially prevent PML-IRIS and subsequently improve IRIS once it occurred. Additional studies of maraviroc in patients with PML are being planned.

PCP

PCP is caused by the fungus *Pneumocystis jirovecii*. In HIV-infected patients, risk factors for PCP include CD4 cell count less than 200/mm^3, CD4 percentage less than 14%, oral thrush, unintentional weight loss, and high plasma HIV RNA levels.[76,77]

The incidence of PCP has declined significantly as a result of prophylaxis and effective ART.[78] At this point, PCP in HIV-infected patients is most commonly seen in those who are unaware of their HIV status or not engaged in care. Nosocomial outbreaks of *P jirovecii* have been seen among patients who underwent renal transplant.[79] Increasing evidence suggests that aerosolization of the fungus can occur from infected patients and may play a role in nosocomial transmission.[80]

Diagnosis

PCP cannot be cultured routinely; therefore, diagnosis requires detection of the organism by microscopic examination of induced sputum, bronchial alveolar lavage (BAL), or tissue. Examination of induced sputum has variable sensitivity (<50%–>90%).[3] BAL has a high sensitivity for PCP; however, it is an invasive procedure with potential morbidity in patients with respiratory compromise. Elevated serum lactate dehydrogenase level is a nonspecific marker, which is often found in cases of PCP.[81] Levels of serum $(1 \rightarrow 3)$-β-D-glucan (β-glucan), a component of the cell wall of *P jirovecii*, may also be elevated in patients with PCP, but there is significant cross-reactivity with other fungal diseases.[82] A recent study evaluated β-glucan testing in 252 HIV-infected individuals with OIs, of whom 173 (69%) were diagnosed with PCP[83]; the overall sensitivity of the test for the diagnosis of PCP was 92%, and the specificity was 65%. In HIV-infected patients with respiratory symptoms, the test performed better (sensitivity, 93%; specificity, 75%; positive predictive value, 96%; negative predictive value, 60%).[84] In the appropriate clinical setting, β-glucan testing can aid in the diagnosis of PCP.

When to start ART in a patient with PCP

ACTG A5164, which evaluated early (within 2 weeks of OI diagnosis) versus deferred ART initiation (after OI therapy was completed) in patients with OIs found a significant decrease in AIDS progression or death with early ART; most patients in this study had PCP.[54] Current guidelines recommend starting ART within 2 weeks of diagnosis of PCP (see **Table 2**).[3]

Recommendations for PCP prophylaxis

Indications for initiating PCP prophylaxis, preferred and alternative therapies, and indications for stopping primary prophylaxis are summarized in **Box 1**.

Vaccine-Preventable OIs

HPV

Epidemiology Infection with oncogenic high-risk HPV types is the major risk factor for the development of cervical cancer in women and anal cancer in both men and women. The oncogenic types include HPV 16, 18, 31, 33, 35, 39, 45, 51, 52, 56, 58, and 59.[85] HPV 16 and 18 cause approximately 70% of all cervical cancers worldwide. All the other types individually contribute less than 5% each to cervical cancers.

HPV vaccine At present, there are 2 HPV vaccines licensed in the United States: the bivalent vaccine protects against HPV 16 and 18; the quadrivalent vaccine protects against HPV 16 and 18 and the nononcogenic HPV 6 and 11 (the most common causes of genital warts). Clinical trials have found both vaccines efficacious in preventing cervical precancer in women; the quadrivalent vaccine has also shown efficacy for preventing vaginal and vulvar precancer in women and in preventing anal intraepithelial neoplasia in men who have sex with men (MSM).[86–88]

Box 1
PCP prophylaxis

Indications for Initiating Primary Prophylaxis:

- CD4 cell count less than 200/mm^3
- Oropharyngeal candidiasis
- CD4 cell percentage less than 14%
- History of AIDS-defining illness
- CD4 cell count greater than 200 but less than 250/mm^3 if CD4 cell count monitoring not feasible

Preferred Prophylaxis Therapy:

- TMP-SMX, 1 DS orally daily
- TMP-SMX, 1 SS orally daily

Selected Alternative Therapies:

- TMP-SMX 1 DS orally 3 times a week
- Dapsone 100 mg orally daily
- Atovaquone 1500 mg orally daily with food

Indication for Discontinuing Primary Prophylaxis:

- CD4 cell count increased from less than 200/mm^3 to 200/mm^3 or more for at least 3 months in response to ART

Abbreviation: TMP-SMX, trimethoprim/sulfamethoxazole.
  Data from Panel on Opportunistic Infections in HIV-Infected Adults and Adolescents. Guidelines for the prevention and treatment of opportunistic infections in HIV-infected adults and adolescents: recommendations from the Centers for Disease Control and Prevention, the National Institutes of Health, and the HIV Medical Association of the Infectious Diseases Society of America. U.S. Department of Health and Human Services; 2013. Available at: http://aidsinfo.nih.gov/contentfiles/lvguidelines/adult_oi.pdf. Accessed February 15, 2014.

The Centers of Disease Control and Prevention's Advisory Committee on Immunization Practices (ACIP) recommends the following[89]:

- Females should receive either the bivalent or quadrivalent HPV vaccine at the age of 11 or 12 years and at 13 to 26 years if not previously vaccinated
- Males should receive the quadrivalent HPV vaccine at the age of 11 or 12 years and at 13 to 21 years if not previously vaccinated. Men aged 22 through 26 years may be vaccinated.
- MSM and immunocompromised persons (including HIV-infected males and females) should be vaccinated through the age of 26 years if not previously vaccinated.

The quadrivalent HPV vaccine is safe and immunogenic in HIV-infected women and men.[90–92]

Varicella and zoster vaccines

Epidemiology Over 95% of US-born adults are immune to VZV. Herpes zoster (HZ) results when latent VZV reactivates. In a study among MSM, the incidence of HZ was much higher in HIV-infected than HIV-negative men (age-adjusted relative risk, 16.9).[93] Risk factors for HZ in HIV-infected patients include a previous zoster episode and CD4 cell count less than 200/mm^3.[94] Use of ART is not necessarily protective against development of HZ, and the risk of HZ may increase soon after ART initiation.[95,96]

Vaccination in HIV-infected patients The live attenuated varicella vaccine is recommended for HIV-infected children with CD4 percentage greater than 15%.[93,97,98] The 2014 ACIP Guidelines and the 2013 Infectious Diseases Society of America (IDSA)/HIV Medical Association (HIVMA) Primary Care Guidelines for HIV-infected Patients recommend varicella vaccination in HIV-infected/VZV-seronegative adults with CD4 cell counts greater than 200/mm^3.[89,99] ACTG A5247 evaluated live attenuated zoster vaccine in HIV-infected adults on ART with CD4 cell count greater than 200 cells/mm^3 and HIV RNA level less than 50 copies/mL; the vaccine was found to be safe and triggered an antibody response.[100] At the current time, however, ACIP does not recommend zoster vaccine in HIV-infected patients. The IDSA/HIVMA guidelines state that zoster vaccine should be considered in HIV-infected patients aged 60 years or older who have a CD4 cell count of 200/mm^3 or more.[99]

ACKNOWLEDGMENTS

We thank Drs Rocio Hurtado, Mark Siedner, Azure Makadzange, and Tracey Cho for their critical reading, thoughtful comments, and assistance with this article.

REFERENCES

1. Buchacz K, Armon C, Palella FJ, et al. CD4 cell counts at HIV diagnosis among HIV outpatient study participants, 2000–2009. AIDS Res Treat 2012;2012: 869841.
2. Mocroft A, Furrer HJ, Miro JM, et al. The incidence of AIDS-defining illnesses at a current CD4 count >/= 200 cells/muL in the post-combination antiretroviral therapy era. Clin Infect Dis 2013;57(7):1038–47.
3. Panel on Opportunistic Infections in HIV-Infected Adults and Adolescents. Guidelines for the prevention and treatment of opportunistic infections in

HIV-infected adults and adolescents: recommendations from the Centers for Disease Control and Prevention, the National Institutes of Health, and the HIV Medical Association of the Infectious Diseases Society of America. U.S. Department of Health and Human Services; 2013. Available at: http://aidsinfo.nih.gov/contentfiles/lvguidelines/adult_oi.pdf. Accessed February 15, 2014.

4. Albalak R, O'Brien RJ, Kammerer JS, et al. Trends in tuberculosis/human immunodeficiency virus comorbidity, United States, 1993-2004. Arch Intern Med 2007;167(22):2443–52.

5. Center for Disease Control. Reported Tuberculosis in the United States, 2012. Atlanta (GA): Department of Health and Human Services; 2013.

6. Ewer K, Deeks J, Alvarez L, et al. Comparison of T-cell-based assay with tuberculin skin test for diagnosis of *Mycobacterium tuberculosis* infection in a school tuberculosis outbreak. Lancet 2003;361(9364):1168–73.

7. Talati NJ, Seybold U, Humphrey B, et al. Poor concordance between interferon-gamma release assays and tuberculin skin tests in diagnosis of latent tuberculosis infection among HIV-infected individuals. BMC Infect Dis 2009;9:15.

8. Mazurek GH, Jereb J, Vernon A, et al. Updated guidelines for using interferon gamma release assays to detect *Mycobacterium tuberculosis* infection - United States. MMWR Recomm Rep 2010;59(RR-5):1–25.

9. Rangaka MX, Wilkinson KA, Glynn JR, et al. Predictive value of interferon-gamma release assays for incident active tuberculosis: a systematic review and meta-analysis. Lancet Infect Dis 2012;12(1):45–55.

10. Targeted tuberculin testing and treatment of latent tuberculosis infection. This official statement of the American Thoracic Society was adopted by the ATS Board of Directors, July 1999. This is a Joint Statement of the American Thoracic Society (ATS) and the Centers for Disease Control and Prevention (CDC). This statement was endorsed by the Council of the Infectious Diseases Society of America. (IDSA), September 1999, and the sections of this statement. Am J Respir Crit Care Med 2000;161(4 Pt 2):S221–47.

11. Efficacy of various durations of isoniazid preventive therapy for tuberculosis: five years of follow-up in the IUAT trial. International Union Against Tuberculosis Committee on Prophylaxis. Bull World Health Organ 1982; 60(4):555–64.

12. Horsburgh CR Jr, Goldberg S, Bethel J, et al. Latent TB infection treatment acceptance and completion in the United States and Canada. Chest 2010; 137(2):401–9.

13. LoBue PA, Moser KS. Use of isoniazid for latent tuberculosis infection in a public health clinic. Am J Respir Crit Care Med 2003;168(4):443–7.

14. Sterling TR, Villarino ME, Borisov AS, et al. Three months of rifapentine and isoniazid for latent tuberculosis infection. N Engl J Med 2011;365(23):2155–66.

15. Monkongdee P, McCarthy KD, Cain KP, et al. Yield of acid-fast smear and mycobacterial culture for tuberculosis diagnosis in people with human immunodeficiency virus. Am J Respir Crit Care Med 2009;180(9):903–8.

16. Boehme CC, Nabeta P, Hillemann D, et al. Rapid molecular detection of tuberculosis and rifampin resistance. N Engl J Med 2010;363(11):1005–15.

17. Barnard M, Albert H, Coetzee G, et al. Rapid molecular screening for multidrug-resistant tuberculosis in a high-volume public health laboratory in South Africa. Am J Respir Crit Care Med 2008;177(7):787–92.

18. Chang K, Lu W, Wang J, et al. Rapid and effective diagnosis of tuberculosis and rifampicin resistance with Xpert MTB/RIF assay: a meta-analysis. J Infect 2012; 64(6):580–8.

19. Van Rie A, Page-Shipp L, Mellet K, et al. Diagnostic accuracy and effectiveness of the Xpert MTB/RIF assay for the diagnosis of HIV-associated lymph node tuberculosis. Eur J Clin Microbiol Infect Dis 2013;32(11):1409–15.

20. Vadwai V, Boehme C, Nabeta P, et al. Xpert MTB/RIF: a new pillar in diagnosis of extrapulmonary tuberculosis? J Clin Microbiol 2011;49(7):2540–5.

21. Porcel JM, Palma R, Valdes L, et al. Xpert(R) MTB/RIF in pleural fluid for the diagnosis of tuberculosis. Int J Tuberc Lung Dis 2013;17(9):1217–9.

22. Hillemann D, Rusch-Gerdes S, Boehme C, et al. Rapid molecular detection of extrapulmonary tuberculosis by the automated GeneXpert MTB/RIF system. J Clin Microbiol 2011;49(4):1202–5.

23. Wood R, Racow K, Bekker LG, et al. Lipoarabinomannan in urine during tuberculosis treatment: association with host and pathogen factors and mycobacteriuria. BMC Infect Dis 2012;12:47.

24. Lawn SD. Point-of-care detection of lipoarabinomannan (LAM) in urine for diagnosis of HIV-associated tuberculosis: a state of the art review. BMC Infect Dis 2012;12:103.

25. Lawn SD, Kerkhoff AD, Vogt M, et al. Diagnostic accuracy of a low-cost, urine antigen, point-of-care screening assay for HIV-associated pulmonary tuberculosis before antiretroviral therapy: a descriptive study. Lancet Infect Dis 2012; 12(3):201–9.

26. Abdool Karim SS, Naidoo K, Grobler A, et al. Timing of initiation of antiretroviral drugs during tuberculosis therapy. N Engl J Med 2010;362(8):697–706.

27. Padayatchi N, Abdool Karim SS, Naidoo K, et al. Improved survival in multidrug-resistant tuberculosis patients receiving integrated tuberculosis and antiretroviral treatment in the SAPiT Trial. Int J Tuberc Lung Dis 2014;18(2):147–54.

28. Havlir DV, Kendall MA, Ive P, et al. Timing of antiretroviral therapy for HIV-1 infection and tuberculosis. N Engl J Med 2011;365(16):1482–91.

29. Abdool Karim SS, Naidoo K, Grobler A, et al. Integration of antiretroviral therapy with tuberculosis treatment. N Engl J Med 2011;365(16):1492–501.

30. Blanc FX, Sok T, Laureillard D, et al. Earlier versus later start of antiretroviral therapy in HIV-infected adults with tuberculosis. N Engl J Med 2011;365(16): 1471–81.

31. Luetkemeyer AF, Kendall MA, Nyirenda M, et al. Tuberculosis immune reconstitution inflammatory syndrome in A5221 STRIDE: timing, severity and implications for HIV-TB programs. J Acquir Immune Defic Syndr 2014;65(4): 423–8.

32. WHO. Consolidated guidelines on the use of antiretroviral drugs for treating and preventing HIV infection. Geneva (Switzerland): WHO; 2013.

33. Torok ME, Yen NT, Chau TT, et al. Timing of initiation of antiretroviral therapy in human immunodeficiency virus (HIV)–associated tuberculous meningitis. Clin Infect Dis 2011;52(11):1374–83.

34. Swaminathan S, Padmapriyadarsini C, Venkatesan P, et al. Efficacy and safety of once-daily nevirapine- or efavirenz-based antiretroviral therapy in HIV-associated tuberculosis: a randomized clinical trial. Clin Infect Dis 2011;53(7): 716–24.

35. Boulle A, Van Cutsem G, Cohen K, et al. Outcomes of nevirapine- and efavirenz-based antiretroviral therapy when coadministered with rifampicin-based antitubercular therapy. JAMA 2008;300(5):530–9.

36. Manosuthi W, Kiertiburanakul S, Sungkanuparph S, et al. Efavirenz 600 mg/day versus efavirenz 800 mg/day in HIV-infected patients with tuberculosis receiving rifampicin: 48 weeks results. AIDS 2006;20(1):131–2.

37. Luetkemeyer AF, Rosenkranz SL, Lu D, et al. Relationship between weight, efavirenz exposure, and virologic suppression in HIV-infected patients on rifampin-based tuberculosis treatment in the AIDS Clinical Trials Group A5221 STRIDE Study. Clin Infect Dis 2013;57(4):586–93.

38. Nijland HM, L'Homme RF, Rongen GA, et al. High incidence of adverse events in healthy volunteers receiving rifampicin and adjusted doses of lopinavir/ritonavir tablets. AIDS 2008;22(8):931–5.

39. Murphy RA, Marconi VC, Gandhi RT, et al. Coadministration of lopinavir/ritonavir and rifampicin in HIV and tuberculosis co-infected adults in South Africa. PLoS One 2012;7(9):e44793.

40. Wenning LA, Hanley WD, Brainard DM, et al. Effect of rifampin, a potent inducer of drug-metabolizing enzymes, on the pharmacokinetics of raltegravir. Antimicrob Agents Chemother 2009;53(7):2852–6.

41. Grinsztejn B, De Castro N, Arnold V, et al. ANRS 12 180 Reflate TB study group. Raltegravir for the treatment of patients co-infected with HIV and tuberculosis (ANRS 12 180 Reflate TB): a multicentre, phase 2, non-comparative, open-label, randomised trial. Lancet Infect Dis 2014;14(6):459–67.

42. Brainard DM, Kassahun K, Wenning LA, et al. Lack of a clinically meaningful pharmacokinetic effect of rifabutin on raltegravir: in vitro/in vivo correlation. J Clin Pharmacol 2011;51(6):943–50.

43. Dooley KE, Sayre P, Borland J, et al. Safety, tolerability, and pharmacokinetics of the HIV integrase inhibitor dolutegravir given twice daily with rifampin or once daily with rifabutin: results of a phase 1 study among healthy subjects. J Acquir Immune Defic Syndr 2013;62(1):21–7.

44. Park BJ, Wannemuehler KA, Marston BJ, et al. Estimation of the current global burden of cryptococcal meningitis among persons living with HIV/AIDS. AIDS 2009;23(4):525–30.

45. Rajasingham R, Meya DB, Boulware DR. Integrating cryptococcal antigen screening and pre-emptive treatment into routine HIV care. J Acquir Immune Defic Syndr 2012;59(5):e85–91.

46. Boulware DR, Rolfes MA, Rajasingham R, et al. Multisite validation of cryptococcal antigen lateral flow assay and quantification by laser thermal contrast. Emerg Infect Dis 2014;20(1):45–53.

47. Kabanda T, Siedner MJ, Klausner JD, et al. Point-of-care diagnosis and prognostication of cryptococcal meningitis with the cryptococcal antigen lateral flow assay on cerebrospinal fluid. Clin Infect Dis 2014;58(1):113–6.

48. Jarvis JN, Percival A, Bauman S, et al. Evaluation of a novel point-of-care cryptococcal antigen test on serum, plasma, and urine from patients with HIV-associated cryptococcal meningitis. Clin Infect Dis 2011;53(10):1019–23.

49. World Health Organization. Rapid advice: diagnosis, prevention and management of cryptococcal disease in HIV-infected adults. Geneva (Switzerland): World Health Organization; 2011.

50. Jackson A, van der Horst C. New insights in the prevention, diagnosis, and treatment of cryptococcal meningitis. Curr HIV/AIDS Rep 2012;9(3):267–77.

51. Perfect JR, Dismukes WE, Dromer F, et al. Clinical practice guidelines for the management of cryptococcal disease: 2010 update by the Infectious Diseases Society of America. Clin Infect Dis 2010;50(3):291–322.

52. Day JN, Chau TT, Wolbers M, et al. Combination antifungal therapy for cryptococcal meningitis. N Engl J Med 2013;368(14):1291–302.

53. Hamill RJ, Sobel JD, El-Sadr W, et al. Comparison of 2 doses of liposomal amphotericin B and conventional amphotericin B deoxycholate for treatment of

AIDS-associated acute cryptococcal meningitis: a randomized, double-blind clinical trial of efficacy and safety. Clin Infect Dis 2010;51(2):225–32.

54. Zolopa A, Andersen J, Powderly W, et al. Early antiretroviral therapy reduces AIDS progression/death in individuals with acute opportunistic infections: a multicenter randomized strategy trial. PloS One 2009;4(5):e5575.

55. Makadzange AT, Ndhlovu CE, Takarinda K, et al. Early versus delayed initiation of antiretroviral therapy for concurrent HIV infection and cryptococcal meningitis in sub-Saharan Africa. Clin Infect Dis 2010;50(11):1532–8.

56. Boulware DR, Meya DB, Muzoora C, et al. Timing of antiretroviral therapy after diagnosis of cryptococcal meningitis. N Engl J Med 2014;370(26):2487–98.

57. Haddow LJ, Colebunders R, Meintjes G, et al. Cryptococcal immune reconstitution inflammatory syndrome in HIV-1-infected individuals: proposed clinical case definitions. Lancet Infect Dis 2010;10(11):791–802.

58. Shelburne SA 3rd, Darcourt J, White AC Jr, et al. The role of immune reconstitution inflammatory syndrome in AIDS-related *Cryptococcus neoformans* disease in the era of highly active antiretroviral therapy. Clin Infect Dis 2005;40(7): 1049–52.

59. Bicanic T, Meintjes G, Rebe K, et al. Immune reconstitution inflammatory syndrome in HIV-associated cryptococcal meningitis: a prospective study. J Acquir Immune Defic Syndr 2009;51(2):130–4.

60. Chang CC, Dorasamy AA, Gosnell BI, et al. Clinical and mycological predictors of cryptococcosis-associated immune reconstitution inflammatory syndrome. AIDS 2013;27(13):2089–99.

61. Boulware DR, Bonham SC, Meya DB, et al. Paucity of initial cerebrospinal fluid inflammation in cryptococcal meningitis is associated with subsequent immune reconstitution inflammatory syndrome. J Infect Dis 2010;202(6):962–70.

62. d'Arminio Monforte A, Cinque P, Mocroft A, et al. Changing incidence of central nervous system diseases in the EuroSIDA cohort. Ann Neurol 2004;55(3):320–8.

63. Lanoy E, Guiguet M, Bentata M, et al. Survival after neuroAIDS: association with antiretroviral CNS penetration-effectiveness score. Neurology 2011;76(7): 644–51.

64. Cinque P, Koralnik IJ, Gerevini S, et al. Progressive multifocal leukoencephalopathy in HIV-1 infection. Lancet Infect Dis 2009;9(10):625–36.

65. Carson KR, Focosi D, Major EO, et al. Monoclonal antibody-associated progressive multifocal leucoencephalopathy in patients treated with rituximab, natalizumab, and efalizumab: a review from the research on adverse drug events and reports (RADAR) project. Lancet Oncol 2009;10(8):816–24.

66. Garvey L, Winston A, Walsh J, et al. Antiretroviral therapy CNS penetration and HIV-1-associated CNS disease. Neurology 2011;76(8):693–700.

67. Hall CD, Dafni U, Simpson D, et al. Failure of cytarabine in progressive multifocal leukoencephalopathy associated with human immunodeficiency virus infection. AIDS Clinical Trials Group 243 Team. N Engl J Med 1998;338(19):1345–51.

68. De Luca A, Ammassari A, Pezzotti P, et al. Cidofovir in addition to antiretroviral treatment is not effective for AIDS-associated progressive multifocal leukoencephalopathy: a multicohort analysis. AIDS 2008;22(14):1759–67.

69. Clifford DB, Nath A, Cinque P, et al. A study of mefloquine treatment for progressive multifocal leukoencephalopathy: results and exploration of predictors of PML outcomes. J Neurovirol 2013;19(4):351–8.

70. O'Hara BA, Atwood WJ. Interferon beta1-a and selective anti-5HT(2a) receptor antagonists inhibit infection of human glial cells by JC virus. Virus Res 2008; 132(1–2):97–103.

71. Moenster RP, Jett RA. Mirtazapine and mefloquine therapy for progressive multi-focal leukoencephalopathy in a patient infected with human immunodeficiency virus. Am J Health Syst Pharm 2012;69(6):496–8.

72. Lanzafame M, Ferrari S, Lattuada E, et al. Mirtazapine in an HIV-1 infected patient with progressive multifocal leukoencephalopathy. Infez Med 2009;17(1):35–7.

73. Yoshida H, Ohshima K, Toda J, et al. Significant improvement following combination treatment with mefloquine and mirtazapine in a patient with progressive multifocal leukoencephalopathy after allogeneic peripheral blood stem cell transplantation. Int J Hematol 2014;99(1):95–9.

74. Tan K, Roda R, Ostrow L, et al. PML-IRIS in patients with HIV infection: clinical manifestations and treatment with steroids. Neurology 2009;72(17):1458–64.

75. Giacomini PS, Rozenberg A, Metz I, et al. Maraviroc and JC virus-associated immune reconstitution inflammatory syndrome. N Engl J Med 2014;370(5):486–8.

76. Kaplan JE, Hanson DL, Navin TR, et al. Risk factors for primary *Pneumocystis carinii* pneumonia in human immunodeficiency virus-infected adolescents and adults in the United States: reassessment of indications for chemoprophylaxis. J Infect Dis 1998;178(4):1126–32.

77. Kaplan JE, Hanson DL, Jones JL, et al. Adult, adolescent spectrum of HIVDPI. Viral load as an independent risk factor for opportunistic infections in HIV-infected adults and adolescents. AIDS 2001;15(14):1831–6.

78. Wolff AJ, O'Donnell AE. Pulmonary manifestations of HIV infection in the era of highly active antiretroviral therapy. Chest 2001;120(6):1888–93.

79. Le Gal S, Damiani C, Rouille A, et al. A cluster of *Pneumocystis* infections among renal transplant recipients: molecular evidence of colonized patients as potential infectious sources of *Pneumocystis jirovecii*. Clin Infect Dis 2012;54(7):e62–71.

80. Damiani C, Choukri F, Le Gal S, et al. Possible nosocomial transmission of *Pneumocystis jirovecii*. Emerg Infect Dis 2012;18(5):877–8.

81. Smith RL, Ripps CS, Lewis ML. Elevated lactate dehydrogenase values in patients with *Pneumocystis carinii* pneumonia. Chest 1988;93(5):987–92.

82. Pisculli ML, Sax PE. Use of a serum beta-glucan assay for diagnosis of HIV-related *Pneumocystis jirovecii* pneumonia in patients with negative microscopic examination results. Clin Infect Dis 2008;46(12):1928–30.

83. Sax PE, Komarow L, Finkelman MA, et al. Blood (1->3)-beta-D-glucan as a diagnostic test for HIV-related *Pneumocystis jirovecii* pneumonia. Clin Infect Dis 2011;53(2):197–202.

84. Wood BR, Komarow L, Zolopa AR, et al. Test performance of blood beta-glucan for *Pneumocystis jirovecii* pneumonia in patients with AIDS and respiratory symptoms. AIDS 2013;27(6):967–72.

85. Castle PE. The evolving definition of carcinogenic human papillomavirus. Infect Agents Canc 2009;4:7.

86. Paavonen J, Naud P, Salmeron J, et al. Efficacy of human papillomavirus (HPV)-16/18 AS04-adjuvanted vaccine against cervical infection and precancer caused by oncogenic HPV types (PATRICIA): final analysis of a double-blind, randomised study in young women. Lancet 2009;374(9686):301–14.

87. FUTURE II Study Group. Quadrivalent vaccine against human papillomavirus to prevent high-grade cervical lesions. N Engl J Med 2007;356(19):1915–27.

88. Palefsky JM, Giuliano AR, Goldstone S, et al. HPV vaccine against anal HPV infection and anal intraepithelial neoplasia. N Engl J Med 2011;365(17):1576–85.

89. Center for Disease Control. Recommended adult immunization schedule: United States. Atlanta (GA): Center for Disease Control; 2014.

90. Kahn JA, Xu J, Kapogiannis BG, et al. Immunogenicity and safety of the human papillomavirus 6, 11, 16, 18 vaccine in HIV-infected young women. Clin Infect Dis 2013;57(5):735–44.

91. Kojic EM, Kang M, Cespedes MS, et al. Immunogenicity and Safety of the Quadrivalent Human Papillomavirus Vaccine in HIV-1-Infected Women. Clin Infect Dis 2014. pii: ciu238. [Epub ahead of print] PMID: 24723284.

92. Wilkin T, Lee JY, Lensing SY, et al. Safety and immunogenicity of the quadrivalent human papillomavirus vaccine in HIV-1-infected men. J Infect Dis 2010; 202(8):1246–53.

93. Buchbinder SP, Katz MH, Hessol NA, et al. Herpes zoster and human immunodeficiency virus infection. J Infect Dis 1992;166(5):1153–6.

94. Engels EA, Rosenberg PS, Biggar RJ. Zoster incidence in human immunodeficiency virus-infected hemophiliacs and homosexual men, 1984-1997. District of Columbia Gay Cohort Study. Multicenter Hemophilia Cohort Study. J Infect Dis 1999;180(6):1784–9.

95. Gebo KA, Kalyani R, Moore RD, et al. The incidence of, risk factors for, and sequelae of herpes zoster among HIV patients in the highly active antiretroviral therapy era. J Acquir Immune Defic Syndr 2005;40(2):169–74.

96. Vanhems P, Voisin L, Gayet-Ageron A, et al. The incidence of herpes zoster is less likely than other opportunistic infections to be reduced by highly active antiretroviral therapy. J Acquir Immune Defic Syndr 2005;38(1):111–3.

97. Son M, Shapiro ED, LaRussa P, et al. Effectiveness of varicella vaccine in children infected with HIV. J Infect Dis 2010;201(12):1806–10.

98. Taweesith W, Puthanakit T, Kowitdamrong E, et al. The immunogenicity and safety of live attenuated varicella-zoster virus vaccine in human immunodeficiency virus-infected children. Pediatr Infect Dis J 2011;30(4):320–4.

99. Aberg JA, Gallant JE, Ghanem KG, et al. Primary care guidelines for the management of persons infected with HIV: 2013 update by the HIV medicine association of the Infectious Diseases Society of America. Clin Infect Dis 2014;58(1): e1–34.

100. Benson C, Hua L, Andersen J, et al. ZOSTAVAX is generally safe and immunogenic in HIV+ adults virologically suppressed on ART: results of a phase 2, randomized, double-blind, placebo-controlled trial. Presented at the 19th Conference on Retroviruses and Opportunistic Infections. Abstract #96. Seattle (WA), March 5–8, 2012.

Index

Note: Page numbers of article titles are in **boldface** type.

Infect Dis Clin N Am 28 (2014) 519–527
http://dx.doi.org/10.1016/S0891-5520(14)00050-6
0891-5520/14/$ – see front matter © 2014 Elsevier Inc. All rights reserved.

id.theclinics.com

Moving?

Make sure your subscription moves with you!

To notify us of your new address, find your **Clinics Account Number** (located on your mailing label above your name), and contact customer service at:

Email: journalscustomerservice-usa@elsevier.com

800-654-2452 (subscribers in the U.S. & Canada)
314-447-8871 (subscribers outside of the U.S. & Canada)

Fax number: 314-447-8029

Elsevier Health Sciences Division
Subscription Customer Service
3251 Riverport Lane
Maryland Heights, MO 63043

*To ensure uninterrupted delivery of your subscription, please notify us at least 4 weeks in advance of move.

Printed and bound by CPI Group (UK) Ltd, Croydon, CR0 4YY

03/10/2024

01040488-0003